PERSONAL HEARING PROTECTION IN INDUSTRY

Personal Hearing Protection in Industry

Editor

P. W. Alberti, M.B., Ph.D., F.R.C.S., F.R.C.S.(C.)
*Departments of Otolaryngology and Occupational and
Environmental Medicine, and Otolaryngologist-in-Chief,
Mt. Sinai Hospital, University of Toronto
Toronto, Ontario, Canada*

Raven Press ■ New York

Raven Press, 1140 Avenue of the Americas, New York, New York 10036

© 1982 by Raven Press Books, Ltd. All rights reserved. This book is protected by copyright. No part of it may be reproduced, stored in a retrieval system, or transmitted, in any form or by any means, electronic, mechanical, photocopying, recording, or otherwise, without the prior written permission of the publisher.

Made in the United States of America

Great care has been taken to maintain the accuracy of the information contained in the volume. However, Raven Press cannot be held responsible for errors or for any consequences arising from the use of the information contained herein.

Library of Congress Cataloging in Publication Data
Main entry under title:

Personal hearing protection in industry.

   Papers presented at an international symposium, University of Toronto, May 1980.
   Includes bibliographical references and index.
   1. Deafness, Noise induced–Prevention–Congresses. 2. Ear–Protection–Congresses. 3. Industrial hygiene–Congresses. I. Alberti, P. W. (Peter W.) II. University of Toronto. [DNLM: 1. Occupational medicine–Congresses. 2. Protective devices–Congresses. 3. Ear protective devices. WV 26 P467 1980]
RF293.5.P45   617.8′052   81–40748
ISBN 0–89004–698–0   AACR2

Preface

Noise is the most ubiquitous of industrial pollutants; there are others more dangerous but none so widespread. Occupational noise is the most common single cause of hearing loss in the developed nations of the world. Although long recognized as harmful to the ears, steps to reduce sound at source and to protect individuals from excessive exposure have become widespread only in the past two decades. There is a great lack of knowledge about hearing conservation programs in the workplace—how to implement them, what to expect of them, how to monitor them, and indeed what equipment to use to protect individuals.

This book was born out of the editor's frustration while delving through a multidisciplinary literature, attempting to find answers to some of these questions. There is an increasing literature on the biological effects of noise on the ear in both biological and medical journals, but information on the design and testing of the hearing protectors is sparsely spread throughout the physical, engineering, and acoustical literature; on the effects of wearing protectors on hearing, in industrial medical, otological, and audiological journals; on the effects on communication, in military manuals and in industrial, medical, and psychological journals; and much information has not been published at all. Many references are to obscure bulletins and government reports, and in general, workers in the field have not had a comprehensive reference source reviewing the state-of-the-art.

To rectify this, an international symposium was hosted at the University of Toronto in May of 1980, in which the acknowledged experts in these fields were asked to discuss existing knowledge and bring new information about personal hearing protection in industry, within a framework of biological and physically based science, but in the context of a total program of hearing conservation. They collated existing information and contributed new research; this book is the end product.

It surveys the biological effect of noise on the ear; the risks to hearing and the effect of intermittent exposure are discussed. There is a thorough discussion of the design of hearing protectors and their theoretical limitations together with several national approaches to methods of testing them. There are chapters on evaluation of protectors performance, both by means of threshold and super threshold testing as well as new techniques involving miniature probe-microphones placed inside the protectors themselves. Legislators need a simple means of describing the performance of protectors—the single number methods of rating protectors are discussed comprehensively. The relative effectiveness of different protectors are discussed in everyday work situations and many practical problems are dealt with, particularly the many reasons why protectors fail to meet published performance standards. Concern has been expressed for many years that the wearing of hearing protectors may be dangerous because of interference with warning sounds and spoken instructions. These matters are addressed, as are problems peculiar to the military and to the mining industry. The final section of the book covers comprehensively the area of hearing conservation programs, their implementation, problems involved in their maintenance, and how to motivate a work force to accept a hearing conservation program and to continue its use. Any such major programs require careful evaluation and this is discussed from an industrial, academic and a government standpoint.

This volume has been edited to serve as a reference source for those working in the area of hearing protector design, and as a practical guide to those involved in hearing conservation programs. The authors come from seven countries and thus contribute further to the expansive scope of the information contained herein, which has never previously been compiled into a reference handbook.

P. W. Alberti

Acknowledgments

I am grateful for the help given in the production of this book by a large number of people and organisations. Pat Rogers of ESS cheerfully bore the brunt of the typing; my daughters Fiona and Kathryn helped with layout and production. Ivan Gareau and his staff of the Department of Medical Photography, Mount Sinai Hospital, did magnificent work with the photographs. The Saul A. Silverman Family Foundation gave generous support to make the book possible; the Workman's Compensation Board of Ontario contributed to our work. Without the unflagging efforts of Mrs. Doris MacBride of the Continuing Education Division of the Faculty of Medicine, University of Toronto, the Symposium on which this volume is based would not have taken place: her help is gratefully acknowledged. My wife and children lived through the vicissitudes of production, and gave support when it was needed.

Contents

Introduction: The Biological Effects of Noise

1. Inner Ear Damage from Acoustic Trauma
   I. M. Hunter-Duvar and M. Suzuki 1

2. Neurological Basis for the Symptoms of Noise-Induced Hearing Loss
   Donald Henderson, Richard J. Salvi and Roger P. Hamernik .. 15

3. Risks to Hearing: The Effect of Intermittent Exposure
   W. Dixon Ward 35

Personal Hearing Protectors: Design and Standards

4. Hearing Protector Design Concepts and Performance Limitations
   Edgar A. G. Shaw 51

5. Hearing Protection Standards
   Charles W. Nixon 69

6. The Canadian Standards Association Classification of Hearing Protectors: History and Practical Problems
   Edgar E. G. Shaw 91

7. A Test Facility for the Objective Measurement of Circumaural Hearing Protector Attenuation
   J. A. Chillery 101

8. Acoustical and Mechanical Properties of Earmuff Type Hearing Protectors and their Testing
   K. Brinkmann and M. R. Serra 133

Personal Hearing Protectors: Evaluation

9. Evaluation of the Comfort of Personal Hearing Protectors
   André Damongeot, Micheal Tisserand, Ghislain Krawsky, Jean-Pierre Grosdemange, and Daniel Lievin 151

10. Measurers' Choices in Standard and Nonstandard Testing of Hearing Protector Effectiveness
    Jerry V. Tobias 163

11. The *In-Situ* Measurement of the Attenuation of Hearing Protectors by The Use of Miniature Microphones
    Graham M. Rood 175

12	Hearing Protector Attenuation in High Noise Levels *Larry E. Humes, Daniel F. Konkle, and Jay W. Sanders*	199
13	Hearing Protectors Attenuation Measurement by Means of Bone Conduction Testing *André Damongeot and Robert Latye*........................	211
14	Single Number Performance Factors for Hearing Protectors *Paul L. Michael*	221
15	Single-Number Noise-Reduction Factor of Circumaural Hearing Protectors by Dosimetry *David Y. Chung, Jorge Menyhart, and R. Patrick Gannon*	237

Noise and Real World Effectiveness of Protectors

16	The Advantages of Supplementing Conventional Static Noise Analysis Measurements with Personalized Sound Exposure Analysis *G. E. Menzies and R. F. Winn*...............................	249
17	The Effective Attenuation of Hearing Protectors As a Function of Wearing Time *Roland Tengling and Rune Lundin*	263
18	How Realistic Are Standard Subjective Test Methods for Evaluating Hearing Protector Attenuation? *Alan Martin*	273
19	Laboratory Estimates of the Real World Performance of Hearing Protectors *E. H. Berger*	299
20	User Fitting of Hearing Protectors: Attenuation Results *S. M. Abel, P. W. Alberti, and K. Riko*	315

Practical Problems with Protectors

21	How Ear Protectors Fail: A Practical Guide *K. Riko and P. W. Alberti*	323
22	The Effects of Hearing Protection on the Perception of Warning Sounds *P. A. Wilkins and A. M. Martin*...............................	339
23	Speech Intelligibility in Noise: With and Without Ear Protectors *S. M. Abel, P. W. Alberti, C. Haythornthwaite, and K. Riko*.....	371
24	Hearing Protector Problems in Military Operations *S. E. Forshaw and J. I. Cruchley*	387

25	Practical Problems of Hearing Protector Use in Canadian Mines M. U. Savich	403
26	New Design Concepts in Personal Hearing Protectors A. G. Gorman	427

Hearing Conservation Programs: Problems of Implementation

27	Personal Hearing Protection: Problems Associated with the Hearing Protection Phase of the Hearing Conservation Program L. H. Royster and S. R. Holder	447
28	Hearing Protector Programme Establishment D. Else	471
29	How to Motivate People in the Use of Their Hearing Protectors H. Lofgreen, M. Holm, and R. Tengling	485
30	Employee Attitudes Towards Hearing Protection as Affected by Serial Audiometry S. J. Karmy and A. M. Martin	491

Hearing Conservation Programs: Evaluation and Effectiveness

31	Methods of Evaluating Hearing Conservation Program Audiometric Data Bases L. H. Royster and J. D. Royster	511
32	The Long-Term Effectiveness of a Hearing Conservation Programme Based Upon Personal Hearing Protection S. Pell, T. A. Dear, and B. W. Karrh	541
33	Hearing Conservation Based on Hearing Protectors: A Provincial Project D. Y. Chung, R. P. Gannon, M. E. Roberts, and K. Mason	559
34	Planning a Provincial Hearing Conservation Program P. L. Pelmear and M. J. Pike	569

Conclusions

35	Summation of Personal Hearing Protection in Industry W. Dixon Ward	577
	Subject Index	593

Contributors

S. M. Abel, Ph.D.: *Assistant Professor of Otolaryngology, Silverman Hearing Research Laboratory, Mount Sinai Hospital, University of Toronto, 200–600 University Avenue, Toronto, Ontario, M5G 1X5 Canada*

P. W. Alberti, M. B., Ph.D., F.R.C.S.: *Professor of Otolaryngology and Environmental and Occupational Medicine, University of Toronto, Otolaryngologist-in-Chief, Mount Sinai Hospital, 405–600 University Avenue, Toronto, Ontario, M5G 1X5 Canada*

E. H. Berger, B.S., M.S.M.E. (acoustics): *Manager, Acoustical Engineering, E-A-R Corporation, 7911 Zionsville Road, Indianapolis, Indiana 46268*

K. Brinkmann, Ph.D.: *Physikalisch-Technische Bundesanstalt, Bundesallee 100, 3300 Braunschweig, Federal Republic of Germany*

J. A. Chillery, Ph.D.: *I.S.V.R., The University of Southampton, currently Ministry of Defence, Royal Aircraft Establishment, Flight Systems Department, Farnborough, Hants GU14 6TD, England*

D. Y. Chung, Ph.D.: *Research Associate, Medical Department, Workers' Compensation Board, 10551 Shellbridge Way, Richmond, British Columbia, V6X 2X1 Canada*

J. I. Cruchley, B.A.: *Research Associate, Behavioural Sciences Division, Defence and Civil Institute of Environmental Medicine, 113 Sheppard Avenue West, Downsview, Ontario, Canada*

A. André Damongeot: *I.N.R.S., Centre de Recherche de Nancy, Avenue de Bourgogne, 54500 Vandoeuvre, France*

T. A. Dear, B.A., B.S., M.S., F.I.O.A.: *Senior Consultant Noise and Acoustics, E du Pont de Nemours and Co., Louviers Building, Wilmington, Delaware 19898*

E. Else, Ph.D.: *Senior Tutor, Department of Safety and Hygiene, University of Aston, Birmingham B4 7ET, England*

S. E. Forshaw, P. Eng.: *Head, Sonics Section, Behavioural Sciences Division, Defence and Civil Institute of Environmental Medicine, 113 Sheppard Avenue West, Downsview, Ontario, Canada*

R. P. Gannon, M.D.: *Director Hearing Branch, Workmens' Compensation Board, 10551 Shellbridge Way, Richmond, British Columbia, Canada*

A. G. Gorman, D.F.H., C. Eng., M.I.E.E.: *Technical Director, Racal Acoustics Ltd., Beresford Avenue, Wembley, Middlesex HAO IRU England*

J.-P. Grosdemange: *I.N.R.S., Centre de Recherche de Nancy, Avenue de Bourgogne, 54500 Vandoeuvre, France*

CONTRIBUTORS

R. P. Hamernick, Ph.D.: Associate Professor of Otolaryngology and Communication Sciences, Callier Centre, Dallas, Texas 75235

C. Haythornthwaite, M.Sc.: Research Associate, Silverman Hearing Laboratory, Department of Otolaryngology, Mount Sinai Hospital, University of Toronto, Toronto, Ontario, M5G 1X5 Canada

D. Henderson, Ph.D.: Associate Professor of Otolaryngology and Communication Science, Callier Centre, Dallas, Texas 75235

S. R. Holder: Department of Psychology, North Carolina State University, Raleigh, North Carolina 27650

M. Holm: Marketing Director, Bilsom, Billesholm, Sweden

L. E. Humes, Ph.D.: Assistant Professor and Director of Research, Division of Hearing and Speech Sciences, Vanderbilt University School of Medicine, and the Bill Wilkerson Hearing and Speech Center, Nashville, Tennessee 37232

I. Hunter-Duvar, Ph.D.: Director, Otologic Research Laboratory, Department of Otolaryngology, Hospital for Sick Children, 555 555 University Avenue, Toronto, Ontario M5G 1X8. Associate Professor, Department of Otolaryngology, University of Toronto, Toronto, Ontario, M5G 1X8 Canada

S. Karmy, B.A., M.Sc., M.I.O.A.: Lecturer (Industrial Audiometry), Institute for Sound and Vibration Research, The University of Southampton, Southampton S09 5NH, England

B. W. Karrh, M.D.: Corporate Medical Director, E du Pont de Nemours and Company, Louviers Building, Wilmington, Delaware 19898

D. F. Konkle, Ph.D.: Division of Hearing and Speech Sciences, Vanderbilt University School of Medicine and the Bill Wilkerson Hearing and Speech Center, Vanderbilt University, Nashville, Tennessee 37232

G. Krawsky: I.N.R.S., Centre de Recherche de Nancy, Avenue de Bourgogne, 54500 Vandoeuvre, France

R. Lataye: I.N.R.S., Centre de Recherche de Nancy, Avenue de Bourgogne, 54500 Vandoeuvre, France

D. Lievin: I.N.R.S., Centre de Recherche de Nancy, Avenue de Bourgogne, 54500 Vandoeuvre, France

H. Lofgreen: Vice President, Bilsom International Ltd., Toronto, Ontario, M4T 2V7 Canada

A. M. Martin, B.Sc., M.Sc., Ph.D.: Head of Audiology Group, Institute for Sound and Vibration Research, The University, Southampton S09 5NH, England

K. Mason, M.S.: Workers' Compensation Board, 10551 Shellbridge Way, Richmond, British Columbia, V6X 2X1 Canada

J. Menyhart, Eng.: Workers' Compensation Board, 10551 Shellbridge Way, Richmond, British Columbia, V6X 2X1 Canada

CONTRIBUTORS

G. E. Menzies, B. Eng., P. Eng.: *Division Foreman, Steel Company of Canada, Stelco Tower, Hamilton, Ontario, G8N 3T4 Canada*

P. L. Michael, B.S., M.S., Ph.D.: *Professor of Environmental Acoustics and Director of the Environmental Acoustics Laboratory, Pennsylvania State University, 110 Moore Building, University Park, Pennsylvania 16802*

C. Nixon, Ph.D.: *Chief, Biological Acoustics Branch, Biodynamics and Bioengineering Division, Air Force Aerospace Medical Research Laboratory (AFSC). Wright-Patterson Air Force Base, Ohio 45433*

S. Pell, Ph.D.: *Manager, Epidemiology Division, E du Pont de Nemours and Co., Louviers Building, Wilmington, Delaware 19898*

P. L. Pelmear, M.D., M.F.O.M., D.I.H.: *Director, Occupational Health Branch, Ontario Ministry of Labour, 400 University Avenue, Toronto, Ontario, M7A 1T7 Canada*

M. Pike, M.A., C.C.C.: *Audiologist, Occupational Health Branch, Ontario Ministry of Labour, 400 University Avenue, Toronto, Ontario, M7A 1T7 Canada*

K. Riko, M.Sc. (App.): *Chief Audiologist, Assistant Professor of Otolaryngology, University of Toronto, Department of Otolaryngology, Mount Sinai Hospital, 201–600 University Avenue, Toronto, Ontario, M5G 1X5 Canada*

M. E. Robert, M.S.: *Audiologist, Workers' Compensation Board, 10551 Shellbridge Way, Richmond, British Columbia, V6X 2X1 Canada*

G. M. Rood, Ph.D., M.Sc., C. Eng., M. I. Mech. E., M.R.A.E.S.: *Principal Scientific Officer, Human Engineering Division, Ministry of Defence, Flight Systems Department, Q153 Building, Royal Aircraft Establishment, Farnborough, Hants GU14 6TD, England*

J. D. Royster, M.S., C.C.C.-Sp/A: *Graduate Student, Department of Psychology, North Carolina State University, Box 5246, Raleigh, North Carolina 27650*

L. H. Royster, B.S., Ph.D.: *Professor, Department of Mechanical and Aerospace Engineering, North Carolina State University, Box 5246, Raleigh, North Carolina 27650*

J. W. Sanders, Ph.D.: *Division of Hearing and Speech Sciences, Vanderbilt University School of Medicine and The Bill Wilkerson Hearing and Speech Center, Nashville, Tennessee 37232*

M. U. Savich, Dipl. Eng.: *Research Scientist, Elliott Lake Laboratory, Mining Research Laboratories, Canada Center for Mineral and Energy Technology, Department of Energy, Mines and Resources, 58 Hirshhorn Avenue, Elliott Lake, Ontario, P5A IN9 Canada*

M. R. Serra, Ing.: *Fellow of the Consejo Nacional de Investigaciones Cientificas y Tecnicas de la Republica Argentina. Physikalisch-Technische, Bundesanstalt, Bundesallee 100, 3300 Braunschweig, Germany*

E. A.G. Shaw, Ph.D.: *Head, Acoustics Section, Division of Physics, National Research Council of Canada, Ottawa, Ontario, K1A 0R6 Canada*

M. Suzuki, M.D.: Research Associate, Hospital for Sick Children, 555 University Avenue, Toronto, Ontario, M5G 1X8 Canada

R. Tengling, M.A.: Product Development Manager, Bilsom AB, S-260 50 Billesholm, Sweden

M. Tisserans: I.N.R.S., Centre de Recherche de Nancy, Avenue de Bourgogne, 54500 Vandoeuvre, France

J. V. Tobias, Ph.D.: Director, Industrial Audiology Consultants, Professor of Psychology, University of Oklahoma, P.O. Box 358, Norman, Oklahoma 73069

W. D. Ward, B.S., Ph.D., D.Sc.: Professor, Department of Otolaryngology, Hearing Research Laboratory, University of Minnesota, 2630 University Avenue, S.E., Minneapolis, Minnesota 55455

P. A. Wilkins, B.Eng., M.Sc., Ph.D.: Institute for Sound and Vibration Research, The University, Southampton, Hants S09 5NH, England

R. F. Winn, B.Sc.: Engineer, Noise and Vibration Laboratory, Steel Company of Canada, Stelco Tower, Hamilton, Ontario, G8N 3T4 Canada

Personal Hearing Protection in Industry, edited by P. W. Alberti, Raven Press, New York ©

1
INNER EAR DAMAGE FROM ACOUSTIC TRAUMA
I. M. Hunter-Duvar and M. Suzuki

INTRODUCTION

Our studies have concentrated on determining the origin and sequence of damage to cochlear structure in acoustic overstimulation. This necessitates the use of animal models since, with human subjects, the damage due to aging is confounded with other damage by the time temporal bones become available for study. Much of our research time has been spent on developing higher magnification techniques and adapting tools used in other areas to the reliable assessment of the cochlea. This paper will demonstrate results from the use of tools such as the scanning and the transmission electron microscope.

Stimulation has generally been done with a pure tone and usually at a frequency of 1000 Hz. This relatively simple stimulus allows us to localize better the area in which damage might be expected from overstimulation.

Preparation of the cochlea for inspection with the electron microscope is a major problem because of the small size, the delicate construction and the difficult location, completely embedded in bone. Knowing the approximate lesion area allows us to use procedures that ensure that particular area will be subjected to a minimum of preparation artifacts. This becomes especially important when we wish to assess damage to such minute structures as sterocilia of sensory cells, using the scanning electron microscope.

METHODOLOGY

The animals used in our research have been monkeys, cats and chinchillas. Data presented in this paper will be from chinchillas. We have exposed over 100 of these animals to a 1kHz pure tone stimulus varying in intensity from 90dB to 120 dB (SPL).

Animals are decapitated at periods ranging from immediately after exposure to 12 weeks post exposure. After decapitation, cochleas are immediately removed and prepared for histological assessment with the scanning electron microscope. Procedures used are fully explained in a previous publication[1]. Briefly, cochleas are fixed with glutaraldehyde; rinsed overnight in buffer and post fixed the next day with osmium tetroxide. They are then dissected in 70% alcohol. Great care is taken during dissection not to disturb the organ of Corti in the lower middle and upper basal turns. It is in this area that a lesion from 1kHz stimulus is most likely to occur. The area is therefore left encased in bone to a level just above the basilar membrane. (Fig. 1.) When this procedure is employed, the spiral ligament above the bone can be removed without placing any stress on the organ of Corti. Reissner's membrane is then removed. The tectorial membrane is left in place as it will turn up during subsequent critical point drying to expose the cilia of the hair cells.

Figure 1. Light micrograph of lower middle and upper basal turn of chinchilla cochlea after dissection prior to critical point drying for inspection with the scanning electron microscope. The spiral ligament has been removed to the level of the bone which has been left just above the basilar membrane so that no stress is placed on the organ of Corti during dissection. Reissner's membrane has been removed but the tectorial membrane remains in place over the stereocilia of the sensory (hair) cells.

Figure 2. A - Scanning electronmicrograph of the area shown in Figure 1 after the specimen has been incubated in osmium tetroxide and thiocarbohydrazide. The tectorial membrane (TM) has lifted up to give full access to the surface of the organ of Corti (OC). Fragments of Reissner's membrane (RM) which was removed during dissection can be seen. Large cracks (arrows) have opened in the organ of Corti due to the shrinkage which occurs during drying. M= modiolus, CC= Claudius cells, SL= spiral ligament, B= bone.

B - Scanning micrograph of a shrinkage crack demonstrating how cracks may be useful in assessment of interior of organ of Corti when they occur in opportune areas. Four outer hair cells which occur occasionally can be clearly seen in this micrograph. TC= tunnel of Corti, HC= Hensen cells, PC= pillar cell.

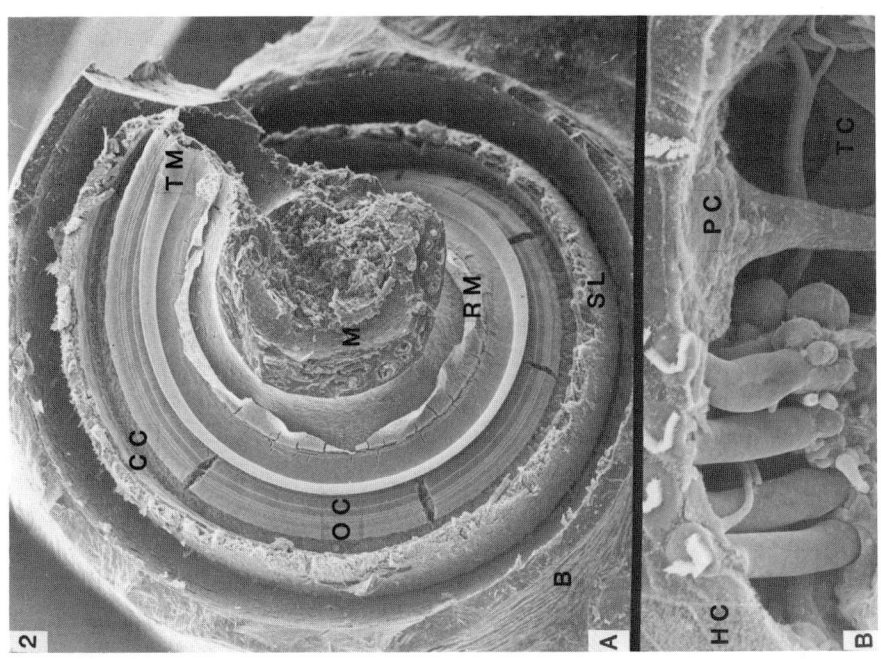
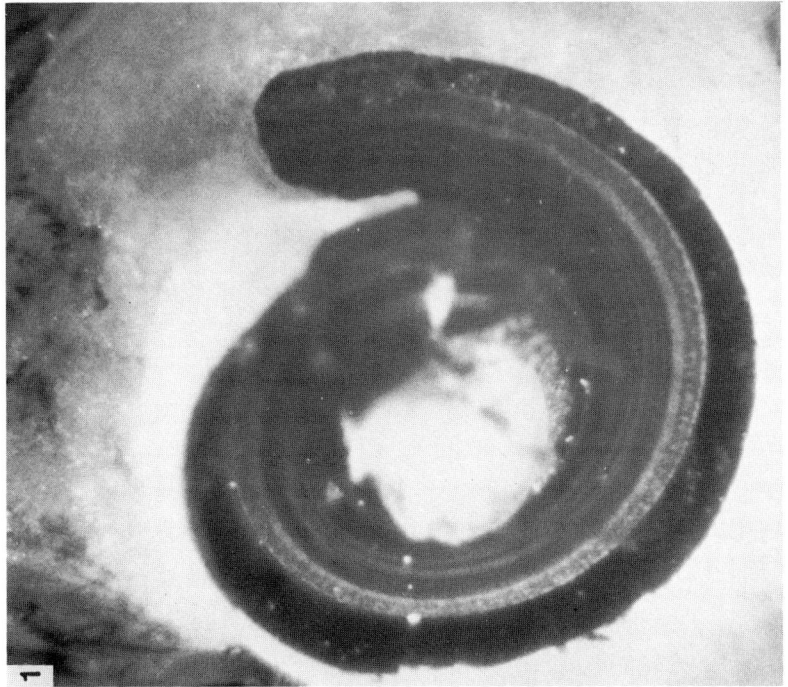

After dissection, specimens are processed with osmium and thiocarbohydrazide[1] then dried from 100% ethanol with CO_2 in the critical point drier. Specimens are viewed in the scanning electron microscope which allows the assessment of all surface details. Drying the specimen causes random cracks to open through the organ of Corti (Fig. 2) and when these cracks appear in opportune places they allow inspection of the interior of the organ of Corti.

In the event that information is desired on the condition of the internal structure, the entire specimen is placed in absolute ethanol and embedded in Spurr. Areas of interest are then prepared for inspection with the transmission electron microscope using routine procedures. The heavy osmification makes staining of the thin sections unnecessary. The combination of scanning and transmission electron microscopes allows for thorough inspection of cochlear ultra-structure.

RESULTS AND DISCUSSION

In humans and in animals, exposure to the same traumatic stimulus may result in large individual differences in the damage sustained. Minimal types of damage appear to be bending of stereocilia on outer and inner hair cells (Fig. 3), distortion of hair cell bodies (Fig. 4) and swelling of hair cells bodies. This type of damage would appear to be reversible if the traumatic stimulus is withdrawn soon enough. Great care must be taken in the interpretation as all three of these phenomena can also occur during fixation.

The great variability in sensitivity makes the sequence of events in damage difficult to follow, however, from looking at the results of a large number of animals killed at various times after exposure we believe that cilia bent over during exposure, and seen bent over when animals are dispatched immediately after exposure, may recover and again become erect. Evidence for this comes from the fact that bent over cilia are not

Figure 4. A transmission electron micrograph showing a horizontal cut through cell bodies of several outer hair cells demonstrating the irregular shapes of the cell bodies several days after exposure to acoustic trauma.

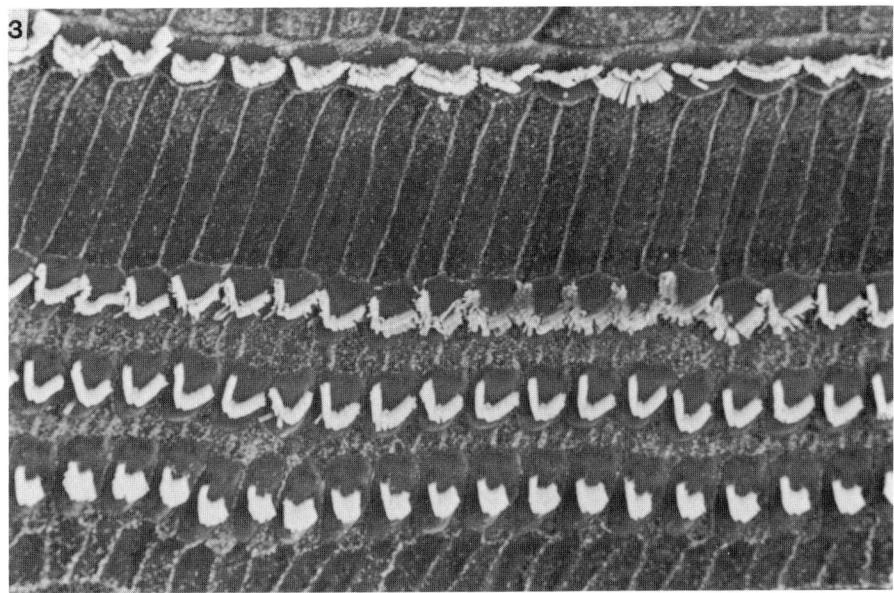

Figure 3. Scanning micrograph showing area where the stereocilia of an inner hair cell and stereocilia of several first outer row hair cells are disrupted in an animal sacrificed immediately after exposure to acoustic trauma.

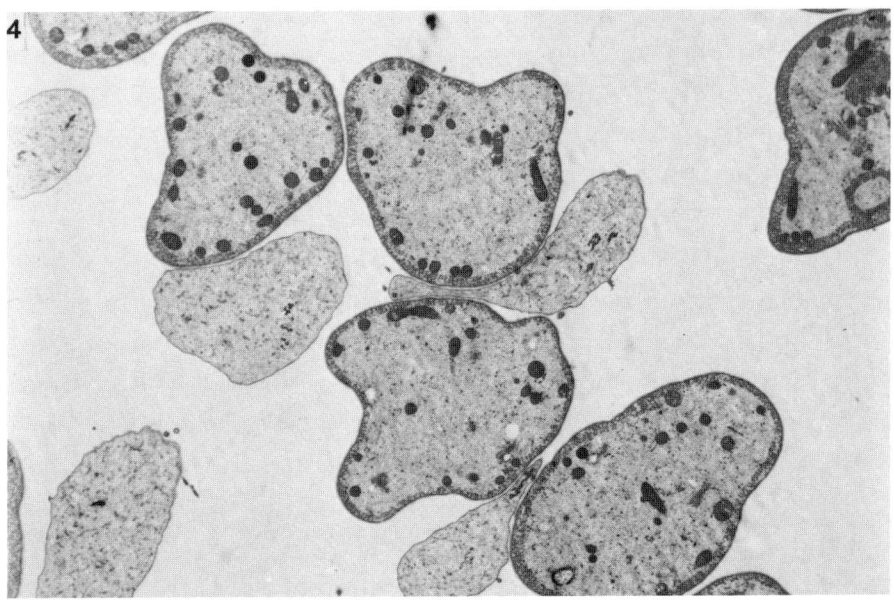

found on hair cells when they are examined several days after exposure. Often areas of expected damage will show hair cells with some cilia missing. Since this phenomenon is not seen in other areas of the cochlea or in the animal's other cochlea which has been protected from the traumatic stimulus, we believe that some stereocilia can be damaged beyond the point of repair and are detached and resorbed by the cochlea while the remainder of the bent cilia presumably return to a normal erect state. Fig. 5 shows some missing stereocilia on first row outer hair cells several days post exposure. Remaining cilia are erect.

Increased surface damage is seen in several forms. Fig. 6 shows the focal point of a lesion of moderate severity. In animals killed immediately after exposure the cuticular plates on the phalangeal processes of Deiter cells can be seen to blister then collapse, leaving indentations in the surface of the organ of Corti (Fig. 7). By the time the cuticular plates of the phalangeal process have collapsed cilia on surrounding hair cells have agglutinated or fused and are undergoing some type of autolysis (Fig. 8).

Inspection of the area under the cuticular plate (Fig.9) shows that the indentations in the phalangeal process do not go through into the interior of the organ of Corti. It is also seen that hair cells with stereocilia in the process of destruction have largely deteriorated beneath the surface and that the contents are errupting into the sub-tectorial space of the scala media through perforations in the area of the basal body. (Fig.9, Fig. 10) The stereocilia on the hair cells at the focal point of the lesion are eventually completely autolysed and leave only stumps giving the impression that they have been broken off (Fig. 10). The gradient of damage indicates that the first row outer hair cells are most susceptible to trauma followed by second and third row outer hair cells respectively. Inner hair cells generally are more resistant to damage from sound than are outer hair cells. There are exceptions to this finding but parameters of the exceptions are not yet defined.

This is the rather messy ongoing picture that is seen when the cochlea is examined immediately after moderate overstimulation. If the stimulation

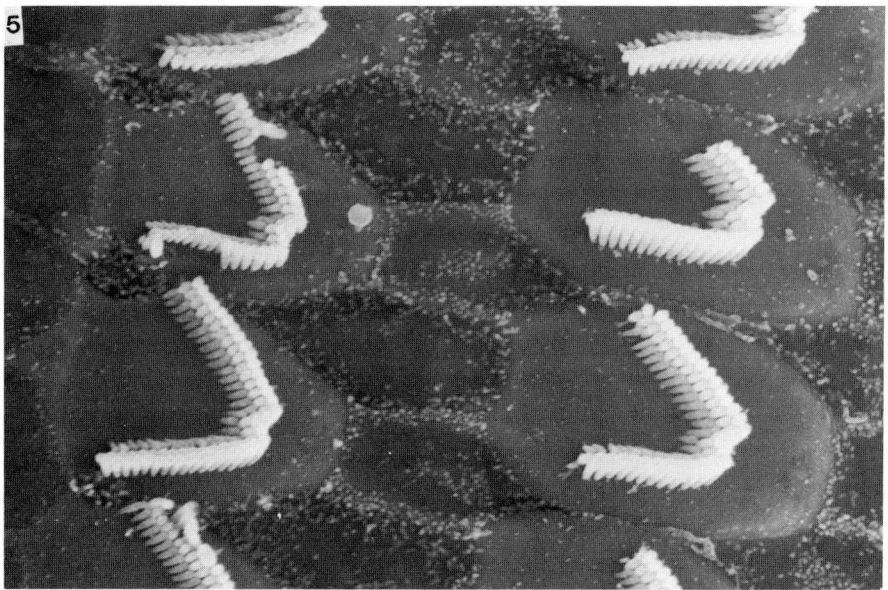

Figure 5. Scanning micrograph of outer hair cells on an animal previously exposed to acoustic trauma showing missing stereocilia. All remaining cilia are erect.

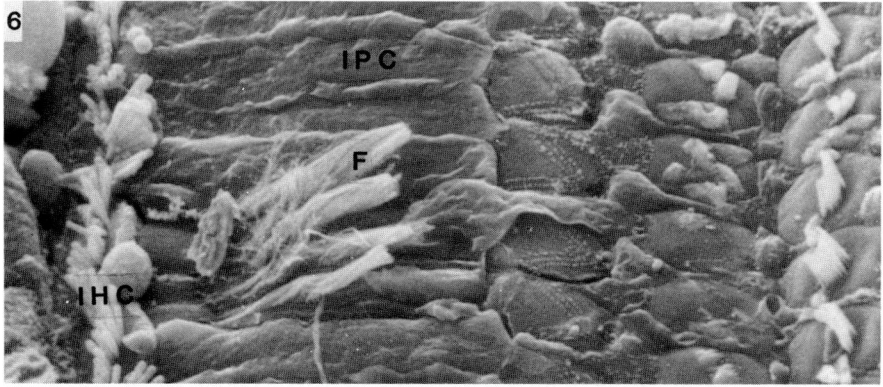

Figure 6. Scanning micrograph showing focal area of lesion in chinchilla exposed to a 1kHz tone of 120 dB for 15 min. and decapitated immediately. Stereocilia of inner hair cells (IHC) are in disarray and some inner pillar cells (IPC) have fibers (F) bursting through the cuticular plates. Stereocilia on outer hair cells are missing or fused.

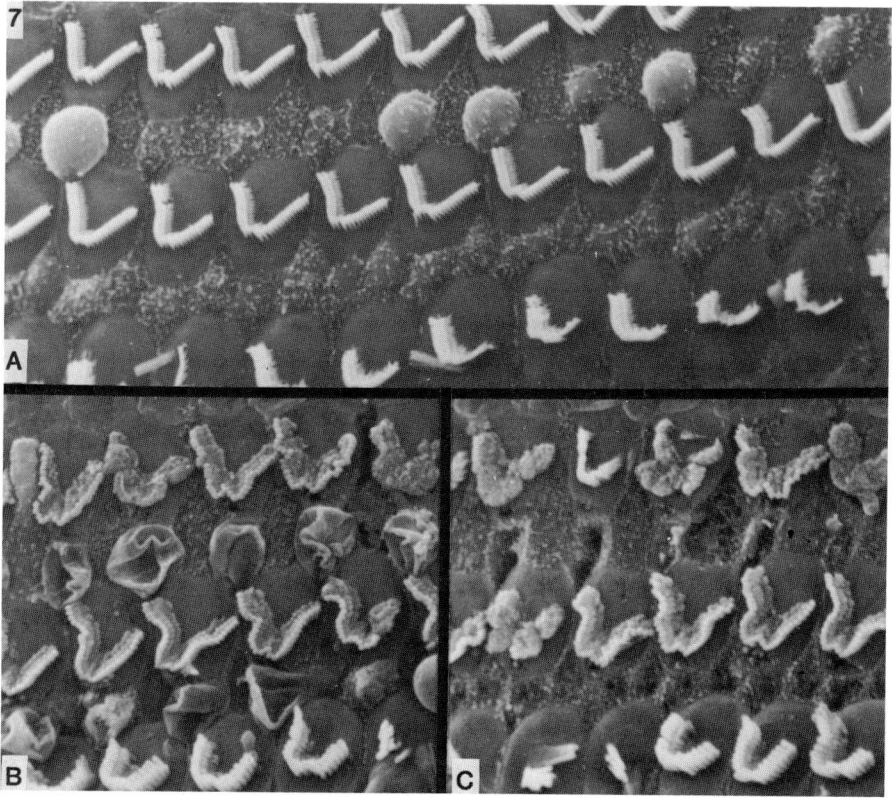

Figure 7.   Scanning micrographs, showing damage areas of different severity, indicate what we believe to be sequence in damage to phalangeal processes of Deiter cells. A - Cuticular surfaces are seen to bubble. B - The bubbled surfaces are seen in a state of collapse.   C - Indentations appear in the cuticular plate in areas of collapse.

Figure 8.   A - Scanning micrograph of outer hair cell from lesion in Figure 6 on which stereocilia have fused. B -Transmission micrograph of section through hair cell in A showing how partial outlines of stereocilia remain.

Figure 9.   A - Higher power scanning micrograph of indentations shown in Figure 7 and showing further deterioration of stereocilia.   B - Transmission micrograph of section through area shown in A indicating the indentations do not extend through to the fluid spaces of the organ of Corti. The deteriorating hair cell is seen to be ejecting its contents into the subtectorial space (arrow).

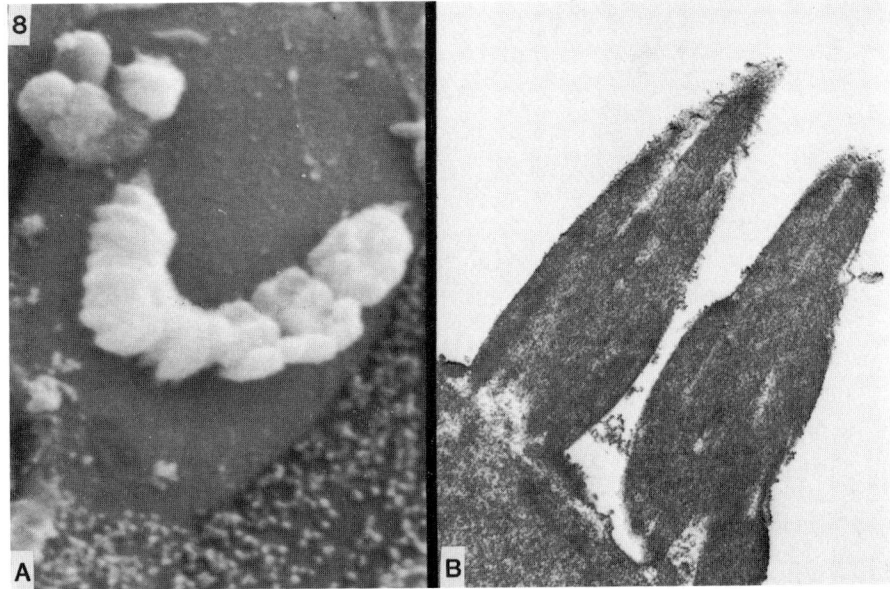

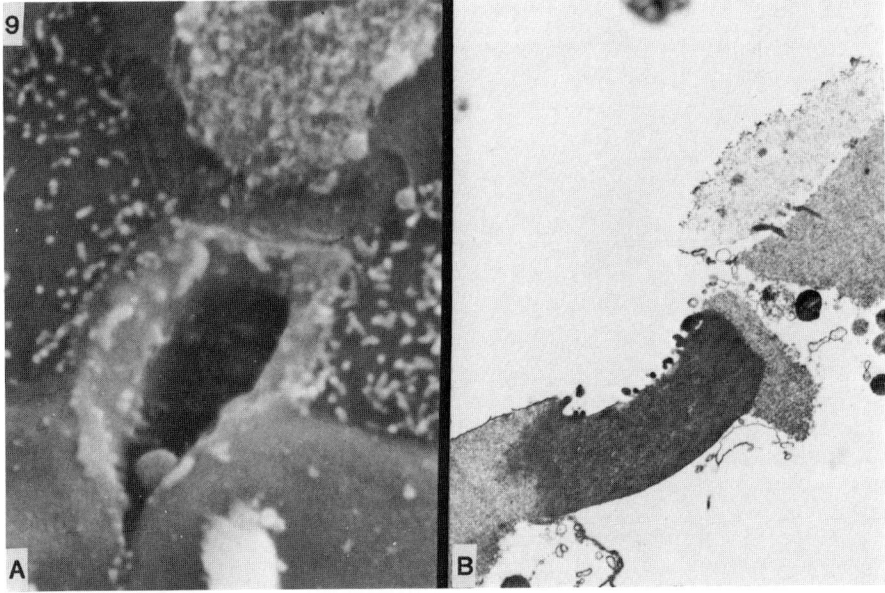

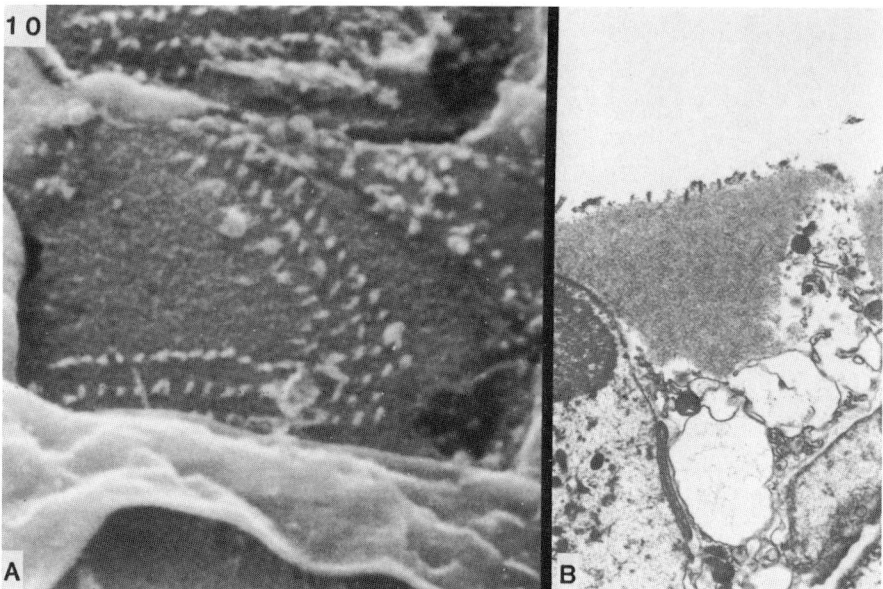

Figure 10. A - Scanning micrograph of hair cell from lesion in Figure 6 after stereocilia have completely gone leaving only stumps. B - Transmission micrograph showing roots of stereocilia remaining in cuticular plate. Contents of hair cell can be seen errupting into the subtectorial space.

Figure 11. Scanning micrograph of acoustic lesion 24 hours post-exposure. Cilia on remaining cells are seen to be relatively erect. First and second outer row hair cells are missing. Cuticular plates from some third outer row hair cells have been ejected onto the surface of the organ of Corti. Some of these have relatively intact stereocilia.

Figure 12. Scanning micrograph of a lesion ten weeks after exposure to acoustic trauma shows area of organ of Corti with scars replacing missing outer hair cells.

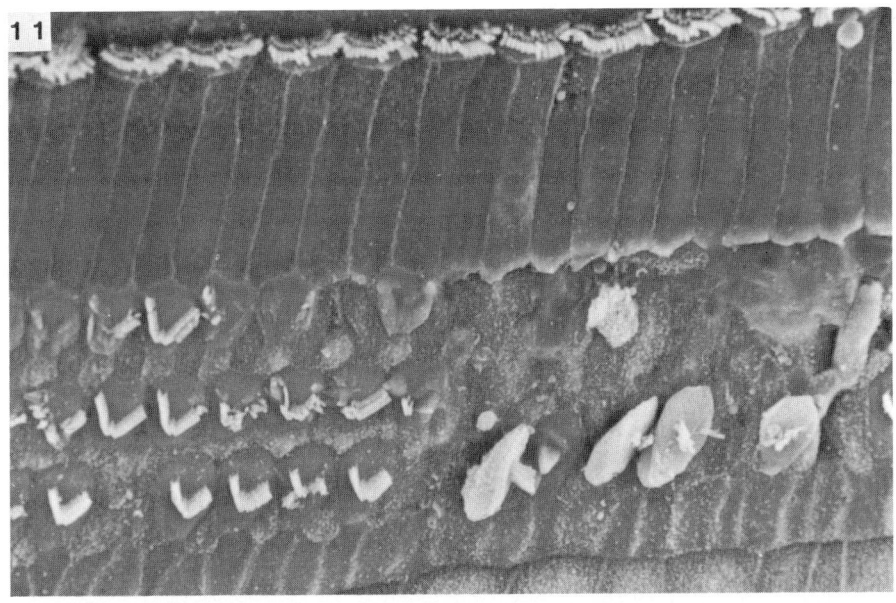

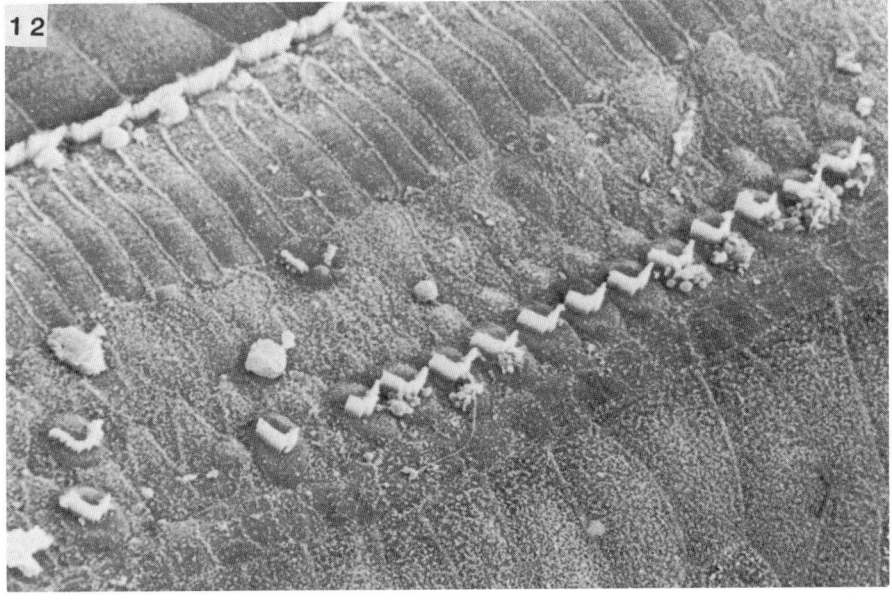

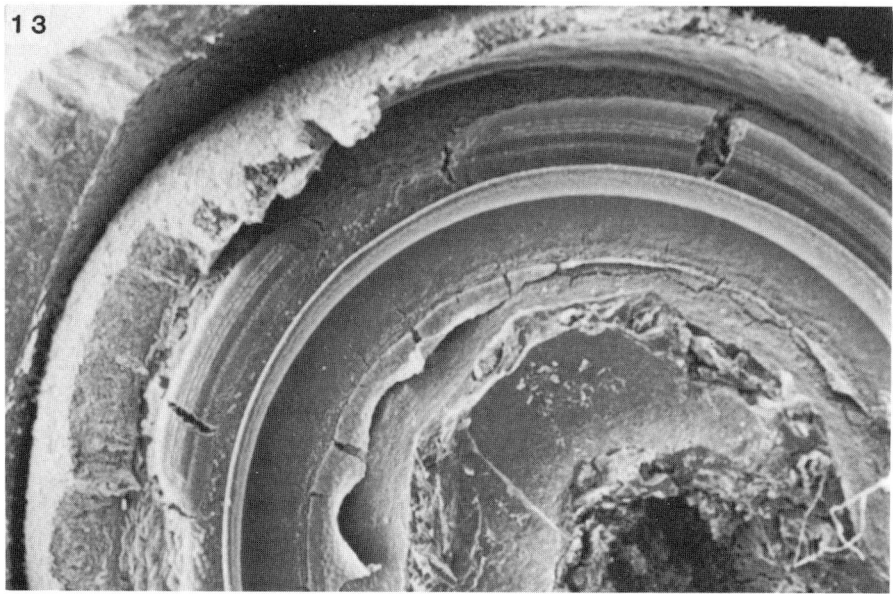

Figure 13. Scanning micrograph shows how ends of lesion have grown over to completely seal the fluid spaces of the organ of Corti when an area is destroyed during acoustic trauma.

time is lengthened with moderate stimulation, or stimuli made more intense, the organ of Corti will be ruptured and damage will be much more severe. This will lessen considerably the inter-subject variability.

The clean up process after exposure to acoustic trauma is very fast. Inspection only 24 hours after cessation of stimulation shows a much tidier surface with erect stereocilia, and lesion borders well defined (Fig. 11). Cuticular plates from deteriorated hair cells may be seen lying on the surface of the organ of Corti, where they have been ejected.

The picture ten weeks after exposure shows a scarred but cleaned up organ of Corti (Fig. 12). In more severe lesions it can be seen that the tunnel and spaces of Nuel of the organ of Corti have been sealed at both ends of the lesion and are no longer continuous over the turn (Fig. 13).

Fused stereocilia may be seen on outer hair cells of animals sacrificed immediately after exposures of only 12 minutes (Fig. 7). It is rare to see them on outer hair cells at long survival times except in the very apex. On inner hair cells the opposite case appears to exist, in that, although stereocilia may be disrupted when the animals are killed immediately after exposure, the cilia are not fused until some time later. Fused and giant cilia on inner hair cells may appear as a product of acoustic trauma, ototoxic drug damage or normal maturation.

This is, in general, the picture seen when chinchillas are exposed to the 1kHz stimulus described. Authors using other species and/or different stimuli have suggested other effects and some of these may be found in the readings included in the bibliography[2,3,4].

REFERENCES

1. Hunter-Duvar, I., Electron Microscopic Assessment of the Cochlea. Acta Otolaryngol. (Suppl). 351, 1978.

2. Bohne, B., Mechanism of Noise Damage in the Inner Ear, in Effects of Noise on Hearing. ed. D. Henderson, R. Hamernick, D. Dosanjh, J. Mills. Raven Press N.Y. 41-67, 1976.

3. Bredberg, G. and Hunter-Duvar I., Behavioral Tests of Hearing and Inner Ear Damage, in Handbook of Sensory Physiology. Vol. V:2, ed. W. Keidel, W. Neff. Springer-Verlag. Berlin, Heidelberg, N.Y.: 261-306, 1975.

4. Spoendlin, H., Anatomical Changes Following Various Noise Exposures, in Effects of Noise on Hearing (ibid.) 69-87, 1976.

ACKNOWLEDGEMENTS

The excellent technical assistance of Richard Mount and the secretarial services of Chris Thomas are sincerely appreciated. This work is supported by the Medical Research Council of Canada, The U.S. National Institute of Occupational Safety and Health and the Research Institute of The Hospital for Sick Children.

Personal Hearing Protection in Industry, edited by P. W. Alberti, Raven Press, New York ©

2 Neurological Basis for the Symptoms of Noise-Induced Hearing Loss

Donald Henderson, Richard J. Salvi, and Roger P. Hamernick

INTRODUCTION

Clinical reports of noise induced hearing loss (NIPTS) are usually limited to a description of the audiogram. However, there are usually other audiological symptoms associated with NIPTS such as the rapid growth of loudness (recruitment), poorer speech discrimination, tinnitus and a reduction in the temporal integration of acoustic signals. These symptoms are thought to be the consequence of pathological changes in the cochlea which modify the neural output going to the central auditory system. Furthermore, the complexity of the audiological symptoms suggests that there are extensive and fundamental changes in the neural output of the cochlea. The purpose of this paper is to relate the audiological symptoms of NIPTS to the changes in the neural code leaving the cochlea. Although understanding the neural basis of the symptoms of NIPTS is a clinical problem, it is currently impossible to study in humans because we are limited to studying gross neurophysiological indices of hearing such as brain stem evoked potentials and electrocochleography and temporal bones of patients with a history of noise induced hearing loss. Animal models provide the opportunity to systematically measure and correlate the psychoacoustic, neurological and anatomical changes brought about by exposure to noise. A fundamental assumption of the animal model is that the animal suffers analagous auditory signal processing problems to man following acoustic trauma.

METHOD

Twenty monaural chinchillas were used as experimental subjects. The chinchilla was chosen because its hearing capabilities are approximately the same as humans; it is possible to measure the chinchilla's hearing reliably with conditioning procedures; the VIII nerve is readily accessable to probing with microelectrodes and the cochlea is easy to dissect.

The animal's hearing is measured using a conditioned avoidance procedure[1,2]. Pre-exposure audiograms were established by averaging the results of 10 days testing at octave steps from .5 to 16 kHz. After reliable estimates of auditory sensitivity had been established, the animals were exposed for five days to an octave band of noise centered at 0.5 kHz and having an SPL of 95 dB. The first group of six animals was tested daily and at 40 days after the exposure. A second group of 6 animals was given the same exposure, then the animals were removed from the noise, anesthetized and the response characteristics of individual auditory nerve fibers were sampled using standard neurological techniques for VIII nerve recording[3,4,5]. The VIII nerve recording sessions lasted approximately 15 hours, then the animal was killed and the cochleas were later analyzed using a surface preparation technique[6]. A third control group of normal animals was also used in single unit studies to establish normative response characteristics of normal VIII nerve neurons in the anesthetized chinchilla.

RESULTS
Normal Response of the VIII Nerve

The normal physiology of individual VIII nerve fibers of the cat has been extensively documented by Kiang and his co-workers[3,7]. Studies by Dallos et al[8] and Salvi et al[9], on the chinchilla show that the VIII nerve responses of chinchilla are essentially the same as in the cat. The next section will describe some of the response properties that are observed in normal neurons in the chinchilla.

In "quiet", the fibers of the auditory nerve show varying amounts of spontaneous activity. Figure 1 shows the distribution of spontaneous activity (S.A.) as a function of the characteristic frequency (CF) of the neuron (the characteristic frequency is the frequency at which the neuron responds with the lowest intensity of stimulation). The S.A. rate ranges

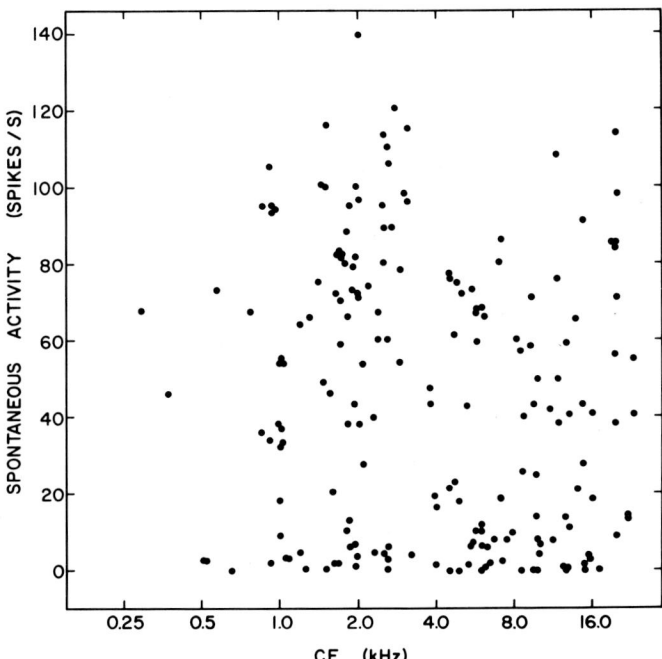

Figure 1: Normal spontaneous activity (spikes/s) as a function of the CF of the neuron in kHz.

from roughly 0 to 120 spikes/s. There appears to be a clustering of units near 1 spikes/s and another group near 40-50 spikes/s.

Another important property of each neuron is its tuning curve, i.e. a plot which describes the unit's threshold as a function of frequency.

The collection of tuning curves in Figure 2 is representative of normal response areas in the chinchilla. The solid dots represent the tips of the tuning curves measured in the normal animals. The tuning curves were measured using 20 msec tone bursts and the criterion for threshold was an increase in firing rate above the level of S.A. using audio-visual methods.

The shapes of the tuning curves in the chinchilla are similar to those in the cat. Above 2 kHz, the tuning curves are asymetrical. There is a low threshold, sharp tip at CF; the high frequency side of the curve is very steep; the low frequency side has a steep section which leads to a broadly

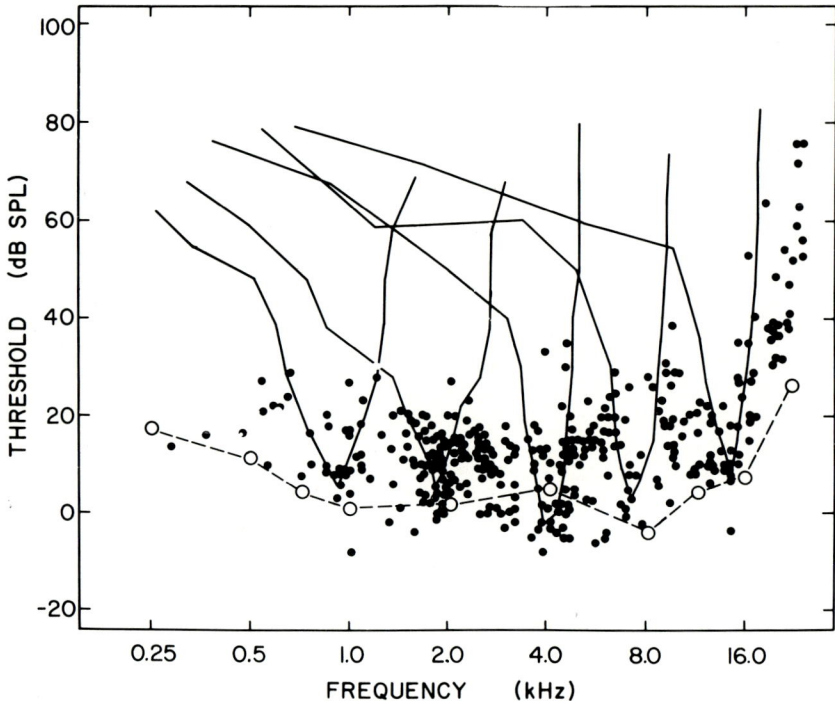

Figure 2: Comparison of tuning curves (solid lines), unit thresholds (●) and behavioral threshold (o--o) from normal chinchillas.

tuned, high threshold, low frequency tail. Below 2.0 kHz the tuning curves are more symetrical and both the high and low frequency segments are not as steep as in units with CF's above 2 kHz. In a sense, the tuning characteristics of individual VIII nerve fibers represent a band pass filter which establishes the frequency selectivity of the auditory system.

The solid points in Figure 2 represent the thresholds at CF for a large population of neurons sampled from 8 normal animals. The dashed line and open circles represent the average behavioral threshold (in dB SPL) at the tympanic membrane. The behavioral threshold includes a transformation to account for the resonance characteristics of the outer ear[10]; thus, the behavioral thresholds and unit thresholds can be compared directly. The most sensitive neurons lie on the behavioral thresholds and the least sensitive are as much as 25 dB above the behavioral threshold. The threshold of units with very high CFs are somewhat greater than

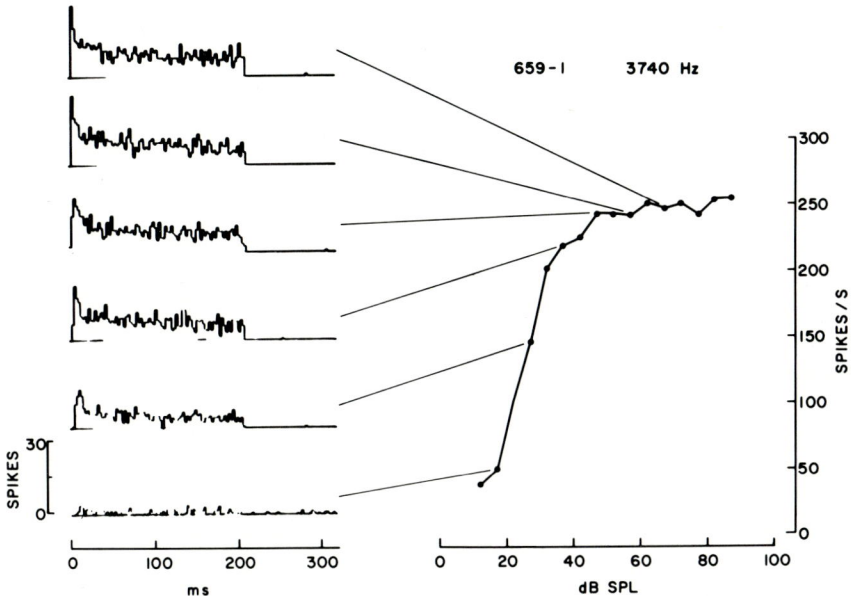

Figure 3: Post-stimulus time (PST) histograms and an input/output function from a normal VIII nerve fiber. The left side of the figure shows a series of PST histograms obtained with 200 ms tone burst at several intensities above threshold. The right side of the figure shows the unit's firing rate as a function of intensity.

behavioral threshold; this may reflect the effects of anesthesia and surgery rather than being a "true discrepancy" between behavioral and neural thresholds[11].

The typical response to tone bursts at several intensities is shown in Figure 3. Near threshold, the neuron responds at a relatively constant rate during the course of the stimulus. At higher intensities, there is a rapid rate of activity at the onset of stimulation that decays to an approximately constant rate of firing. The pattern of response during stimulation by the tones is relatively invariant 30 dB above threshold.

The general relationship between the intensity of stimulation and firing rate is illustrated in the right panel of Figure 3. Most of the neurons have a limited dynamic range*. In the population of normal VIII nerve fibers, the discharge rate typically increases over a 30-50 dB range above threshold then levels off to a saturation rate which varies from 100 to 430 spikes/s.

In summary, the group of 361 neurons sampled from 8 normal chinchillas illustrates certain characteristics of the afferent code leaving the cochlea. Most of the neurons have some spontaneous activity; each of the neurons has a frequency to which it is most sensitive (CF); the response area of each neuron has essentially band pass characteristics; each of the neurons has a limtied dynamic range and they all respond in essentially the same way to tone bursts at CF. The homogeneity in the response properties of normal VIII nerve fibers and the similarities across different mammals enables norms to be established that can be used in studying the response properties of units in noise-treated animals

Auditory Nerve Responses After Noise Exposure
The relationship between behavioral threshold and the sensitivity of the individual neurons is shown in Figure 4. The two solid lines represent the average behavioral threshold shifts from six chinchillas during the noise exposure and at fifteen hours after the exposure. To estimate the amount of threshold shift in an individual neuron, the population of normal neurons was partitioned into octave bands and the average threshold at CF was computed for each octave band between 0.5 and 16 kHz. The threshold shift of a neuron from a noise-exposed animal was the difference between the threshold for the noise-treated neuron at CF and the average normal threshold in that CF region. The threshold shifts for the 209 neurons sampled from six chinchillas approximate the behavioral threshold shifts below 2 kHz and above 8 kHz. In the region between 2 to

---

* An increase in firing rate is not necessarily the first sign that a neuron is affected by sound. At mid and low frequencies, the S.A. of the neuron shifts from random firing to basically a phase-locked response without actually increasing the rate of firing above the neuron's spontaneous rate.

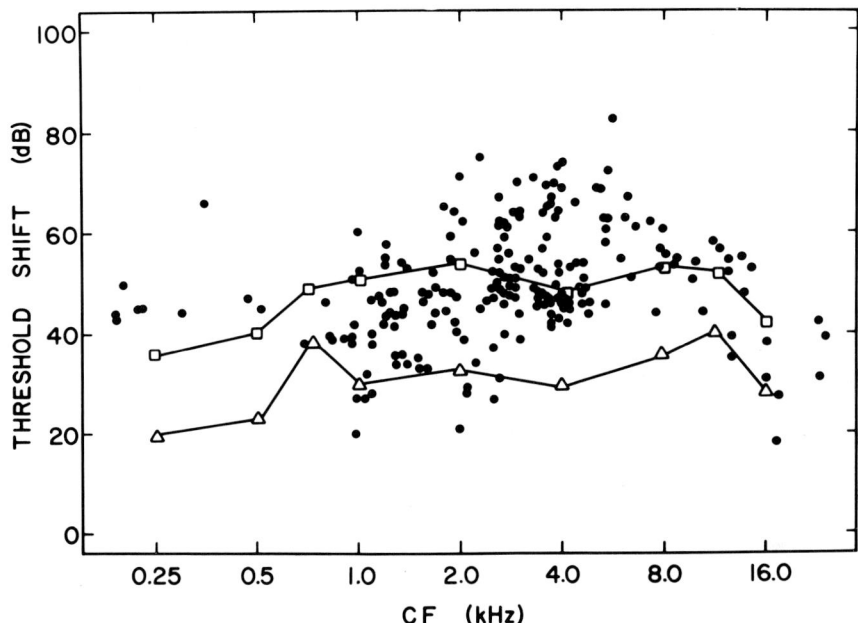

Figure 4: Average behavioral threshold shift during the noise exposure (□) and at 15 hours after the exposure (△). Threshold shifts (•) for 209 auditory nerve fibers obtained from noise-treated chinchillas between 2-15 hours post-exposure.

8 kHz, the neural threshold shifts are 10 to 15 dB higher than the behavioral threshold shifts. Other studies of the relationship between behavioral and neural threshold shifts have shown that the individual neurons have larger losses in sensitivity than would be expected from the behavioral threshold shift[5,8]. There are a number of possible reasons for this discrepancy between 3 and 8 kHz but rather than focus on the discrepancy, the trend of the data suggests that for most of the frequency regions sampled, the sensitivity of the VIII nerve neurons from the noise exposed animals mirrors the behavioral threshold shift.

Hearing Loss and Cochlear Tuning

The top panel of Figure 5 contains several tuning curves from normal chinchillas. In addition, Figure 5 contains 3 general types of tuning curves found in the noise exposed animals. The units shown in the top panel of Figure 5 are examples of the broad "V" shaped tuning curves. The "V" shaped tuning curves resemble those from normal animals, except that the

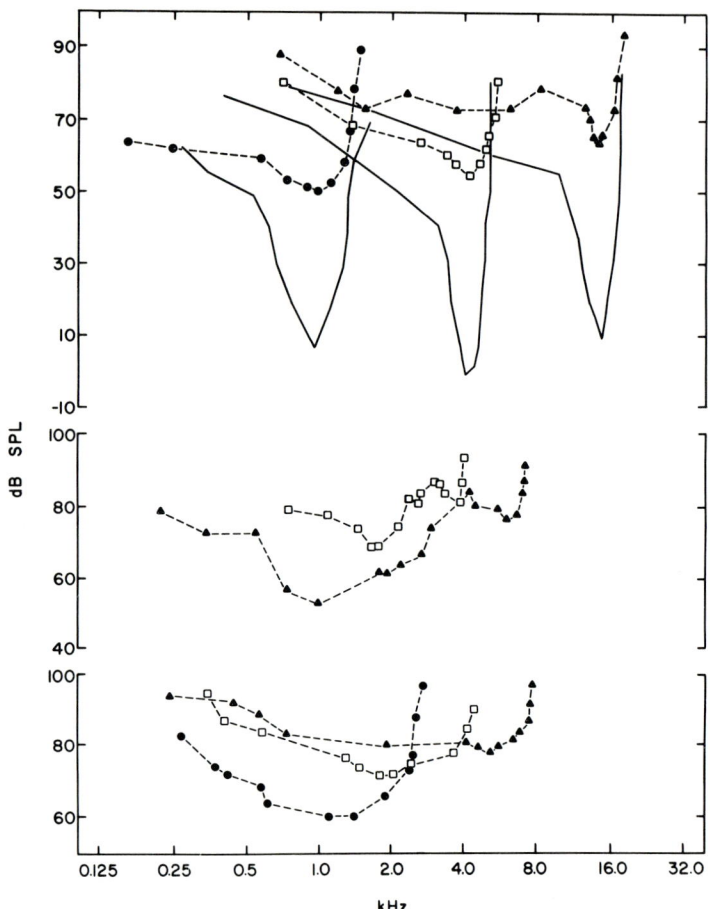

Figure 5: Normal tuning curves (solid line, top panel) and tuning curves from noise-treated chinchillas (symbols) having a blunt "V" shape (top panel), "W" shape (middle panel) and broad "U" shape (bottom panel).

tip of the tuning curve near CF is shorter and wider than the tip of the tuning curves obtained from normal animals. The great majority (75%) of the units in the sample had "V" shaped tuning curves. The "V" shaped tuning curves had CFs that spanned the entire range of CFs and their threshold shifts ranged from 18 to 76 dB with a mean threshold shift of 47 dB.

The units shown in the middle panel of Figure 5 are examples of the "W" shaped tuning curves. The "W" type of tuning curve has two distinct tips. The first tip was located near the high frequency cut off of the tuning curve and was designated as the CF of the unit. This tip was difficult to detect because the tip was relatively narrow and often less than 10 dB in depth. Consequently, frequency and intensity had to be carefully varied so that the tuning curve would be adequately defined. The second tip of the tuning curve, which had the lowest threshold, was located at a frequency below that of the first. Only 17% of the units in the noise-treated group had "W" shaped tuning curves and most of these had CFs between 2 and 8 kHz, i.e., in the region of greatest threshold shift. The mean threshold shift at CF for the units with "W" shaped tuning curves was 57 dB or roughly 10 dB greater than those of "V" shaped tuning curves.

The frequency-threshold curves shown in the bottom panel of Figure 5 are extremely wide in the region of greatest sensitivity and are examples of "U" shaped tuning curves. In some cases, the slope of the high frequency leg of the tuning curve was extremely shallow, consequently, there was some ambiguity in assigning CF using the high frequency cut off criterion discussed earlier. In the examples shown in Figure 5, our best estimates of CF for the 3 units are 2.4, 3.6 and 6.9 kHz. Much lower CFs would have been assigned if the choice of CF had been based strictly on a minimum threshold procedure. It is conceivable that the "U" shaped tuning curves actually represent the residual tails of "W" shaped tuning curves since they are similar in appearance. The high frequency tips of the "W" shaped tuning curves might have been missed because the stimulus intensities were below those necessary to excite the units. If the tips had been overlooked, the actual CFs of the units would have been grossly underestimated[8]. Fortunately, only a small proportion (6%) of the units had "U" shaped tuning curves and their CFs were between 0.5 and 7 kHz. The mean threshold shift was 57 dB or roughly 10 dB greater than units with "V" shaped tuning curves.

Regardless of the type of tuning curve, the general finding across all the neurons sampled is that there is a broadening of the bandwidth of the neuron. Rather than being tuned to one frequency, the pathological units respond with almost the same sensitivity to a wide range of frequencies. Poor speech discrimination in listeners with noise induced hearing loss[12] may be related to the increased bandwidth of auditory nerve fiber tuning curves in a way that was found in this study. As suggested by Evans[13], these impaired neurons will respond both to the signal and noise rather than to just the signal alone. Complex sounds may be heard, but the frerquency components may not be selectively discriminated. Thus, a hearing aid which amplifies both the signal and noise may actually prove to be detrimental to speech discrimination in noise background[12].

Psychological Temporal Integration and Neural Adaption

The response pattern of a typical unit from a noise-exposed animal to tone bursts is shown in the right panel of Figure 6. In virtually all the units from noise-treated animals, the pattern of response to tone burst was the same as in normal units. At low levels of stimulation, the unit fires uniformally during the course of the signal. At high levels of stimulation, the familiar pattern is seen, i.e., rapid firing at the onset of the stimulus which drops off to a constant rate of firing.

The neural behavior from noise-treated units is in contrast to what one might expect from psychophysical data. It is well known that acoustic trauma modifies the process of auditory temporal summation. This change in temporal summation is illustrated in the upper left of Figure 6 using the relationship between the threshold of a tone and its duration. In normal listeners, the threshold to a long duration tone is approximately 12 dB lower than that of a short duration tone; however, the threshold difference for the hearing impaired listener is reduced; in this case to roughly 5 dB[14,15,16]. Explanations of the reduction in temporal summation have assumed that cochlear trauma causes an abnormally rapid decay in the output of the cochlea at intensities near threshold[15]. The normal discharge pattern and the abnormally rapid decay pattern "predicted" for a hearing impaired listener are illustrated in the lower left panel of Figure 6. Presumably, long duration signals are less effective because the

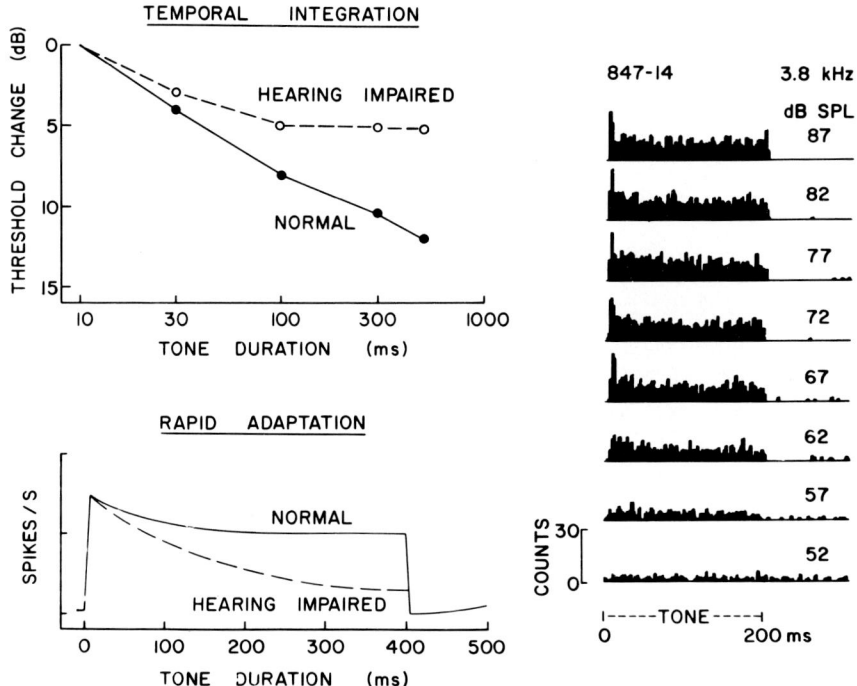

Figure 6: The top left panel shows typical psychophysical data which illustrates the improvement in threshold with increasing signal duration for normal and hearing impaired listeners. The bottom left panel illustrates the firing rate over time near threshold in normal auditory nerve fibers and the firing rate which is "presumed" to occur in hearing impaired ears. The right panel shows a series of PST histograms from a unit in a noise-treated animal with a threshold shift of approximately 50 dB.

physiological summator has fewer neural discharges to integrate over time. Examination of the PST histograms to tone burst stimulation in noise-treated animals shows normal PST histograms and there is no support for an abnormally rapid neural decay in units from noise-treated animals. Such findings are paradoxical because acoustic trauma damages the cochlea and reduces temporal summation, yet it does not seem to significantly alter the temporal firing patterns of peripheral auditory neurons during TTS or PTS[17,18]. Perhaps the reduction in temporal summation is the result of some other change in the neural code, such as a change in the bandwidth of spatial summation at the periphery or at higher auditory centers.

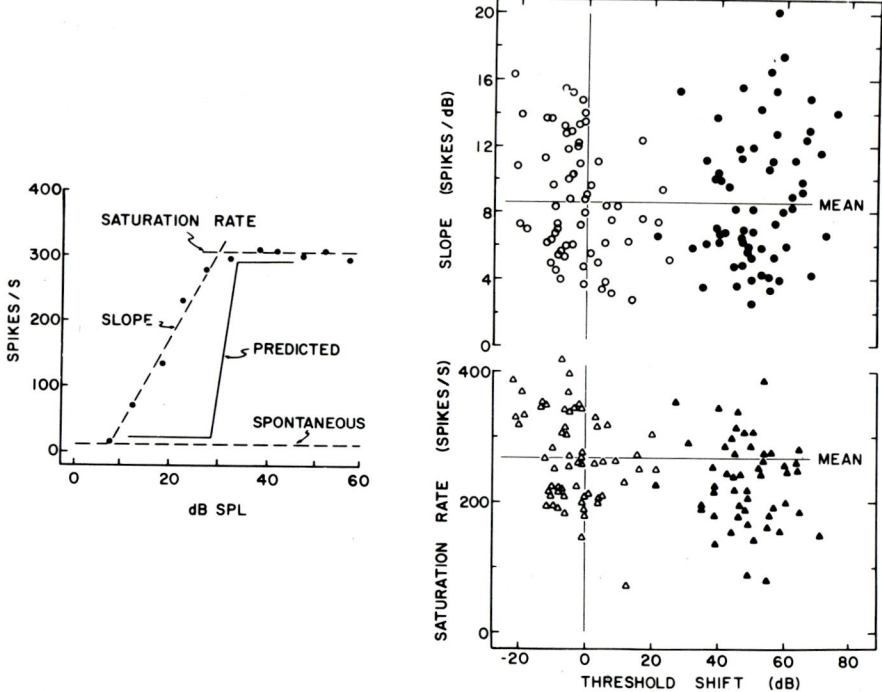

Figure 7: The left panel shows the slope and saturation rate of the input/output function of a normal unit (---) and the "predicted" input/output for a neuron in a hearing-impaired ear (———). The predicted increase in the slope of the input/output would presumably account for loudness recruitment. The right panel shows the slopes and saturation rates obtained from units in normal (open symbols) and noise-treated (filled symbols) animals using 20 ms tone bursts.

Recruitment and Neural Input-Output (I/O) Functions

The function relating neural firing rate to intensity was measured with 20 msec tone bursts at the characteristic frequency of the neuron. The slopes and saturation rates for the units from normal and noise-treated neurons are plotted as a function of threshold shift in Figure 7. The thresholds of the units from the noise-treated animals are elevated approximately 50 dB above the normal thresholds; however, the distribution of the slopes and saturation levels were nearly the same for units in the normal and noise-treated groups (two-tailed t test, = 0.1). Thus,

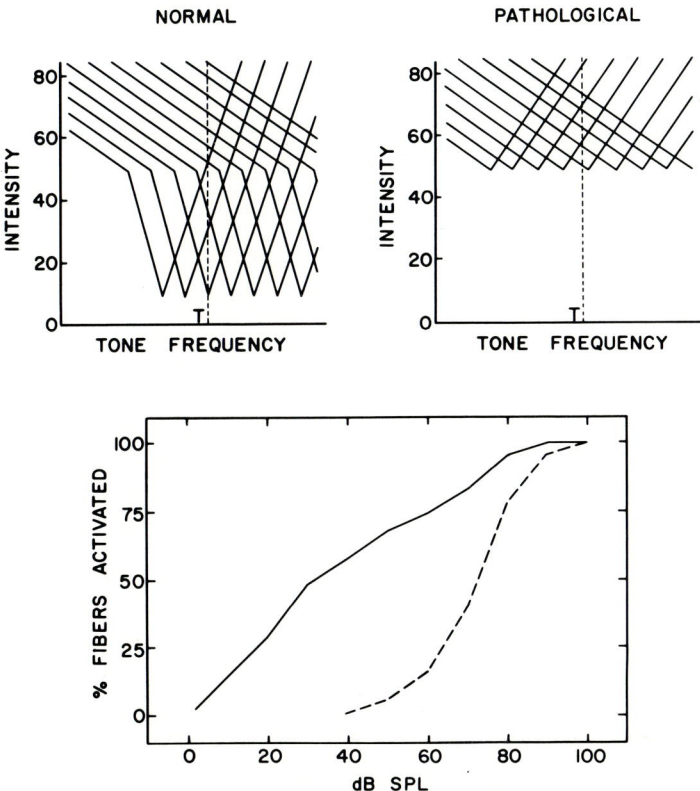

Figure 8: Idealized tuning curves in normal and pathological animals according to Evans (1976). Units begin to respond to the tone (dashed line) at the intensity where the dashed line cuts across the tuning curve. The bottom panel shows the percentage of units in the normal (——) and noise treated (---) chinchillas that were activated as the intensity of a 2 kHz was increased.

the lack of a change in the slope of the neural I/O function for the neurons is difficult to reconcile with the well documented changes in the growth of loudness with hearing loss[19,20].

Another explanation of loudness recruitment suggested by Kiang, et al.[21], and Evans[13] is based on the number of active units in the population of auditory nerve fibers. Each unit has a tuning curve with a low threshold sharply tuned tip near CF and a high threshold, broadly tuned tail below

CF. At low intensities, only a few neurons can respond to tones near the tips of their tuning curves. The difference in sensitivity between the tips and tails of the tuning curves influences the rate at which units are activated with increasing intensity and this in turn presumably influences the rate of loudness growth. Figure 8 illustrates the theoretical model proposed by Evans[13]. The dashed line in Figure 8 indicates the frequency of the stimulus. An individual unit begins to contribute to the population of active neurons when the intensity of the tone exceeds the threshold for that point on the tuning curve. As the stimulus level is increased more neurons respond; however, for a given increment in intensity, a larger percentage of units will become activated in the pathological group than in the normal population. Figure 8 shows the results of applying Evan's model to our data. The solid line represents the percentage of normal units (N = 144) in our sample that responds to a 2 kHz tone as intensity is increased, the dashed line shows similar results for units (N = 96) in the noise-treated group. A comparison of the two curves shows that units in the noise-treated group begin to respond at a level which is roughly 40 dB higher than in the normal sample. Within the first 20 dB of "threshold", the slope of the function of the noise-treated group is shallower than normal; however, at higher intensities the slope becomes steeper than normal so that the function catches up with that of the normal group. Thus, the population response of the noise-treated group appears to parallel the psychophysical finding of loudness recruitment.

Spontaneous Activity and Tinnitus

Subjective tinnitus is another symptom of noise-induced hearing loss. Most physiological explanations of tinnitus have involved the concept of a lesion in the cochlea which presumably gives rise to high rates of spontaneous activity in individual auditory neurons[22,23,24]. The frequency of the tinnitus is presumably correlated with CFs of the units with high spontaneous activity while the loudness of the tinnitus is apparently related to the level of spontaneous activity in these units.

The data from this experiment do not support the hypothesis of an irritative lesion in the cochlea. Spontaneous activity was essentially

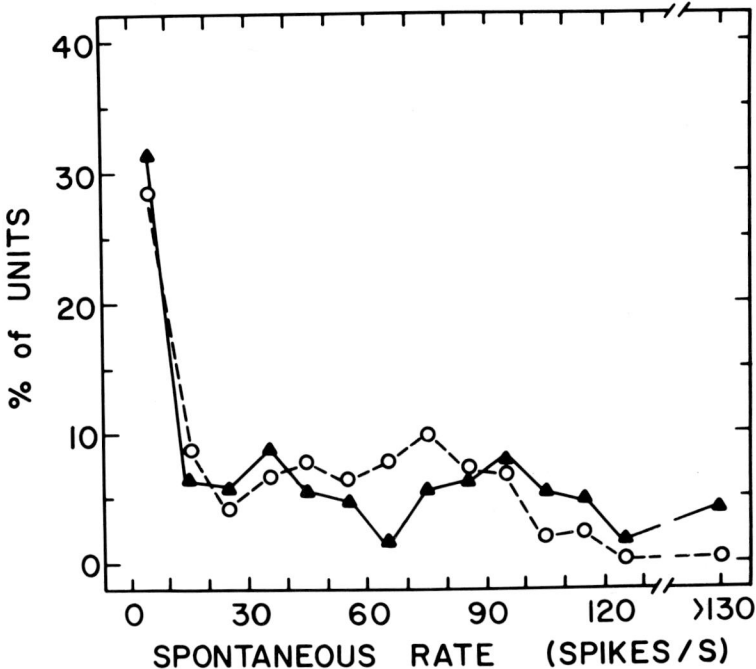

Figure 9: Percent of units in the normal (o) and noise-treated group ( ) with the indicated rates of spontaneous activity.

normal in the population of neurons damaged by noise. A comparison of S.A. in normal (N = 192) and noise treated (N = 125) neurons is made in Figure 9. There is no systematic differences between the two groups. Other studies of S.A. following noise damage have been equivocal. Two studies report a general decline of spontaneous activity in neurons with high thesholds[21,25]. Dallos, et al[4], however, reported that spontaneous activity remains essentially normal in units which innervate areas of the cochlea devoid of outer hair cells, but that have apparently normal inner hair cells. In a TTS experiment[26], the spontaneous activity in auditory nerve fibers was actually depressed after noise exposure.

The preceding studies point out that there may be no simple relationship between spontaneous activity and tinnitus at the level of the auditory

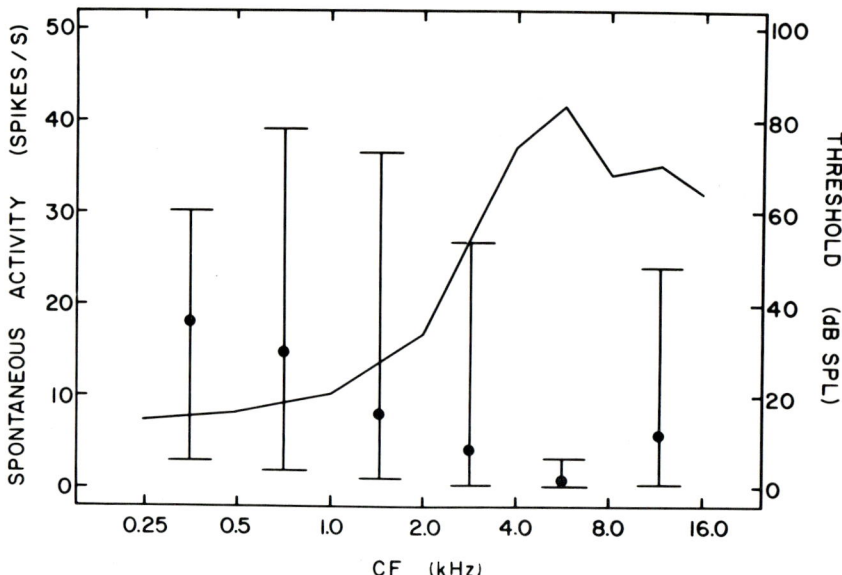

Figure 10: Comparison of the octave band distribution of spontaneous activity (median o; interquartile range I) of units in the cochlear nucleus (left axis) and the average behavioral audiogram (———) of chinchillas exposed to an octave band of noise centered at 4 kHz.

nerve. A possible suggestion for the neurological basis of tinnitus comes from a previous study of TTS in the cochlear nucleus of the chinchilla[17]. In this study, the exposure was an 86 dB octave band of noise centered at 4 kHz. As shown in Figure 10, the noise produced a high frequency loss and a marked depression in S.A. in units with CFs between 4 to 8 kHz. Kiang et al[21], has suggested that the pitch of tinnitus is related to a point in the distribution of spontaneously active neurons where the average spontaneous rate changes rapidly as a function of CF and in so doing creates an "edge" effect in the distribution. This hypothesis is consistent with psychophysical measurement which indicate that when the hearing loss is produced by a band of noise, as in the present study, the pitch of the tinnitus is matched to a frequency which is near the low frequency cutoff of the noise band[23,27]. This is approximately the region where there is a tonotopic boundary between low frequency units that are spontaneously active and high frequency units that are relatively inactive. While these boundary effects may provide a basis for tinnitus, we cannot rule out other patterns of neural activity at more central auditory locations[24].

ACKNOWLEDGEMENTS

This research was supported by the National Science Foundation Grant No. BN 76-18913, National Institute of Environmental Health Sciences Grant No. 1-K04-ES-00011 and National Institute of Neurological and Communicative Disorders Grant No. IR01 NS 16761. The technical assistance of P. Blaisdell and L. Wimer is greatly appreciated. We especially thank G. Pavek for the creative illustrations.

REFERENCES

1. Miller, J.D., Audibility curve of the chinchilla. J. Acoust. Soc. Amer., 48, 513-523, 1970.

2. Blakeslee, E.A., Hynson, K., Hamernik, R.P., Henderson, D., Asymptotic threshold shift in chinchillas exposed to impulse noise, J. Acoust. Soc. Amer., 63, 876-882, 1978.

3. Kiang, N.Y.S., Watanabe, T., Thomas, E.C., Clark, L.G., Discharge patterns of single fibers in the cat's auditory nerve, Res. Monograph 35, Cambridge, MIT Press, 1965.

4. Dallos, P., Harris, D., Properties of auditory nerve responses in the absence of outer hair cells, J. Neurophysiol., 41, 365-383, 1978.

5. Salvi, R., Hamernik, R., Henderson, D., Auditory nerve activity, and cochlear morphology after noise exposure. Arch-Otorhinolaryngol. 224, 111-116, 1979.

6. Engstrom, H., Ades, H.W., Andersson, A., Structural Pattern of the Organ of Corti, Almquist and Wiksell, Stockholm, 1966.

7. Liberman, M.C., Kiang, N.Y.S., Acoustic trauma in cats, Acta Otolaryngol., Suppl. 358, 1978.

8. Dallos, P., Harris, D., Ozdamar, O., Ryan, A., Behavioral, compound action potential and single unit thresholds: relationship in normal and abnormal ears, J. Acoust. Soc. Amer., 64, 151-157, 1978.

9. Salvi, R.J., Henderson, D., Hamernik, R.P., Single auditory nerve fiber and action potential latencies in normal and noise-treated chinchillas, Hearing Res. 1, 237-251, 1979.

10. Bismark, G. von, The sound pressure transformation from free-field to the eardrum of the chinchilla. M.S. Thesis, Massachusetts Institute of Technology, 1967.

11. Hawkins, J.E., Cazals, Y., Erre, J.P., Aran, J.M., Selective evaluation of cochlear whole-nerve thresholds for high frequencies recorded acutely in guinea pigs, J. Acoust. Soc. Amer., 64, Suppl. 1, 1978.

12. Olsen, W.P., Tillman, T.W., Hearing aids and sensorineural hearing loss, Ann. Oto-Rhino-Laryng., 77, 717-726, 1968.

13. Evans, E.F., Temporary sensorineural hearing losses and 8th nerve changes, in Effects of Noise on Hearing. Eds., D. Henderson, R.P. Hamernik, D. Dosanjh, and J.H. Mills, Raven Press, New York, 1976.

14. Jerger, J.F., Difference of stimulus duration on the pure tone threshold during recovery from auditory fatigue, J. Acoust. Soc. Amer., 27, 121-124, 1955.

15. Wright, H.N., Clinical measurement of temporal auditory summation, J. Speech Hear. Res., 11, 109-127, 1968.

16. Henderson, D., Temporal summation of acoustic signals by the chinchilla, J. Acoust. Soc. Amer., 46, 474-475, 1969.

17. Salvi, R.J., Hamernik, R.P., Henderson, D., Discharge patterns in the cochlea nucleus of the chinchilla following noise-induced asymptotic threshold shift, Exp. Brain Res., 32, 301-320, 1978.

18. Henderson, D., Cochlear nucleus firing patterns during asymptotic threshold shift. In Hearing and Davis: Essays Honoring Hallowell Davis. Eds., S.K. Hirsh, D.H. Eldredge, I.J. Hirsh, E.M. Silverman. Washington Univ. Press, St. Louis, 1976.

19. Davis, H., Morgan, C.T., Hawkins, J.E. Jr., Galambos, R., and Smith, F., Temporary deafness following exposure to loud tones and noise. Acta Otolaryng. Suppl. 88., 1950.

20. Hickling, S., Hearing test patterns in noise-induced temporary hearing loss, J. Aud. Res., 7, 63-76, 1967.

21. Kiang, N.Y.S., Moxon, E.C., Levine, R.A., Auditory-nerve activity in cats with normal and abnormal cochleas, In: Sensorineural Hearing Loss Eds., G.E.W. Wolstenholme and J. Knight, London; J. & A. Churchill, 1970.

22. Sataloff, J., Jr., Hearing Loss, Lippincott, Philadelphia, 1966.

23. Atherley, G.R.C., Hempstock, T.I., Noble, W.G., Study of tinnitus induced temporarily by noise, J. Acoust. Soc. Amer., 44, 1503-1506, 1968.

24. Feldman, H., Tinnitus and contralateral masking, Audiol., 10, 138-144, 1971.

25. Schmiedt, R.A., Single-tone and two-tone effects in normal and abnormal cochleas: A study of cochlear microphonics and auditory nerve

units. Ph.D. Thesis, Syracuse University, Syracuse, New York, 1977.

26. Lonsbury-Martin, B.L., Meikle, M.B., Neural correlates of auditory fatigue: Frequency-dependent changes in activity of single cochlear nerve fibers, J. Neurophysiol., 41, 987-1006, 1978.

27. Loeb, M., and Smith, R., Relation of induced tinnitus to physical characteristics of the inducing stimuli, J. Acoust. Soc. Amer., 42, 453-455, 1967.

Personal Hearing Protection in Industry, edited by P. W. Alberti, Raven Press, New York ©

3 Risks to Hearing: The Effect of Intermittent Exposure

W. Dixon Ward

Industrial noise exposures are not steady, generally being interrupted or at least grossly time-varying, either because of intermittence of the noise source per se or due to rest and lunch breaks during the day, or in any event by 14 or 16 hours of some kind of a different noise. What effect do these variations of level with time have on the hazard associated with noise exposure?

The total-energy theory, in its simplest form, must answer "none". In this view of the auditory system as a phonon collector, all that matters is the A-weighted energy that has entered the ear over the lifetime of the individual being tested. Working for 40 years in an 80 dBA area (40 h/wk) is no less hazardous than living in a constant 80 dBA (24 h/day) for 10 years, or in a constant 130 dBA for nearly an hour, according to this theory. And by the same token, this one hour of exposure at 130 dBA is assumed to be no more hazardous than 60 1-min exposures, each separated by a week from its predecessor. Now, this could in fact be the case, if hearing loss involved processes that are completely irreversible. But we know that damage to many biological systems is reversible. If the total-energy theory were true for vision, for instance, we would all be quite blind after a few years of life, as eventually the visual exposure would add up to the same as watching an eclipse without sunglasses.

The most obvious example of the partial reversibility of hearing damage is auditory adaptation, of whose manifestations temporary threshold shift (TTS) has been the most intensively studied. Immediately after a noise exposure, tonal stimuli must be more intense in order to be perceived, but this effect disappears with time, unless the exposure has been so severe that some residual threshold shift (permanent threshold shift, or PTS) remains. The total-energy theorist must argue that the threshold has never returned to its former state, although the amount of sensitivity it has lost may have been too small to measure.

For 25 years, beginning with the birth of AFR 160-3[1] (1956), we have been arguing this point. Is the effect of intermittence in ameliorating hearing damage really negligible, or does it act in the same way as it does in reducing auditory fatigue? By and large, the voices raised on both sides have tended to emphasize only the inherent weaknesses of the opposing viewpoint, as if one extreme position or the other must be completely correct. In such situations, the truth generally lies somewhere between the extreme positions. I shall first discuss the effect of intermittence on TTS in humans, and then describe some experiments on chinchillas in which auditory damage is in fact diminished by intermittence, but not to the extent predicted by analogy from TTS.

As a rather gross first approximation, the TTS_2 (TTS 2-min after exposure) from a time-varying exposure is proportional to the average effective level over the total duration of the exposure. "Effective level" is defined as the number of decibels by which the level exceeds effective quiet. Effective quiet, in turn, is defined as that SPL that will neither produce a TTS_2 that grows with continued exposure nor retard the recovery from a TTS produced by a higher level; effective quiet is around 70 dB for the octave bands centered at 1, 2, or 4 kHz, and 75 dB for those centered at 250 and 500 Hz[2]. Average effective level is the integral of the effective level over the entire exposure period divided by the duration (negative values of effective level are treated as zero). Note that this is not the "equivalent level" $L_{eq(t)}$ of the exposure: if an exposure consists of equal periods of time at 80 and 100 dB SPL, the effective level will be 90 dB, although the equivalent level will be 97 dB.

Figure 1: Temporary threshold shifts measured 2 min (solid symbols) or 32 min (open symbols) after 6-hr. exposures to magenta noise whose level alternated among 90-X, 90, and 90+X dB, as a function of X. From top to bottom, panels show results for test frequencies of 500, 1400, and 4000 Hz. The mean level is constant; equivalent level is indicated in the second line of the abscissa, in parentheses. Data points enclosed in parentheses indicate TTSs following exposure to 95 dB SPL continuously.

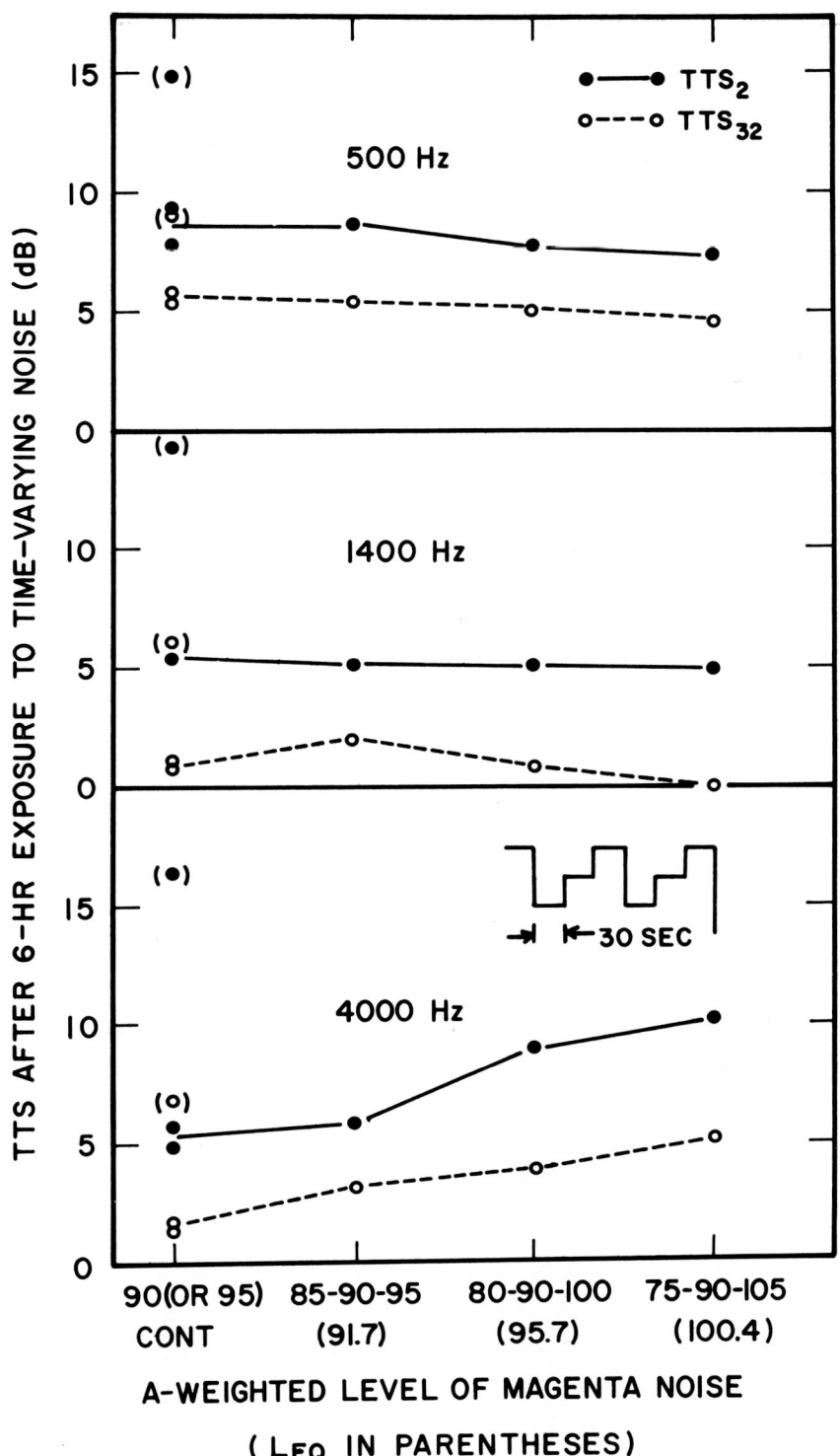

This general relation has been established in a variety of experiments. Figure 1, for example, shows the results of experiments in which the level of "magenta" noise (a noise whose octave-band spectrum has a slope of -5 dB/octave, designed to produce about equal values of TTS at all frequencies) alternated among three values symmetrically spaced around 90 dBA[3]. That is, the level was at (90-X) dBA for 30 sec, then went to 90 dBA for 30 sec, and finally to (90+X) dBA for 30 sec, and then repeated the cycle. X was 0, 5, 10, or 15 dB. In all cases, the average effective level is 90 dBA, although $L_{eq(6h)}$ progresses as shown on the abscissa from 90 to 91.7 to 95.7 to 100.4 dBA. The mean TTS_2 (solid curves) or TTS_{32} (dashed curves) from 10 listeners after 6 h of exposure should remain completely constant, if average effective level were the governing factor, but should increase sharply for the two rightmost points if $L_{eq(t)}$ were dominant. It is clear that at 500 and 1400 Hz (top two panels) all exposures produce the same TTS. Only at 4000 Hz is there any suggestion that the 75-90-105 condition is somewhat more hazardous. However, the TTS_2 has increased only from 5 dB to 10 dB, a value that would be expected from a 92-dBA continuous exposure (Notice that a 95-dBA continuous exposure gives a TTS_2 of 16.5 dB).

Another illustration that total energy fails to predict TTS is shown in Fig. 2. Here the total integrated exposure was 110 dBA of magenta noise for 30 min (the maximum duration allowed at this level by American OSHA regulations). It was presented either in a single 30-min period (CONT) or in 40 bursts of 45 sec duration separated by quiet intervals of either 15 sec (in which case, the on-fraction R was 0.75, so the exposure required 40 min to administer), 45 sec (R=0.5, exposure 1 hour total), 135 sec (R=0.25, 2 h), 345 sec (R=0.125, 4 h), or 495 sec (R=0.075, 6 h). The TTS_2 at 4 kHz (measured 2 min after the end of the final noise burst) clearly declines as the on-fraction decreases, and a similar trend is seen for 500 Hz as well. That this difference persists throughout the period of recovery is indicated by the TTSs at 4 kHz 90 min after exposure. On-fraction therefore plays a significant role in determining TTS; for this particular burst duration, the TTS is about proportional to the on-fraction down to R=0.2 or so, a relation first observed some time ago[4].

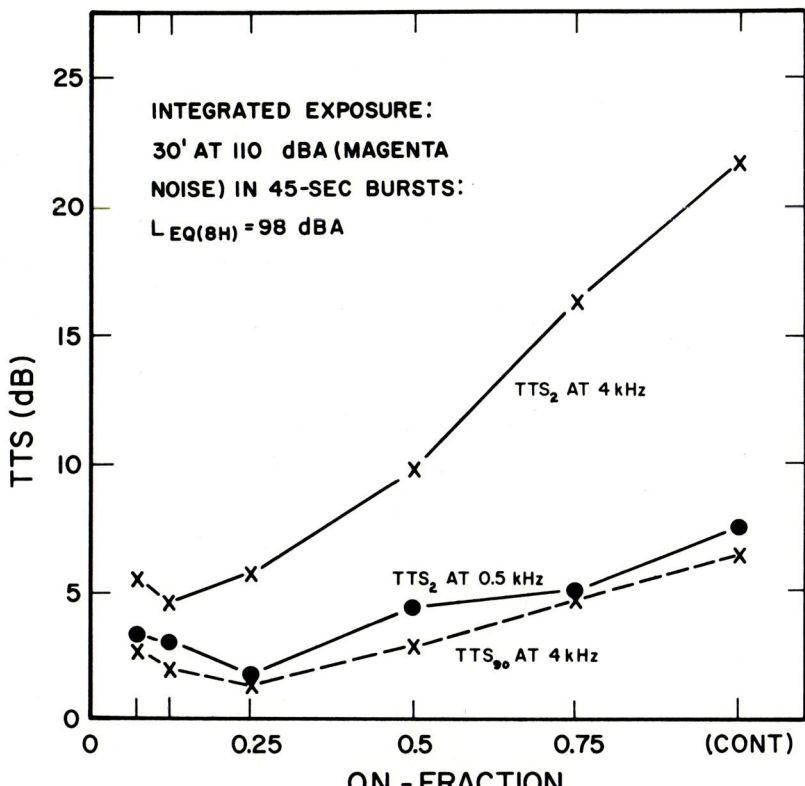

Figure 2: Temporary threshold shifts following exposure to 40 45-sec bursts of magenta noise with interposed quiet periods ranging from 0 to 495 sec. The abscissa is the ratio of the 30 min of cumulative exposure (on-time) to the total duration of the experimental session (sum of on- and off-times).

Other studies[5] have confirmed the validity of the on-fraction rule and the average-effective-level principle. Indeed, a study by Dieroff and Meissner[6], in which they compared the TTSs produced by a steady noise with those generated by three industrial noises (steel pipe falling into a bin, automatic hammer on a steel pipe, steel polishing machine), all of which, as far as one can tell, had an average effective level of 100 dBA, showed the intermittent noises to produce even <u>less</u> TTS than the steady noise. A recent report by Hetu and Tremolieres[7] concludes that TTS from a time-varying noise is proportional to the L_{eq}; however, their noise only alternated between 93 and 98 dBA, so the difference between L_{eq} and average effective level was less than a decibel, and their study is simply irrelevant to the issue.

However, not only the ratio of burst duration to total duration is important; burst duration per se is also a salient factor. A long series of experiments has been performed in our laboratory in which 6- and 8-h intermittent exposures to various octave bands of noise were given to our 10 subjects. For each specific value of noise level and on-fraction, three different values of total period were used: 1.5 min, 9 min and 40 min. Thus, for example, when the on-fraction was 0.5, exposures were given as follows: 45 sec on, 45 sec off; 4.5 min on, 4.5 min off, and 20 min on, 20 min off. Table I shows typical results at 4 kHz for the 4-kHz octave band[8]. It can be seen that the TTS_2 more than doubles as one goes from the 1.5-min to the 40-min cycle. (Incidentally, this Table illustrates that an increase in level of 5 dB can nearly exactly be compensated by a reduction of total exposure time by one-half, as the present OSHA regulations require.)

The point here is that TTS depends not only on on-fraction, level, and overall duration of the exposure, but also on the burst duration. Since 4 kHz is the octave band that produces the greatest magnitude of TTS, for a given noise level, I have been trying to devise a simple equation that will embrace all of the data of Table I. Beginning with the assumption that the TTS should be proportional to the on-fraction, since that assumption would be correct if the TTS_2 was proportional to the average effective level under all conditions, expected values of TTS_2 for the various exposures were calculated, and then the ratio of the actual TTS_2 to this expected value was determined for each of the three different burst durations. Unfortunately, this ratio is a complicated function of burst duration, total period, and level, and a simple equation is yet to be wrestled from the data. So at the moment, the best that can be done is to simply list the ways in which TTS is affected by fluctuations in the exposure level:

1. The TTS is roughly proportional to the on-fraction, if the noise drops at times below effective quiet, or to the average effective

Table I

Temporary Threshold Shift 2 min after Final Noise Burst in 8-hr exposures to 4000-Hz Octave Band Noise with Various on-fractions R and on-off periods T (in min) at SPLs from 75 to 100 dB. Each Datum Represents the Average of 20 ears (10 normal-hearing subjects) at 2 Test Frequencies: 400 and 5600 Hz. The pre-exposure Threshold used in calculated TTS_2 was the mean of the Threshold Measured on the day in question and the Average Threshold over a period of three months or more.

R	T	75	80	85	90	95	100
			4000-Hz Octave Band SPL (dB)				
1	Cont.	6.0	12.2	24.4			
0.5	1.5		5.8	8.2	14.7		
0.5	9			14.2			
0.5	40			16.2			
0.25	1.5				7.7	13.8	
0.25	9				14.0		
0.25	40			10.0	18.5		
0.125	1.5					8.2	17.5
0.125	9					9.6	
0.125	40				14.6	17.5	

level if it does not.

2. However, this holds only for on-fractions between 0.2 and unity; further reduction of on-fraction does not result in corresponding diminution of TTS.

3. The reduction is greatest for burst durations of a minute or less; lengthening the noise bursts will give higher TTSs, even when the quiet periods are lengthened as well, so that on-fraction remains constant.

Now, however, let us turn to the evidence concerning the permanent effects of noise exposure. Basically, the issue reduces to this: Does cutting in half the noise energy absorbed by the ear by making the noise intermittent with an on-fraction of 0.5 result in a reduction of damage by 50%, as the average-effective-level principle would predict, or merely result in a reduction to what would have been produced by a continuous exposure of the same duration but at an intensity 3 dB weaker?

Human studies bearing on the issue of intermittent exposure are becoming more numerous, but the problem with all of them is the difficulty of determining what the noise exposures really were--in <u>any</u> terms, L_{eq}, average effective level, or whatever--for the average worker (to estimate it for any individual is a hopeless goal). One can seek out evidence that can be used as support for either of our hypotheses. Alan Martin[9] has earlier reviewed much of the evidence on the role of impact noise components, and $L_{eq(8h)}$ does appear to be an adequate measure of the daily noise dose for such conditions. However, it must be emphasized that alternative explanations for the agreement of immission level with hearing levels, which of course is only approximate, can be suggested. That is, it could still be the case that at low SPLs (below 120 dB, perhaps), the average level is the determining factor rather than equivalent level, but that the peaks of energy involved in forging operations have an inordinate effect, so that the final result is damage whose extent is nearly that of a continuous exposure at the indicated $L_{eq(8h)}$ or immission level. Such a theory, of course, involves the assumption of a "critical level"--a level at which the rules governing the relation between level and duration abruptly change. This level is unlikely to be completely independent of duration; the longer the transient (impulse or impact) lasts, the lower will be the critical level. Evidence for such a critical level in the 140-145dB-peak area for one specific shape of impulse has already been advanced[10]. That impact peaks of 50 to 100 msec B-duration might be associated with a critical intensity of 120-130 dB is certainly not outside the realm of possibility, although none of the experimenters who use the hammer-on-plate apparatus seem to have looked specifically for it.

Furthermore, certain studies still suggest that damage from intermittent sound is considerably less than predicted by L_{eq}. For example, Sataloff et al[11] studied men from two iron mines, in which bursts of 115-122 dBA drilling noise whose mean duration was 3 min were separated by periods of "relative quiet" of about the same duration. The $L_{eq(8h)}$ can be presumed to be 115 dBA in this situation, while the average level would be around 95 dBA. Daily levels of 115 dBA for 10 years or more would be expected to produce over 60 dB of NIPTS at 4 kHz, and about 25 dB at 1000 H_3[12]. Unfortunately, Sataloff et al do not present their data in terms of years of exposure but give only a breakdown by age group; however, it is clear from their median audiograms that while the Hearing Levels at 4000 Hz are some 40 dB worse than controls comparable in age, those at 1000 Hz are only on the order of 10 to 15 dB worse, which would be a result to be expected from exposure to around 105 dBA of steady noise .. i.e., about halfway between the L_{eq} and average-level predictions.

In view of the uncertainty of measurement of industrial exposures and the problem of eliminating sociacusic and nosoacusic influences from human survey data, the use of experimental animals to determine the effect of intermittence is mandatory, even though we may in the end be frustrated by species differences that render extrapolation to man invalid. The animal we have been using for this purpose is the chinchilla. After a dozen years of work with this animal, some results are finally available that bear on the role of total energy in determining damage, in the form of either PTS or hair-cell destruction caused by a particular 2-octave-wide noise (700-2800 Hz).

Our first goal was to determine the growth of damage with level, in order to establish a "threshold" dose, if possible. Groups of at least 4 chinchillas each were exposed for 220 min at 105, 108, 111 and 114 dB SPL. The number of absent outer hair cells (AOHC) associated with these exposures is shown in Fig. 3. Solid points indicate animals whose thresholds were measured. The scatter of the results is unfortunate, but the trend is clear: 105 dB gives no more damage than one finds in normal animals (anything under 100 AOHC), while 114 dB produces massive destruction. The points marked L and D are data from Lipscomb et al[13] and Dolan et al[14]. Notice that the slope of the line that has been drawn

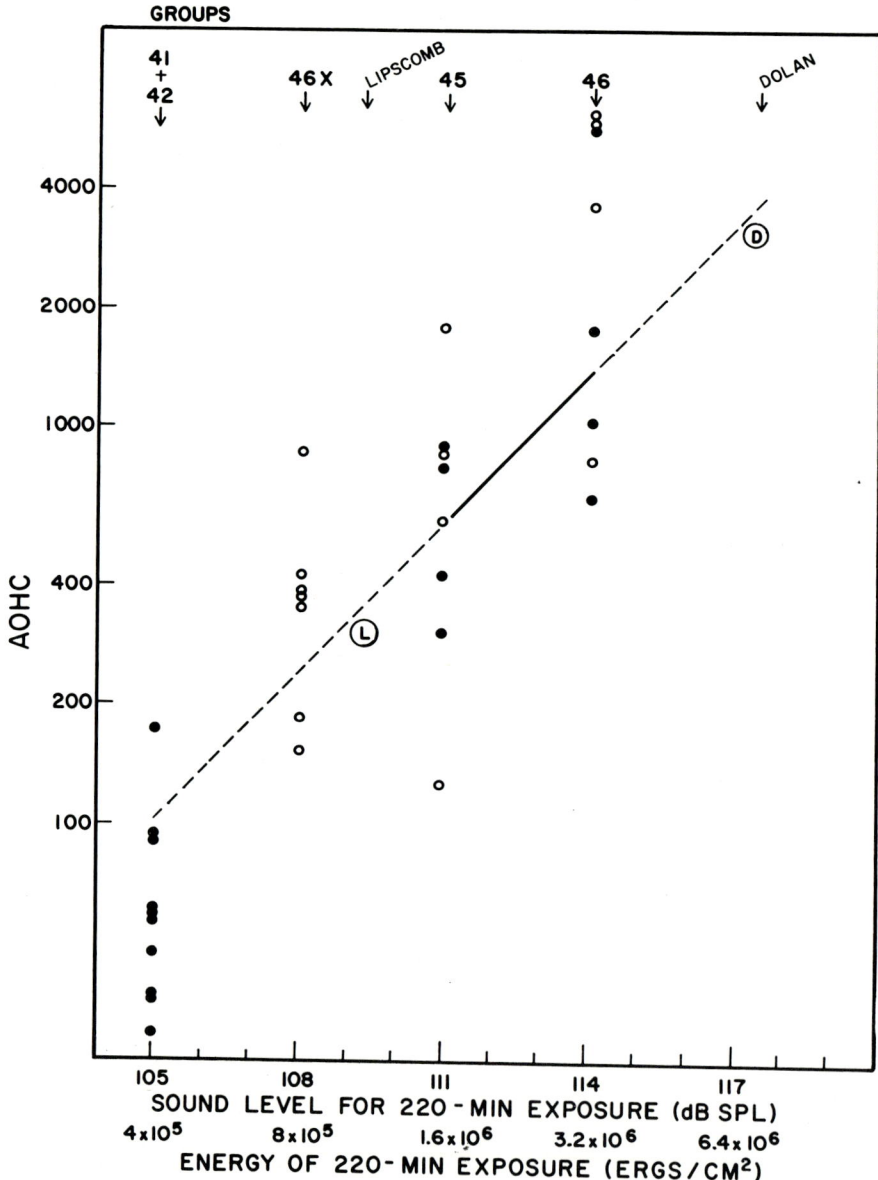

Figure 3: Absent outer hair cells in the cochleas of chinchillas exposed for 220 min to 700-2800-Hz noise at levels indicated on the abscissa. Closed symbols represent animals tested behaviorally, open symbols those not so tested. For information on the points marked L and D, see text.

eye, through medians as far as possible, is not far from unity, which would imply that doubling the energy doubles the damage, with 4×10^5 ergs/cm^2 being the just-safe dose.

To test the total-energy theory (equal energy gives equal effect), groups were also exposed to 102 dB for 220 min (1.5 days) or 92 dB for 15 days. Since these exposures gave average OHC losses of about 800, just what would be produced by 220 min of 112 dB, the total-energy principle seems firmly established for dealing with single continuous exposures.

It does not necessarily follow, though, that this is also true of intermittent exposures. To date, the following groups have been given the same total exposure but with varying temporal patterns:

Group 46: 114 dB, 220 min continuous
Group 49: 114 dB, 440 min of 0.5 min on, 0.5 min off (R=0.5)
Group 52: 114 dB, 2200 min of 0.5 min on, 4.5 min off (R=0.1)
Group 47: 114 dB, 22 10-min exposures separated by half a week

Table 2 summarizes the results obtained from these four groups, as well as the two longer continuous exposures equal in energy to 220 min of 112 dBA that were mentioned earlier. Let us compare Groups 46 and 49 first. Recall that an R of 0.5 in the human TTS experiments would cut TTS in man by half, which, since TTS is proportional to the effective level, would imply a reduction in effectiveness of 20 dB or more, thereby making the exposure completely innocuous. In our chinchillas, however, the average TTS_{60} at 1, 2, 4 and 8 kHz dropped only from 79 dB to 74 dB rather than being reduced 50%, and although the "damage", in terms of either PTS at 1, 2, 4 and 8 kHz or AOHC, was indeed about cut in half, that is equivalent to only about a 2.5 dB reduction in effectiveness, which is not statistically significant. Even dropping the on-fraction to 0.1 (Group 52) added only 1 or 2 dB to the protective effect. It appears, then, that for the chinchilla, a correction to the daily exposure, as expressed in terms of $L_{eq(8)}$, of 3 or 4 dB for intermittence is the most that need be applied.

The results with the 22 10-min exposures (Group 47) indicate that the total-energy theory is slightly farther off the mark when dealing with the

Table 2: Temporary Threshold Shifts, Permanent Threshold Shifts, and Absent Outer Hair Cell Counts for 6 Groups of 4 Chinchillas given a 220-min Exposure to 700-2800-Hz Noise at 114 dB SPL or its Energy Equivalent

Group Exposure	AVE TTS_{60} (1,2,4,8 kHz)	AVE PTS (1,2,4,8 kHz)	MEDIAN AOHC
114 dB:			
46: 220' CONT	79	23	1400
49: 440' INT, R=0.5	74	11	750
52: 2200' INT, R=0.1	60	4	550
47: 22x10' SEMIWEEKLY	32	3	300
48: 102 dB, 2200' CONT	61	3	800
51: 92 dB, 22000' CONT	56	11	800

<u>cumulative</u> effect of exposures, but certainly not as far off as I had expected. This particular breakdown of the 220-min total exposure was chosen in order to test the notion that if the daily TTS is kept moderate and enough time for full recovery from TTS is allowed, no damage will cumulate. Unfortunately, however, the chinchilla is so much more susceptible to TTS than man that even a 10-min exposure to 114 dB produces a TTS_{60} of 40 to 50 dB at one frequency or another, and half a week does not always suffice for full recovery, as was observed during the 11 weeks that this experiment required. At any rate, it can be seen that although no significant hearing loss developed, there was nevertheless some hair-cell destruction, which implies a reduction in effective level of only 5 or 6 dB despite making the on-fraction about 0.002 or so.

This, indeed, is a far cry from the reduction of 20 dB expected if the average-level principle held, and one cannot avoid the conclusion that

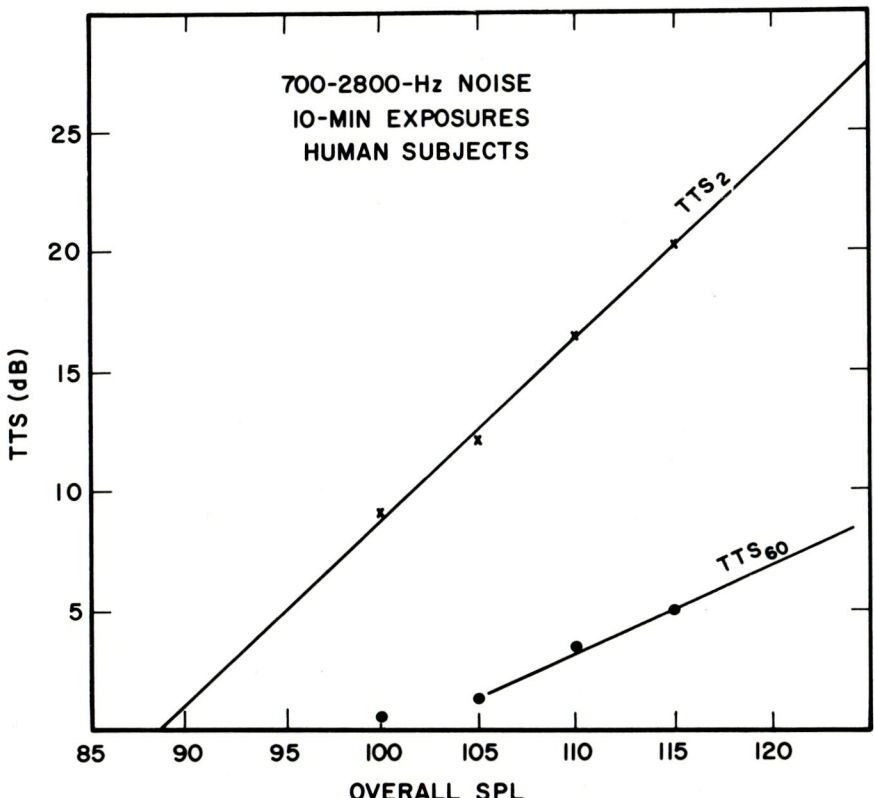

Figure 4: Temporary threshold shifts 2 and 60 min after 10-min exposures to 700-2800-Hz noise as a function of noise level, in humans. Subjects were 10 young normal-hearing adults.

total energy comes closer to the facts at very high intensities for the chinchilla. The only hope for survival of the equal-TTS theory apparently lies in appeal to species differences or to the existence of a crtical level, or both. Figure 4 serves to underscore the difference in susceptibility to TTS between man and chinchilla; shown here are average TTS_2 and TTS_{60} measured after 10-min exposures to the chinchilla noise at levels from 100 to 115 dB SPL. Extrapolation implies that to develop a TTS_{60} of 30 dB in man, which is what the chinchillas show after a 10-min exposure to 95 dB (routinely administered at the late stages of training as a test for individual susceptibility), some 170 dB would be required, and for even a TTS_2 of that value, 130 dB would be needed. Extrapolation is obviously not justified, because eventually the TTS_{60} curve will ascend sharply, when TTS_2 reaches the stage that "delayed recovery" (recovery linear in time instead of exponential) sets in. However, this "critical level", if it exists, is clearly above 115 dB for man, whereas delayed recovery is found in the chinchilla even after the 95-dB exposure just mentioned.

In summary, therefore, the total-energy principle seems to describe the equivalence of daily exposures in producing permanent damage better than the equal-TTS (or equivalent average level) theory. Intermittence can, however, reduce the effect of a given energy by an amount equal to a reduction in level of 5 dB. Whether or not this effective reduction will be greater for exposures more analogous to the real-life situation in industry (i.e., lower levels but longer exposures) remains to be determined by future research.

ACKNOWLEDGEMENT
The research reported here was supported by Grants NS 12125 and OH 00350 from the National Institutes of Health, Public Health Service.

REFERENCES
1. Anon., Hazardous Noise Exposure. Air Force Regulation 160-3, Department of the Air Force, 1956.

2. Ward, W.D., Cushing, E.M., Burns, E.M., Effective quiet and moderate TTS: Implications for noise exposure standards. J. Acoust. Soc. Amer., 59, 160-165, 1976.

3. Ward, W.D., TTS from time-varying noise: A function of average level, not equivalent level. In: Proceedings, 9 International Congress on Acoustics, Madrid, 4-9 July, 1977. Spanish Acoustical Society, Madrid, Spain. P. 344.

4. Ward, W.D., Glorig, A., Sklar, D.L., Dependence of temporary threshold shift at 7 kc on intensity and time. J. Acoust. Soc. Amer., 30, 944-954, 1958.

5. Schmidek, M., Henderson, T., Margolis, B., Evaluation of proposed limits for intermittent noise exposure with temporary threshold shift as a criterion. Am. Ind. Hyg. Assoc. J., 33, 543-5, 1972.

6. Dieroff, H.G., Meissner, W., Zur Erfassung impulshaltiger gehörschädigender Industriegeräusche durch Wirkpegelangaben. Arch. klin. exp. Ohr-Nas-Kehlk.Hlk., 197, 245-253, 1970.

7. Hetu, R., Tremolieres, C., Effects of temporal distribution of sound energy on temporary threshold shift produced by intermittent and varying noise exposures. J. Acoust. Soc. Amer., 61, 1278-1287, 1977.

8. Ward, W.D., A comparison of the effects of continuous, intermittent, and impulse noise. In: Effects of Noise on Hearing, Eds., D. Henderson, R. Hamernik, D. Dosanjh, and J. Mills, Raven Press, New York, 1976.

9. Martin, A.M., The equal energy concept applied to impulse noise. In: Effects of Noise on Hearing. Eds., D. Henderson, R. Hamernik, D. Dosanjh, and J. Mills. Raven Press, New York, 1976.

10. McRobert, H., Ward, W.D., Damage-risk criteria: The trading relation between intensity and the number of nonreverberant impulses. J. Acoust. Soc. Amer., 53, 1297-1300, 1973.

11. Sataloff, J., Vassallo, L., Menduke, H., Hearing loss from exposure to interrupted noise. Arch. Env. Health, 18, 972-981, 1969.

12. Ward, W.D., Effects of noise exposure on auditory sensitivity. In: Handbook of Physiology, Vol. 9: Reactions to Environmental Agents, Ed., D.H.K. Lee, Am. Physiol. Soc., Bethesda, Md., 1977b. Pp. 1-15.

13. Lipscomb, D.M., Axelsson, A., Vertes, D.I., Roettger, R., Carroll, J., The effect of high level sound on hearing sensitivity, cochlear sensorineuroepithelium and vasculature of the chinchilla. Acta Oto-Laryngol., 84, 44-56, 1977.

14. Dolan, T.R., Murphy, R.J., Ades, H.W., A comparison of the permanent deleterious effects of intense noise on the chinchilla resulting from either continuous or intermittent exposure. In: Effects of Noise on Hearing, eds. D. Henderson, R.P. Hamernik, D.S. Dosanjh and J.H. Mills, Raven Press, New York, 1976.

Personal Hearing Protection in
Industry, edited by P. W. Alberti,
Raven Press, New York ©

4 Hearing Protector Design Concepts and Performance Limitations

Edgar A. G. Shaw

INTRODUCTION

As we trace the history of hearing protectors, it is hard to escape the conclusion that limitations in performance have loomed larger, in recent years, than advances in design. With the spreading of protector use from the highly disciplined aviation, military and scientific fields through industry in all its diversity we are brought face to face with difficulties which were hardly considered important twenty years ago or were thought to be solved.

BODY-CONDUCTED SOUND

Hearing protectors reduce the transmission of airborne sound from the free-field to the eardrum but, with few exceptions, provide little protection against body-conducted sound. In fact, the reduction in hearing sensitivity brought about by the total elimination of airborne sound provides an objective standard of performance against which the attenuation of practical hearing protectors can be judged. This parameter, the free-field air-conduction to body-conduction ratio, was carefully estimated in a classical study by Zwislocki many years ago[1]. The principal findings are presented in Figure 1. To attain the degree of sound attenuation indicated by the curve Z2 it is necessary to place a solid earplug in the bony meatus and cover the external ear with a massive circumaural hearing protector of optimum design. It may, in fact, be necessary to adjust the design to suit the sound frequency. When a shallow earplug is placed in the cartilaginous meatus the ear becomes more sensitive to body-conducted sound. This "occlusion effect" has been taken into account in the curve Z1 to provide a plausible estimate of the attenuation limit for conventional earplugs.

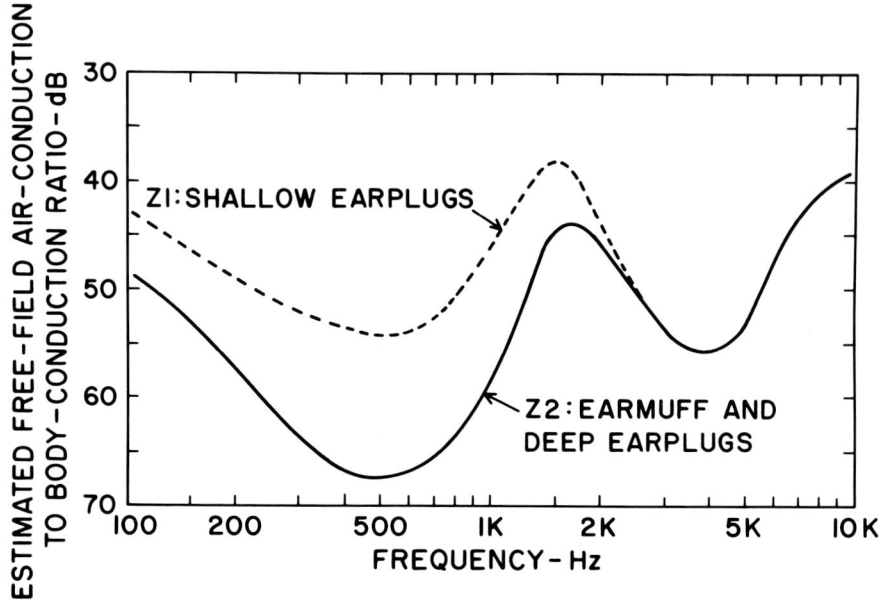

Figure 1. Free-field air-conduction to body-conduction ratio as estimated by Zwislocki (see reference 1). Curve Z2 requires a massive circumaural protector of optimum design and a solid earplug in the bony meatus. Curve Z1 allows for the "occlusion effect" associated with the presence of an earplug in the cartilaginous meatus.

A SIMPLE ACOUSTICAL MODEL

Figure 2a shows an ideal circumaural hearing protector with a rigid cup of mass M which encloses a volume of air V, is sealed to the head by a cushion of spring constant K_2 and mechanical resistance R_2, and covers an area A. Assuming for the moment that the enclosure is completely airtight (Z_L infinite) and the supporting surface both airtight and rigid, the sound pressure p_2 inside the cavity is entirely dependent on the displacement of the cup under the pressure p_1 of the external sound field. Strictly speaking there is also a small contribution due to lateral cushion displacement but this is generally negligible[2,3].

The acoustical behaviour of this system can be represented by the simple acoustical circuit network shown in Figure 2. As can be seen, the inertance L_M, the acoustical resistance R_K, the acoustical capacitance

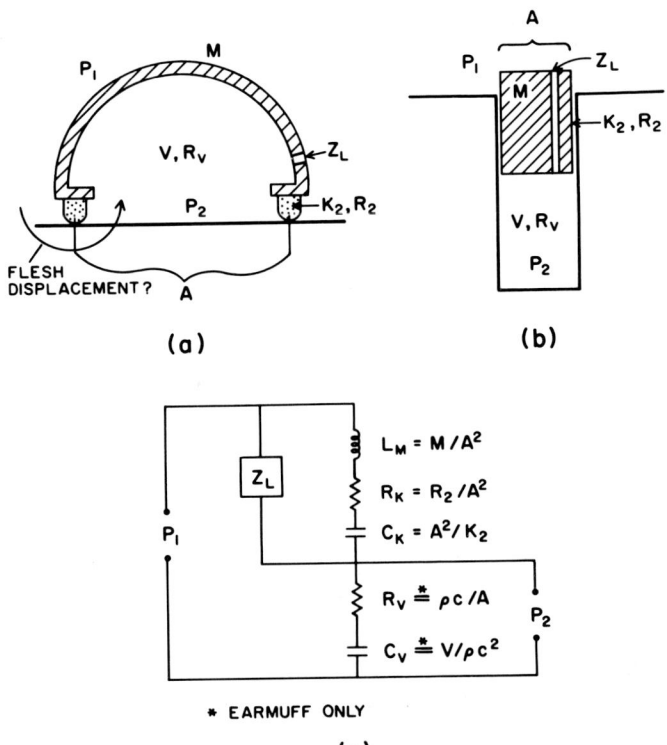

Figure 2. (a) Ideal circumaural hearing protector supported by rigid airtight surface; hypothetical transmission path (flesh displacement) is also indicated; (b) ideal rigid earplug vibrating in rigid ear canal; (c) acoustical circuit network representing ideal protector.

C_K and the capacitance C_V are dependent on M, R_2, K_2 and V, respectively. At frequencies greater than 2000 Hz, where the wavelength of sound is comparable with the cup dimensions, there will be strong air resonances in the cavity unless it is damped with suitable porous sound absorbing material. The resistance R_V is included in the network to represent, in a simple but approximate manner, the effect of this material (which usually occupies most of the cavity volume) on the high-frequency performance. A more advanced treatment is given elsewhere[4]. The acoustic impedance Z_L, which shunts the branch containing L_M, R_K and C_K, represents whatever air leakage there may be through the cup or under the cushion.

The behaviour of an earplug inserted into the ear canal (Figure 2b) can also be represented fairly well by the network of Figure 2c provided that the values of V and R_V are chosen to take into account the volume of the occluded ear canal, the compliance of the eardrum and the resistive component of eardrum impedance.

TYPICAL CHARACTERISTICS

The solid graph lines in Figure 3 show the calculated curves of transmission loss

$$TL = 20 \log_{10} /P_1/P_2/ dB \qquad (1)$$

for an earmuff and an earplug which are representative of high quality hearing protectors in current use. In both cases it is taken for granted that the protector is properly fitted and adjusted. The mechanical and acoustical parameters used in the calculations are given in Tables 1 and 2.

For the earmuff, the chosen value of A (44 cm^2) is the arithmetic mean of the area of head (A_1 = 15 cm^2) in contact with the air cavity and the total area (A_2 = 73 cm^2) enclosed by the outer boundary of the cushion[3]. The value of M (0.12 kg) includes the mass of the cushion which appears reasonable for earmuffs with liquid-filled cushions. The value of R_V (ρ/A) is consistent with optimum cavity damping at frequencies greater than 2000 Hz. The experimental points in the upper panel of Figure 3 are the average values of attenuation[3] for high quality circumaural hearing protectors from ten manufacturers as measured in various laboratories and reported in the 1975 NIOSH List[5]. These average values are considered more reliable than the data for specific hearing protectors. As can be seen, there is good agreement between the experimental attenuation data and the calculated transmission loss up to about 1000 Hz. At the higher frequencies the transmission loss is limited by the elastic properties of the cup especially its rigidity and mechanical damping[3]. This limitation is clearly indicated in the experimental attenuation data in the upper panel of Figure 3 which show a significant loss in performance between 4 and 8 kHz. As can be seen the high-frequency performance is also limited by the body-conduction curve Z2 especially in the vicinity of

Table 1: Mechanical and Acoustical Parameters of Earmuffs

Device	Mechanical Parameters	Acoustical Parameters
1. Earmuff A1 (Standard)	$M=0.12$ kg $K_2=1.63 \times 10^5$ N/m $R_2=145$ N.s/m $V=1.7 \times 10^{-4}$ m^3 (170 cm^3) $A=4.4 \times 10^{-3}$ m^2 (44 cm^2)	$L_M=6200$ Pa.s^2/m^3 $C_K=1.19 \times 10^{-10}$ m^3/Pa $R_K=7.5 \times 10^6$ Pa.s/m^3 $C_V=1.19 \times 10^{-9}$ m^3/Pa $R_V=9.4 \times 10^4$ Pa.s/m^3 $Z_L=\infty$
2. Earmuff A2 (Volume:x2)	M,K_2,R_2,A:see 1 $V=3.4 \times 10^{-4}$ m^3 (340 cm^3)	L_M,C_K,R_K,R_V,A_L:see 1 $C_V=2.38 \times 10^{-9}$ m^3/Pa
3. Earmuff A3 (Mass:x0.5)	K_2,R_2,V,A:see 1 $M=0.06$ kg	C_K,R_K,C_V,R_V,Z_L:see 1 $L_M=3100$ Pa.s^2/m^3
4. Earmuff A4 (Cushion stiffness x0.5, Cushion resistance x0.5)	M,V,A:see 1 $K_2=8.1 \times 10^4$ N/m $R_2=73$ N.s/m	L_M,C_V,R_V,Z_L:see 1 $C_K=2.38 \times 10^{-10}$ m^3/Pa $R_K=3.75 \times 10^6$ Pa.s/m^3
5. Earmuff A5 (Area:1.41)	M,K_2,R_2,V:see 1 $A=6.2 \times 10^{-3}$ M^2 (62 cm^2)	C_V,Z_L:see 1 $L_M=3100$ Pa.s^2/m^3 $C_K=2.38 \times 10^{-10}$ m^3/Pa $R_K=3.75 \times 10^6$ Pa.s/m^3 $R_V=6.65 \times 10^4$ Pa.s/m^3 $Z_L=$
6. Earmuff A1-A ("ventilation aperture")	M,K_2,R_2,V,A:see 1 Aperture dimensions: diameter=3mm cup thickness=3mm	L_M,C_K,R_K,C_V,R_V:see 1 $L_L=940$ Pa.s^2/m^3 $R_L=8700 \times$(frequency)$^{0.5}$ Pa.s/m^3
7. Earmuff A1-S (Slot-like opening under cushion)	M,K_2,R_2,V,A:see 1 Slot dimensions: length=27mm width=10mm height=1mm	L_M,C_K,R_K,C_V,R_V:see 1 $L_L=3200$ Pa.s^2/m^3 $R_L=5 \times 10^4 \times$(frequency)$^{0.5}$ Pa.s/m^3
8. Earmuff A1-E (Eyeglass leakage)	M,K_2,R_2,V,A:see 1	L_M,C_K,R_K,C_V,R_V:see 1 $L_L=6200$ Pa.s^2/m^3 $R_L=5 \times 10^6$ Pa.s/m^3

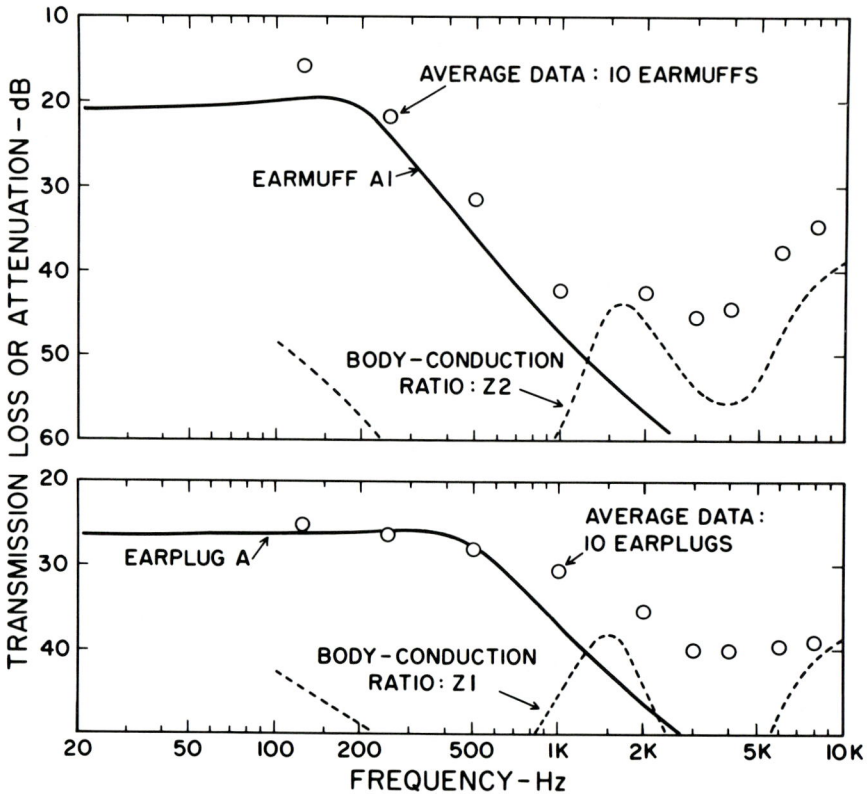

Figure 3. Calculated transmission loss curves for ideal Earmuff A1 and ideal Earplug A (See Tables 1 and 2) compared with (a) body-conduction ratios Z2 and Z1 from Figure 1 and (b) average measured mean values of attenuation from reference 3 which are based on data for 10 earmuffs and 10 earplugs included in the 1975 NIOSH List (reference 5).

2000 Hz.

The value of A (0.44 cm^2) adopted for Earplug A is the value now widely accepted as the standard (median) cross-sectional area of the human earcanal. The value of M (0.5g) is the mass of the widely used V51R rubber earplug. The assumption that the plug vibrates as a rigid body appears reasonable up to at least 500 Hz but is probably invalid at high frequencies. No independent data are available for K_2 and R_2 but these parameters are clearly dependent on the fit of the earplug in the earcanal and the properties of the tissue. The values in Table 2 have therefore

Table 2: Mechanical and Acoustical Parameters of Ear Plugs

Device	Mechanical Parameters	Acoustical Parameters
1. Earplug A	$M=0.5g$ $K_2=4300N/m$ $R_2=1.74N.s/m$ $V=1.3\times10^{-6}m^3$ (1.3 cm^3: occluded canal + eardrum) $A=4.4\times10^{-5}m^2$ (0.44 cm^2)	$L_M=2.56\times10^5 Pa.s^2/m^3$ $C_K=4.5\times10^{-13} m^3/Pa$ $R_K=9\times10^8 Pa.s/m^3$ $C_V=9\times10^{-12} m^3/Pa$ $R_V=1.2\times10^7 Pa.s/m^3$ $Z_L=\infty$
2. Earplug B (non-linear aperture)	M, K_2, R_2, V, A: see 1 Aperture dimensions: diameter=0.7mm disc thickness=0.04mm	L_M, C_K, R_K, C_V, R_V: see 1 $L_L=1850 Pa.s^2/m^3$ $R_1=1.3\times10^6 Pa.s/m^3$ $R_2=7.5\times10^4$(frequency)$^{1/2}$ Pa.s/m^3 $R_3=1.09\times10^{13} U_L$ Pa.s/m^3(see text)

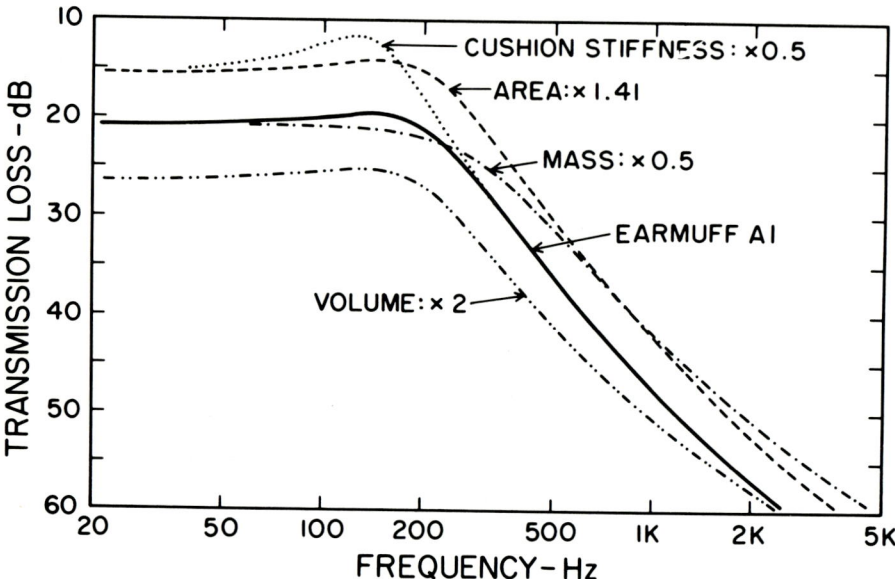

Figure 4. Calculated transmission loss curves for four variants of Earmuff A1 (See Table 1 for parameter values): Earmuff A2 (volume increased 100%), Earmuff A3 (mass reduced by 50%), Earmuff A4 (cushion stiffness and resistance reduced by 50%), Earmuff A5 (protector area increased by 41%).

been chosen to make C_K one twentieth of C_V and to provide substantial damping as indicated by the experimental attenuation data. The experimental points in the lower panel of Figure 3 are the average values of attenuation[3] for ten earplugs reported in the 1975 NIOSH List[5]. Strictly speaking, since the presence of an earplug in the ear canal changes the acoustical characteristics of the external ear, it is the insertion loss rather than the transmission loss which should be compared with the "real-ear" attenuation data. The distinction is unimportant below 1500 Hz (see Figure 6).

Calculated transmission loss curves for four variants of Earmuff A1 are presented in Figure 4. These curves show how each of four major design parameters affects the transmission loss calculated in accordance with Figure 2c. As can be seen, doubling the enclosed volume V while leaving all other parameters unchanged (Table I, Earmuff A2), increases the transmission loss by nearly 6 dB up to approximately 500 Hz where the cavity resistance R_V begins to take control. Reducing the mass by a factor of two (Table I, Earmuff A3) reduces the transmission loss by 6 dB at high frequencies but has little effect below 250 Hz where the cup motion is controlled by the cushion. Conversely, reducing the cushion stiffness (and, to be consistent, the cushion resistance also) by a factor of two reduces the transmission loss by nearly 6 dB at low frequencies but has no effect above 250 Hz where the motion is mass-controlled. As shown in Figure 2c, increasing the area by the factor $\sqrt{2}$ adversely affects all of the acoustical parameters except C_V and Z_L. As a consequence there is approximately 6 dB reduction in transmission loss over most of the frequency range.

The acoustical network of Figure 2c and the ideal circumaural hearing protector which it represents excludes from consideration certain aspects of human physiology. In particular, it is unrealistic to suppose that the circumaural region of the head is perfectly rigid. In well-designed earmuffs such as A1 it is, in fact, the finite mechanical impedance of the flesh which determines the values of the cushion constants K_2 and R_2. Hence, it would be unrealistic to suppose that a firmer cushion would produce significantly greater low-frequency transmission loss than the 20 dB indicated in Figures 3 and 4. Similarly, at somewhat higher frequencies there is evidence of a sound transmission path which is independent of cup motion[2]. Hence it would be unrealistic to suppose that an increase in cup mass would, by itself, significantly improve the performance between 200 and 1000 Hz. This second mechanism has been described as a flow of flesh under the cushion[3] (see Figure 2a) but has not yet been adequately treated in the scientific literature. New work to be presented at this Symposium should shed fresh light on this question[6].

AIR LEAKAGE
Perhaps the thorniest problem of all is air leakage especially leakage due to the misuse of hearing protectors. Earplugs are frequently loosely fitted or poorly inserted and, according to one report, hearing protective

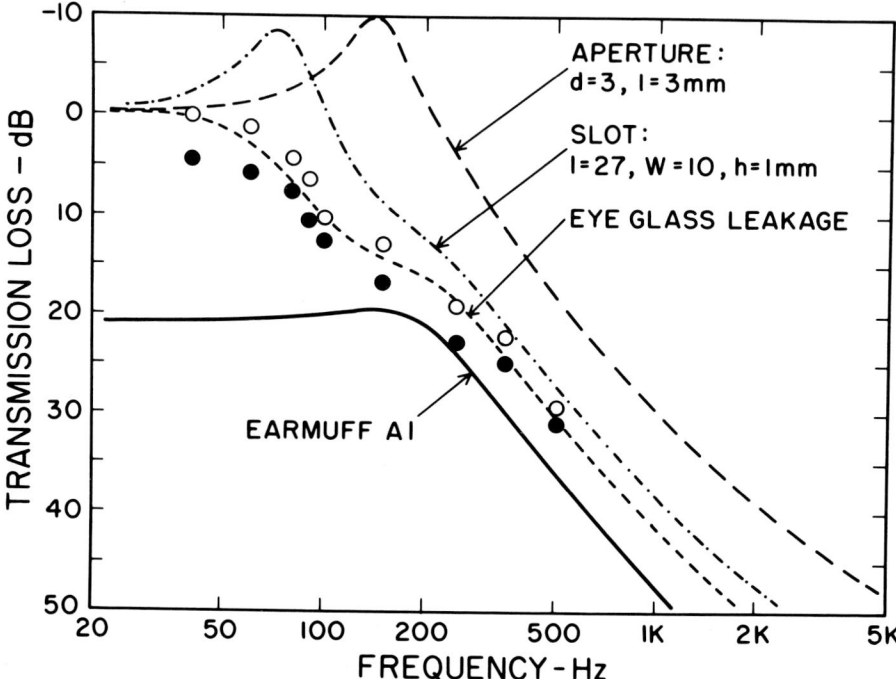

Figure 5. Calculated transmission loss of Earmuff A1 degraded by three degrees of air leakage (See Table I, Earmuffs A1-A, A1-S and A1-E).

devices may be mutilated to relieve the pressure they exert against the ears or to provide for air circulation particularly when worn in work areas of high heat and humidity[7].

The first curve in Figure 5 shows the loss of performance due to a "ventilation aperture" 3 mm in diameter drilled through the cup of Earmuff A1. The aperture produces a leakage impedance

$$Z = 2\pi \iota \upsilon L_L + R_L$$

where υ is the frequency and L_L and R_L have the values given in Table I (see Earmuff A1-A). As can be seen this leakage turns the hearing protector into a pressure amplifier below 200 Hz and reduces the transmission loss by 18 dB at higher frequencies. Acoustically, the leakage is equivalent to a total loss of cushion stiffness and an eight-fold decrease in cup mass.

The second curve shows the effect of a hypothetical leakage slot which might be created by placing an obstacle such as an eyeglass frame under the cushion. The experimental points (open and solid circles) show the results of a simple objective experiment in which the performance of a circumaural hearing protector similar to Earmuff A1 was measured with and without an eyeglass frame passing under the cushion. The measurements were made on a male subject with well-trimmed hair wearing eyeglasses with a plastic frame fitting tightly against the head. A probe microphone was used to measure the sound pressure near the pinna. The third curve ("eyeglass leakage") has been fitted to the experimental data (open circles) by adjusting the values of L_L and R_L (see Table I, Earmuff A1-E).

Experiments performed many years ago indicated that, in most cases, air leakage due to the presence of hair under the cushion was unlikely to cause much loss of performance. More recent measurements[8] by an objective method seem to indicate that losses of the order of 5 dB over the frequency range 100 - 1000 Hz may be fairly common but the mechanism is not entirely clear. Further objective measurements on real heads appear warranted.

Since the leakage impedance Z_L shunts the upper branch of the network (that which contains L_M, C_K and R_K), substantial leakage (Z_L small, as in Earmuff A1-A) destroys the benefits gained by large mass M, large cushion stiffness K_C and small effective area A. In the presence of such leakage it is the cavity volume V alone which determines the protector attenuation at frequencies below 1 or 2 kHz. It follows that the protector whose performance is primarily dependent on an usually large volume is intrinsically less vulnerable to degradation due to leakage than a protector whose performance is primarily dependent on the choice of mass, stiffness or area.

ACOUSTICAL PERFORMANCE: A BROADER VIEW

So far we have limited our attention to the primary aspect of protector performance: the sound transmission loss, and two classes of hearing protector: earmuffs and earplugs. Other aspects of acoustical performance which clearly deserve attention are the gains and losses in perception, especially the ability to hear speech sounds and warning signals and the ability to localize sound sources in noisy environments. Other classes of hearing protector which clearly deserve attention are those which have significant non-linearity in their acoustical behaviour and those which employ active elements such as transducers and electronic amplifiers. A comprehensive classification of hearing protectors which includes such devices is given in Table 3.

Non-Linear (Amplitude-Dependent) Hearing Protectors

An earplug with an aperture of the order of 0.5 mm in diameter provides excellent protection against intense high-frequency impulsive noises such as gunfire but transmits speech without appreciable attenuation. Such non-linear earplugs have been studied in several laboratories[9-11] at various times and at least two types are now in production. A brief theoretical account of their mode of operation is given here since no similar treatment of non-linear performance seems to be readily available.

The classical V5IR earplug is, in essence, a moulded rubber tube closed at one end. In the typical non-linear earplug, the end wall is replaced by a thin steel disc of thickness t with an aperture of radius a. This produces a leakage impedance

$$Z_L = R_L + 2 \quad L_L, \tag{2}$$

as indicated in Figure 2, where

$$R_L \simeq (R_1^2 + R_2^2 + R_3^2)^{1/2}, \tag{3}$$

$$R_1 \simeq 3 \ /a^3, \tag{4}$$

$$R_2 \simeq (4\rho\nu\mu/\pi)^{1/2}(1.7a+t)/a^3, \qquad (5)$$

$$R_3 \simeq 1.34\rho U_L/\pi^2 a^4, \qquad (6)$$

$$L_L \simeq \rho(1.7a+t)/\pi a^2, \qquad (7)$$

ν is the sound frequency (Hz), ρ the air density (1.2 kg/m^3), μ the viscosity (1.85 x 10^{-5} Pa.s) and U_L the rms velocity of airflow through the orifice (m^3/s). The first and second components of orifice resistance R_1 and R_2 are simply the dc flow resistance and the low-level acoustic damping resistance. The third component R_3 increases with the volume velocity U_L and hence becomes predominant at sufficiently high sound levels. The orifice inertance L_L is essentially independent of the sound level. To calculate the transmission loss (Eqn. 1) at any given sound pressure level it is necessary to find the value of U_L which simultaneously satisfies Eqns 3 - 6 and the acoustical network equations appropriate to Figure 2c. This is readily accomplished with a computer.

The aperture diameter chosen for Earplug B (0.7 mm, see Table 3) is the same as that recommended by Forest for military use but the disc is thinner (0.04 mm compared with .13 mm). The corresponding values of resistance and inertance, calculated from Equations (4) - (7), are given in Table 2. Figure 6 shows the calculated pure tone transmission loss curves for Earplug B at input SPL between 110 and 190 dB. Also shown are the low-level limit and the curve for Earplug A which is a hypothetical high-level limit. As can be seen, at low sound levels the transmission loss is slightly negative below 1.5 kHz and not very large at higher frequencies. It should, however, be remembered that at 3000 Hz in a free sound field the SPL at the eardrum with the canal open is approximately 10 dB greater than the SPL near the canal entrance with the canal closed[12] as shown by the dotted line in Figure 6. To obtain the insertion loss (c.f. attenuation) this difference must be added to the transmission loss[11]. At approximately 110 dB SPL amplitude-dependent attenuation begins to be noticeable for frequencies around 1 kHz, and at 130 dB this non-linear attenuation amounts to approximately 7 dB. At yet higher levels

Table 3:   Classification of Devices

Mode of operation	Mode of Engagement with Ear	Linear Devices	Non-Linear (Amplitude-Dependent) Devices
Passive	Intra-aural	Conventional Earplug	Earplug with aperture (for intense impulses only)
Passive	Supra-aural	Traditional earphone (Transmission loss usually small)	
Passive	Circumaural	Conventional earmuff	
Passive	Complete enclosure of head	Space helmet	
Active	Intra-aural	Earplug with electronic sound absorption *	Conventional low-gain hearing aid with airtight earmold, 0 dB insertion (see text) loss at low sound levels and automatic gain control
Active	Supra-aural		
Active	Circumaural	Earmuff with electronic sound absorption *	Earmuff with built-in "hearing aid" (amplifier, external microphone, internal earphone)

* Linearity limited by power-handling capacity of amplifier and earphone.

additional attenuation is gained at the rate of 5 dB per 10 dB increase in level. The experimental values of amplitude-dependent attenuation obtained by Forest[11] and Martin[13] with an earplug similar to Earplug B are in reasonable agreement with Figure 6.

A low-gain hearing aid with automatic gain control and an airtight earmold could, in principle, serve as an active amplitude-dependent hearing protector. With the insertion gain set at 0 dB for low-level sounds, such a device could offer unimpeded speech communication against a quiet background while providing perhaps 20 dB of sound attenuation at high sound levels. Circumaural hearing protectors based on this idea were described in the patent literature approximately fifteen years ago[14-16] and several practical devices for military use and for the mining industry have been designed in Britain, the U.S.A., Canada and elsewhere[17,18].

Electronic Sound Absorption

In 1953 it was shown that a microphone, an electronic amplifier and a loudspeaker suitably connected would act as a sound absorber[19]. In a typical application the loudspeaker and microphone were placed immediately above the head of an operator thereby reducing the local level of low-frequency machinery noise. Close to the microphone reductions in level as great as 25 dB over one octave and 10 dB over three octaves were reported but the performance fell sharply when the distance exceeded a fraction of the wavelength. Three years later[20] further progress was reported in an oral paper which included a preliminary account of a circumaural hearing protector embodying electronic sound absorption. This application seemed particularly promising since the microphone could be placed close to the ear. Furthermore, comparatively little sound power would be required to control the acoustical environment in such a small space. The oral paper also enunciated more clearly the nature of electronic sound absorption which was shown to be equivalent to a reduction in acoustical impedance in the vicinity of the absorber. In terms of Figure 2 one can infer that electronic sound absorption would increase the effective volume of the hearing protector V (and hence the

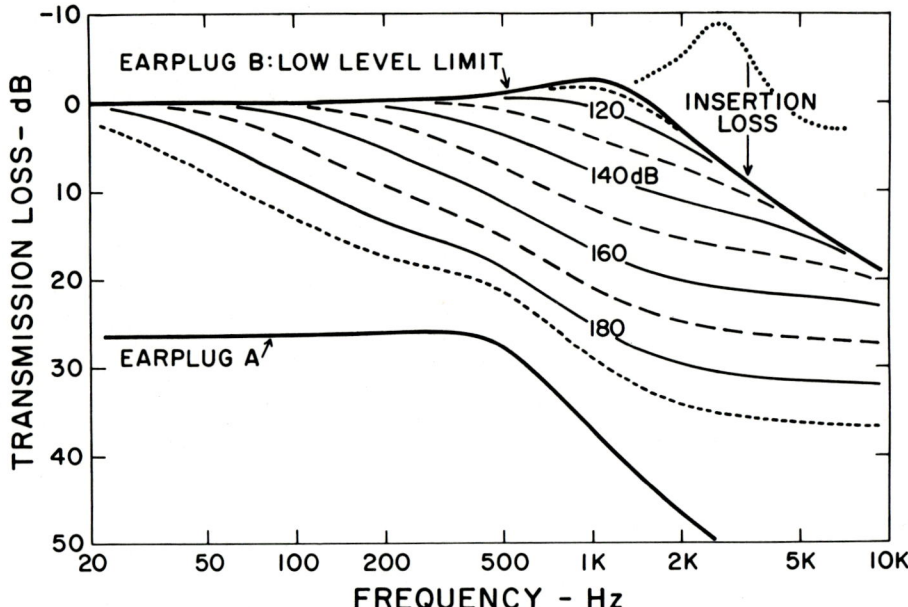

Figure 6. Calculated pure-tone transmission loss curves for earplug with 0.7 mm aperture (Table 2, Earplug B) at sound pressure levels up to 190 dB. Curve for Earplug A is taken from Figure 3. Dotted line shows estimated transfer function from centre of plug closing ear canal entrance to eardrum position with ear canal open.

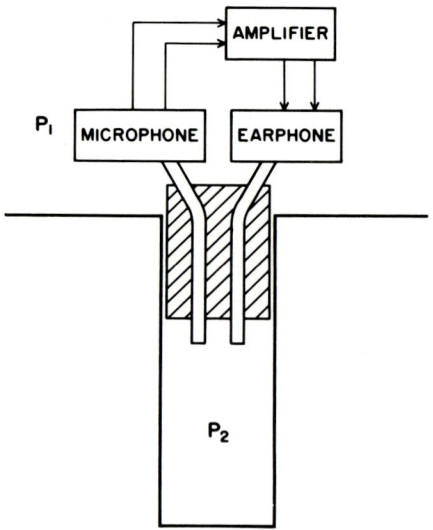

Figure 7. Earplug with electronic sound absorption. Microphone amplifier and earphone form a negative feedback loop which reduces p_2.

value of C_V) and/or decrease the effective value of R_V.

Since the magnitude of the space to be controlled is so important in electronic sound absorption, it seems likely that it would be easier to obtain substantial increases in attenuation with earplugs than with ear muffs. Figure 7 shows the essential elements of such a system. With the development of high performance hearing aid transducers and miniature integrated circuits during the past decade it is clear that we now have at our disposal far greater technological resources than were available when electronic sound absorption was first proposed nearly thirty years ago. The field now seems ripe for the development of various non-linear and linear hearing protectors with active elements which could alleviate some of the more subtle limitations of current passive devices.

REFERENCES

1. Zwislocki, J., In search of the bone-conduction threshold in a free sound field. J. Acoust. Soc. Amer. 29, 795-802, 1957.

2. Shaw, E.A.G., Thiessen, G.J., Improved cushion for ear defenders. J. Acoust. Soc. Amer. 30, 24-36, 1958.

3. Shaw, E.A.G., Hearing protector attenuation: A perspective view. Applied Acoustics 12, 139-157, 1979.

4. Shaw, E.A.G., Thiessen, G.J., Acoustics of circumaural earphones. J. Acoust. Soc. Amer. 34, 1233-1246, 1962.

5. Kroes, P., Fleming, R., Lempert, B., List of personal hearing protectors and attenuation data, U.S. National Institute for Occupational Safety and Health, Cincinnati, Ohio, 1975.

6. Gorman, A.G. Private Communication, 1980.

7. Mellard, T.J., Doyle, T.J., Miller, M.H., Employee Education - The Key to Effective Hearing Conservation. Sound and Vibration, 12, 24-29, January 1978.

8. Russell, M.F., May, S.P., Objective test for earmuffs. J. of Sound and Vibration, 44, 545-562, 1976.

9. Zwislocki, J., New types of ear protectors. J. Acoust. Soc. Amer., 24, 762, 1952.

10. Allen, C.H., Bolt, Beranek and Newman unpublished report. (Private Communication) 1975.

11. Forest, M.R., Summary report on the development of an improved amplitude-sensitive earplug (INM-Modified V51R), Report HeS135, RNPRC, MRC of Great Britain, 1969. (See reference 3 for other relevant information.)

12. Shaw, E.A.G., Acoustic response of external ear replica at various angles of incidence. J. Acoust. Soc. Amer., 55, 432(A), 1974.

13. Martin, A.M., Dependence of acoustic attenuation of hearing protectors on incident sound level. Brit. J. Industr. Med., 36, 1-4, 1979.

14. Wood, H.J., Protective Hearing Aid. United States Patent 3,306,991, February 1967.

15. Kahn, L.R., Dispositif de protection des organes de l'ouie ne diminuant pas le pouvoir auditif. Brevet d'Invention No. 1,512,289, Paris, February 1968.

16. Barker, P.J. and Livermore, R.A., Ear defenders. Patent Specification 1,160,341, The Patent Office, London, August 1969.

17. Michael, P.L., Private communication, 1980.

18. Forshaw, S. and others. Private Communications, 1980.

19. Olson, H.F., Electronic sound absorber. J. Acoust. Soc. Amer., 25, 1130-1136, 1953.

20. Olson, H.F., Electronic Control of Noise, Vibration and Reverberation. J. Acoust. Soc. Amer., 28, 156(A), 1956.

5
HEARING PROTECTION STANDARDS
Charles W. Nixon

INTRODUCTION

The accurate description of the performance of personal equipment intended to provide protection against the adverse effects of acoustic energy is critical to programs dedicated to insuring public health and welfare in our daily living activities. National and international procedures to provide performance descriptors of hearing protection devices have existed for some time. Individual national policies and programs differ in guidelines and in criteria which govern allowable acoustic exposures and in methods for controlling them. Nevertheless, it is of scientific and technical as well as practical importance that the provisions of a sound protection descriptor be generally agreeable among user agencies and nations. This agreement is becoming more urgent as international standardization is extending to such practices as hearing conservation and as hearing protection devices manufactured in one nation are sold and used in others. It is the intent of this paper to address some aspects of achieving uniformity or standardization in the area of hearing protection. It will not be exhaustive on any subject nor will it yield to the temptation to discuss interesting elements of various national standards now in use throughout the world. Among the matters presented are the concept of standardization and its implementation as it has evolved in hearing protection, the status of the International Standards Organization hearing protection standards, representative measurement methods, calculation of sound reduction values and the identification of standards that are needed by governments, manufacturers and users of hearing protection.

CONCEPT OF STANDARDIZATION

The general concept of standardization familiar to most of us is one that results in uniformity, compatability or interchangeability of components, procedures or operations. It is something considered by general consent or by an authority as a basis for comparison; an approved measurement or model. This standardization is assured because the measurement or model is based on the latest state of knowledge at the time the document is prepared. Standards may consider such factors as terminology, fabrication, measurement, performance, quality and use. Their application includes manufacture, selection, care and use of products and services. Products and activities accomplished in accordance with standards are expected to reflect similar and compatible results within the tolerances associated with the specific standard.

In the United States a few decades ago, the number of individuals and testing facilities interested and active in hearing protection work was very small. Hearing protection research and development was generally confined to these few independent facilities with little need for intercommunication or cross-fertilization of ideas. In the late 1940's and early 1950's an increase in hearing protection activity was stimulated by a more widespread use of jet engines in military and commercial aircraft. The number of different hearing protectors available at that time was small, consequently the various testing facilities measured the performance of the same hearing protectors. Interactions among these groups gradually increased and subsequent comparisons of the performance of the same hearing protector often revealed significant variations. Further communications indicated that each of the testing laboratories was using measurement procedures that differed substantively from one another. It was in this climate that the small community of researchers, most of whom were active in the Acoustical Society of America, promoted the need for standardized measurement procedures in the hearing protection and hearing conservation arenas. The subsequent result was the standard for the measurement of the Real-Ear Attenuation of Ear Protectors at Threshold, Z24.22, 1957. The use of Z24.22 increased as hearing conservation practices were adopted more widely by industry, the military and other noisy activities. Its application continued for over 15 years until its revision in 1974 to the current US standard ANSI S3.19-1974 (ASA STD 1-1975), Method for the Measurement of Real-Ear Protection of Hearing

Protectors and Physical Attenuation of Earmuffs. A similar evolution of hearing protection standards in the United States took place in other nations in a similar time frame. Today, the number of private, educational, industrial and governmental organizations active in some area of hearing protection is quite large throughout the world.

STANDARDS DEVELOPMENT

The standardization process, whether at the national or international level, is intended to provide a set of firm, clearcut guidelines for accomplishing a specific task. These guidelines are formulated by personnel most knowledgeable and experienced with the task on the basis of the most current and appropriate data base. The process includes provisions for numerous technical reviews by persons ranging from the potential users of the standards to bodies that govern and control the promulgation of such instruments. Yet, it appears that only a small percentage of those involved in hearing protection work have any significant familiarity with the standardization process or the standards themselves.

There is no mystery or magic associated with hearing protector standards, although an inexperienced person may comment that only a magician could implement some of them. Hearing protector standards are formulated in response to particular needs as requested by any individual or group with special interests in the matter to be standardized, members of the standards organizations, users of the standard or its product and governmental agencies. A working group is formed with a membership comprised of representative knowledgeable and experienced persons in that technical area who are willing to devote time and to work on the problem. The problem is addressed by the group on the basis of state-of-the-art technology and a consensus draft standard is formulated. The working group does not conduct research even in areas where data and experience may be lacking. During this developmental process the working group recognizes available technology, identifies limitations and attempts to formulate the draft standard accordingly.

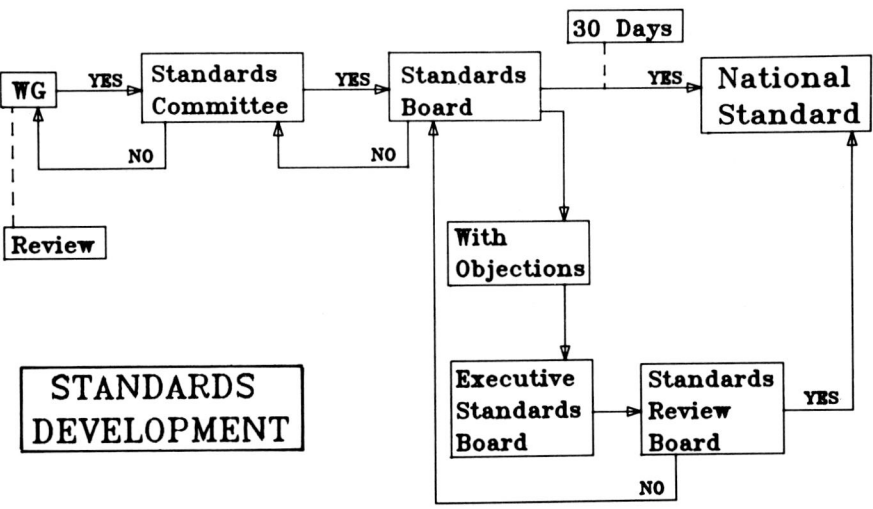

Figure I. General Development of a Standard and the Review Process

The general development of a standard and the critical review process to which it is subjected is exemplified in Figure I which depicts the process followed in the American National Standards Institute for standards on bio-acoustics. A draft standard agreeable to the working group is submitted to the next higher review level for action. This action usually involves a balloting of the draft but may consist only of a request for technical comments with the vote to be taken after incorporation of the comments. At the present time the proposed standard must be acceptable to at least 80% of the standards committee for approval. Draft documents approved by the Standards Committee are submitted to the Acoustical Standards Board.

Approval by the Acoustical Standards Board, with no objection, results in a standard. An approved draft standard with objections requires further review by the Executive Standards Board and then the Standards Review

Board, where an affirmative vote results in a standard. As indicated in Figure I, disapproved draft standards are referred back to appropriate lower level groups for necessary action. Unresolved negative comments and objections are always accompanied by explanatory and supportive materials to assist reviewers in their evaluation of the proposed document. Although various nations have different review procedures, the process described herein represents the general operation of standards development.

The intended purpose of a standard and the national structure in which it is to be implemented may strongly influence its contents. For example, in some nations a single laboratory staffed with highly experienced technical personnel and equipped with modern instrumentation is responsible for all hearing protector research and evaluations. Since no other facility in that nation will be using the standard, it can contain strict, complex requirements that need high level technical skills and sophisticated instrumentation for accomplishment. In other nations, standards may be intended for widespread use by government, industry, professional consultants, universities and even private citizens. In this setting, the measurement standard would address the least strict requirements and procedures needed to satisfy the purpose of the standard. It would contain guidelines and specifications that might be readily understood and practiced by university students as well as industrial and government laboratories. These factors have contributed to differences between some of the national hearing protection standards that exist today. However, a working group has been established (WG 17, Hearing Protection) under ISO Technical Committee 43/ SC 1, "Noise," to develop international standards for hearing protection.

STATUS OF INTERNATIONAL STANDARDS

The international working group has dealt with three proposed standards for the measurement of hearing protector performance (Table I). The first proposed standard contained both subjective and physical measurement methods and was circulated to Technical Committee 43, Sub Committee I in December 1975. As a consequence of the member body

Table 1: Status of International Standards Organization Hearing Protection Standards

DOCUMENT		STATUS
ISO 4869	Measurement of Sound Attenuation of Hearing Protectors - Subject Method	International Standard
- -	Physical Measurement of Attenuation	Tabled
ISO 6290	A Simplified Method for A Measurement of Insertion Loss of Hearing Protectors of Earmuff Type for Quality Control Purposes	Draft International Standard

comments, the two methods were then prepared as separate documents. The subjective method, ISO 4869 received major support during the subsequent member body voting and was issued as a standard in 1979. The physical measurement method was discussed at length and subsequently tabled because of inadequate data in certain areas. This physical method intended for research, development, certification testing, quality control, and the like, has not been abandoned but only set aside for the present until more technical information relevant to the method is available. A third document was prepared as an interim physical measurement method, a Simplified Method For A Measurement of Insertion Loss of Hearing Protectors of Ear-Muff Type For Quality Control Purposes (ISO 6290). The first draft of this proposed method was revised in accordance with comments received during its review by member bodies early in 1979. The second draft was approved as a Draft International Standard at the meeting of Technical Committee 43 in Stockholm, Sweden in May 1979. This simplified measurement method is intended for quality control purposes only and is not applicable to engineering, design, development, research and other similar activities.

ISO 4869, Measurement of Sound Attenuation of Hearing Protectors - Subjective Method, has been established as an international standard. However, at this time it is unlikely that many nations have adopted the new international standard as a replacement for their own national standard. This retention of national guides is necessary in most situations because laws, regulations, guidelines and even other standards are based on performance data from the national standard. Although this dilemma exists whenever any international standard is established, efforts should be made to resolve differences, develop conversion factors for application of data and eventually to adopt international standards - especially by nations that vote affirmative on the draft proposal. Recent emphasis on the adoption of ISO 4869 by various nations, pointed out problems encountered today by hearing protector manufacturers who distribute their product in several nations of the world. The product may require repeat evaluations, in the nation in which the protector is manufactured as well as in every other nation where it is used. This single problem as well as others would be resolved, in large degree, if all nations involved utilized the same measurement/performance standard, namely ISO 4869. the ISO working group will continue to work for standards that are both practical as well as international in scope.

The concept of standardization is such that standards are not permanent documents but instead are based on the current state of knowledge and that they should be revised whenever new knowledge allows the procedure to be improved. The standards development process appears to move slowly, however, it must be recognized that a substantial amount of work and coordination is required to produce a draft proposal. Also, the critical review process is accomplished at several levels to insure that the final document is both reasonable and accurate. Finally, an organization or nation must process an approved standard according to its established procedures to determine if it is to be adopted and put into practice. Although these various actions cannot be accomplished quickly, standards organizations encourage the updating of standards. Some require that all standards be reviewed at specified time intervals, such as every four years, and be confirmed, revised or even eliminated if appropriate. All actions of this nature by standards organizations are intended to insure that established documents are contemporary, accurate and in the most practical form for prospective users.

REPRESENTATIVE MEASUREMENT METHODS

Over the years many different methods have been and are being used for the evaluation of hearing protection devices (Table 2). Perhaps the most widely used are various forms of the real ear attenuation at threshold method. All measurement methods have both advantages and disadvantages. However, the real ear attenuation at threshold method satisfies many of the requirements of a "standard" procedure without being seriously invalidated by its disadvantages and weaknesses. Various other measurement procedures have applications or features that also satisfy important requirements, however, some of their features have prohibited their standardization.

Table 2: Representative Measurement Methods for Hearing Protector Attenuation

* Real Ear Attenuation at Threshold

* Loudness Balance
    - Air-to-Air Loudness Balance
    - Bone-to-Air Loudness Balance
    - Insert Receiver to Air Loudness Balance
    - Null Procedures

* Temporary Threshold Shift

* Aural Reflex

* Subjective Comparison

* Miniature Microphone or Subjective - Objective

* Masked-Threshold

* Hearing Loss for Speech

* Cadaver Measurements

Several measurement methods will be briefly explained in the following discussion, however, it is beyond the scope of this paper to address the pros and cons of each method. At some time, almost all of these have been proposed as candidate standard procedures. The reader will recognize from the descriptions why many of them have not been promulgated. Characteristics most often responsible for rejection as a standard include time required to run the test, level of difficulty for the subject, reliability of measures, safety of the subject and costs that apply to the facility as well as the evaluation.

Real Ear Attenuation At Threashold (REAT)

The REAT method generally involves the measurement of the hearing threshold levels of unoccluded ears for selected test signals. The measurements are repeated with the subject wearing the hearing protector under evaluation. The difference between the open ear threshold values and the occluded (with hearing protector) ear threshold values is described as the protection or attenuation of the device. This method is used to evaluate all types of hearing protection equipment (except perforate and other nonlinear devices) ranging from insert earplugs to fire fighters helmets to space suits.

Loudness Balance Methods

The basic loudness balance method involves the measurement of the perceived loudness of a reference signal (in nontest ear) and of a comparison signal (in test ear) judged by an observer to be equal in loudness to the reference. Placement of the reference signal under the protector, (unoccluded ear) and the comparison signal outside the protector (occluded ear), allows the attenuation of a protector to be quantified. The difference between the reference test signal and the comparison test signal judged to be equal in loudness is described as the attenuation of the hearing protector. This method may be used with the test signals at hearing threshold level or at any other higher level within the safety limits of the volunteers and the range of the signal processing equipment. It also allows the use of different types of signals for the reference and comparison signals. A pure tone can be balanced with a tone of different frequency, with a narrow band of noise, with a broad band of noise, or one band of noise can be compared to a different band of noise, etc.

Air-To-Air Loudness Balance

In air-to-air loudness balance the subject is presented test signals via air conduction hearing. The subject attends to a signal with unoccluded ears, then dons the protector and attempts to adjust the level to that which he heard open ear. This can be done binaurally (both ears) or monaurally by occluding the ear not under test with earplugs and earmuffs. An earphone is sometimes used for the reference signal when earmuffs or helmets are evaluated.

Bone-To-Air Comparison

In bone-to-air loudness balance either the reference or comparison signal is presented via bone conduction hearing. Conventionally, the bone conducted signal is used as the reference signal and is considered an open or unprotected ear condition. In this operation a reference signal is presented via bone conduction and a loudspeaker produced air conduction signal is adjusted to be equal to the reference tone by a subject wearing the hearing protector.

One national standard utilizes this air-to-bone loudness balance. Pulsed pure tones are presented to the subject via the bone conduction vibrator. An octave band of noise is presented via loudspeakers at a high intensity level. The subject wearing the hearing protector adjusts the pulsed tone until it just emerges from the ambient noise. The hearing protector is removed and the subject adjusts the level of the ambient noise until the pure tone bone conducted signal again just emerges from the noise. The difference in the levels of the airborne octave bands of noise between the two trials is described as the attenuation of the device.

Insert Receiver to Air Comparisons

Another form of loudness balance uses an insert receiver as the source of the reference signal. A comparison signal from a loudspeaker source is balanced with the reference signal while wearing protectors other than inserts. In addition, the ear contralateral to the one containing the insert must be fit with an excellent noise excluding device to insure that lateralization to that ear does not occur under high intensity testing conditions.

Null Procedures

One variation of the loudness balance method which may use either air-to-air or bone-to-air signal presentation requires the subject to adjust the comparison signal to cancel or null the reference signal. This method is not common because of difficulties encountered with the instrumentation and in actually achieving the null. The same pure tone signal must be used as both reference and comparison signals. The subject must adjust two controls, phase and amplitude, if the frequency of the signals does not drift, otherwise frequency adjustments are also required. With appropriate instrumentation and experienced subjects most test signals can be cancelled so long as the protector does not produce distortion in the comparison signal that cannot be compensated by frequency, intensity and phase adjustments. Testing sessions are very long because of numerous repeated adjustments of the signal variables required to achieve a null condition. Although very interesting from a scientific point of view, this method does not lend itself to standardization.

Temporary Threshold Shift Methods

There are two general categories of temporary threshold shift (TTS) methods of assessing hearing protector performance. The first method measures the amount of TTS produced in an unprotected ear by a noise exposure. The measurement is repeated with the subject wearing the hearing protector. Performance is described in terms of the amount of TTS reduction provided by the protector. The second method measures the amount of TTS produced by a specific noise exposure while the subject wears the hearing protector under test. Performance is described in terms of the capability of the hearing protector to reduce or prevent TTS in the specific exposure used. This method assesses the hazard to hearing of the noise exposure as well as the performance of the protector.

The first threshold shift method described has become increasingly unpopular in today's research environs where experimental protocols must be reviewed, usually by committee, and approved prior to test initiation. Studies that purposefully induce TTS in humans are highly undesirable in most situations and totally unacceptable in others. The second method, on the other hand, is generally more acceptable. It is used primarily when the adequacy of a particular hearing protector is evaluated in a specific noise environs. A hearing protector determined to be acceptable by this method is used as a criterion, that is, hearing protectors that provide equal or greater protection than the unit tested are also considered adequate for the noise environment of concern.

Aural Reflex Method
The aural reflex is a sudden contraction of the muscles of the middle ear system in response to loud sound. The muscle contractions cause a retraction of the eardrum membrane and an increase in the resistance of the middle ear system which results in less sound transmission to the inner ear. An average aural reflex threshold for pulsed tones is about 90 dB sensation level. The aural reflex response is consensual, that is, the middle ear muscle contractions occur in both ears, even when the adequate stimulus is presented to only one ear. It is the simultaneous response in both ears that allows the reflex to be used to assess hearing protectors at above threshold levels.

The technique of tympanomanometry is one means of measuring the aural reflex. A sealing plug is inserted in one external auditory canal trapping a small volume of air between the plug and the tympanic membrane. The reflex causes a deflection of the tympanic membrane and change in the trapped air pressure. Pressure changes are reflected as deflections of the normal baseline of an oscilloscope trace, and with appropriate instrumentation, appear superimposed on the trace of the stimulus. The difference in decibels between the open ear and occluded ear (with protector) aural reflex threshold levels is described as the protection provided by the device.

Subjective Comparison Methods

A rather simple method for judging the performance of hearing protectors involves comparing untested protectors with one whose performance has been quantified. The known and the untested protectors are worn in the same test signals and a paired comparison judgement is made. When the various protectors are judged to be equal or better than the known protector in an appropriate number of test signals they are treated as being equal in performance to the protector measured by some quantitative means. The result of these assessments allows protectors judged as inferior to the criterion to be avoided and those judged equal to be used. Neither absolute attenuation values nor rankings can be assigned to the protectors on the basis of the paired comparison judgements.

Miniature Microphone or Subjective-Objective Methods

Many laboratories use miniature microphones located under headsets, helmets and ear protectors for measuring the level of the acoustic energy near the entrance to the external auditory canal. Hearing protection is measured by positioning a microphone usually in the concha and measuring the test signal level at the microphone with and without the hearing protector in place over the ear. Another version of this method employs two microphones, one inside and one outside the protector, and takes simultaneous measurements of the noise. The difference between these two measures describes the performance of the hearing protector. Insert devices cannot be evaluated with this type of measurement. Results obtained with this method do not necessarily agree with those obtained using standard procedures. The contribution of tissue and bone conduction hearing with this general method remains to be fully described. Nevertheless, it has many positive features including extremely brief testing periods when various real time analysers are used as part of the system. Miniature microphone methods for evaluating hearing protectors are expected to be even more common in the future.

Masked-Threshold Method

The masked-threshold method employs an earphone for presentation of the test signal. Hearing threshold levels are plotted for the test signals in the presence of an ambient noise. The muff type or helmet protector is donned over the earphones and a second set of hearing threshold levels are measured in the same ambient noise condition. The difference between the two masked hearing threshold level measurements is the sound protection of that device in the ambient noise employed. This method is not used with inserts or earmuffs. It does measure attenuation in the particular noise field of interest.

Hearing Loss For Speech
The hearing loss for speech measurements are essentially the same as the second temporary threshold shift method described earlier. Volunteers wearing hearing protectors are exposed to noise conditions and then tested for speech reception following the exposure. This measurement, as with several others described above, is useful for evaluating specific protectors in designated noise fields. Hearing loss for speech is sometimes reported as the threshold shift in decibels for the conventional discrete frequencies in the speech frequency range.

Cadaver Measurements
A few investigations of hearing protector performance have been accomplished using freshly prepared and instrumented cadaver ears. These studies primarily investigated principles of hearing protection rather than attenuation performance only. The studies were very interesting and very well done, providing insight into critical questions of the functioning of protectors. However, this method is clearly not appropriate for standardization and widespread application.

Measurement Method Criteria
Several Methods used for evaluating hearing protection features of personal equipment have been described. Few have been found suitable for standardization, usually because of their inability to satisfy adequately the following general criteria.

1. Relatively simple
2. Universal application

3. Results generalized to total population
4. Not time consuming
5. Not too costly

HEARING PROTECTION PERFORMANCE DESCRIPTOR

The various methods of measuring hearing protector attenuation are intended to provide a numerical descriptor that can be used to indicate protector performance in noise. The numerical description of the protector is subtracted from a corresponding numerical description of the noise. The difference or noise reduction values relate to effective attenuation and are used to estimate allowable exposure of the wearer in terms of some hearing damage risk criteria. This concept of obtaining noise reduction values for use in estimating hearing risk is not the result of a comprehensive research effort. Instead, it appeared in much the same manner that an American English slang word may eventually appear in the dictionary as acceptable, simply through widespread and continued use. The concept is logical and certainly no better approach has been presented, however, it is a subject that deserves more scientific and technical scrutiny than it has received to date.

Among the first estimations of noise reduction of protectors, and still recognized as the most accurate, is the octave band method based on the actual noise environment. The method is straightforward and simply involves subtraction of the attenuation values of the protector from the corresponding octave band levels of the noise in which it will be worn. The result is an octave band description of the noise at the ear of the wearer. Octave band descriptions were appropriate for early noise exposure standards which were also formulated using octave bands. However, with the swing to simplification, the single number A-weighted sound level replaced spectrum and band level descriptions in the hearing conservation and noise control areas, except for noise control engineering. Damage risk criteria, speech communication criteria, work space criteria, and the like, were defined in terms of A-weighted sound level. Development of the single number noise reduction description for hearing protectors soon followed. Today it is commonly used in slightly varying forms throughout the world.

The single number reduction value of a hearing protector, frequently called dBA reduction, may be calculated in several ways but all deal with essentially the same parameters. The attenuation values for a protector are obtained from a measurement method, hopefully standardized. These values are subtracted from the octave band values of the noise. When the actual noise spectrum is unknown, a "representative" spectrum is employed with pink noise being commonly used today. At some point in the procedure the calculation is corrected for A-weighting and this can occur at one of several points. The resulting values subtracted from the noise and corrected for A-weighting are added logarithmically to provide a single number noise reduction value.

A critical requirement in the calculation procedure is that the spectrum of the noise be incorporated. The two general treatments of spectra are to include the C-weighted values and the A-weighted values of the noise in the calculation procedure or to construct a table which contains the different dBA reduction values as a function of the C-weighted minus A-weighted values of the noise. The measured dBA reduction value for a single protector may vary more than 20 dB simply as a function of the spectrum of the noise in which it will be used. The spectrum of the noise must be an integral part of the hearing protector noise reduction calculation.

Except for rare situations where measurement is accomplished for an individual worker with his protector in the noise environment that he works, dBA reduction values should be generalized to most of the using population. In view of the numerous sources of variance in the evaluation and calculation procedures, results must be treated statistically. Measures of central tendency and variance are commonly used for this task. It is accepted practice to subtract either one or two standard deviations from the mean values, presumably to estimate the protection received by about 84% or 98% of the population. It is recognized that this is not a totally acceptable method, but instead is an interim solution to be used until more and better information is known about effective attenuation.

One comment is in order concerning the size of the standard deviation. Standardized measurement procedures are formulated to keep the variance associated with subjects, psychophysical procedure and the like, constant as much as is practical. It is intended that the measurement procedure discriminate between those protectors with small variances and those with large variances. It is assumed that prediction of performance with the smaller variances will be more accurate and reliable. It is inappropriate for an evaluator to key on the size of the standard deviation as an indicator of the quality of a facility or an evaluation. It is not the objective of the standard measurement to strive for small standard deviations but instead it is to measure the actual variances associated with that protector in use. When measurements are conducted in full compliance with standard procedures differences in standard deviation are expected among protectors. Standard deviations are employed in calculating dBA reduction values; the importance of accurately measuring and obtaining valid measures of variances for predictive purposes is obvious.

AREAS IN WHICH STANDARDS ARE NEEDED

Current ISO and various national hearing protector standards are not appropriate for evaluating all types of personal sound excluding devices.

Table 3: Some Areas in which Standards are Needed

* Physical Measurement Method for Insert Devices
* Non-Linear Hearing Protector Evaluation
* Active Hearing Protectors
* Correlation Between Physical and Real Ear Methods
* Detection of Warning and Communication Signals
* Laboratory vs. Field Performance
* Total or Comprehensive Protector Evaluation

It is clear that additional guidelines are needed by manufacturers, government agencies, industry, universities and users to accommodate these exceptions (Table 3). However, in almost all of the cases to be cited below, more research is required to provide technology that will allow these needed standards to be developed. Even with full resources some of them may require many years for completion, if at all, because the technological problems are so difficult. Generally, few resources have been dedicated to hearing protection research in recent years and little appears planned for the future. This absence of financial support for research activities offers very little encouragement that the needed standards will be realized in the near future. The following are among the more important guidelines which would be used today, if available; they are not prioritized or rank ordered.

Physical Method for Insert Protectors

There is no known physical measurement method for evaluating insert hearing protectors that is a likely candidate for standardization. Several independent systems have been fabricated that contain a measurement microphone housed in a sound excluding fixture containing a small hole for positioning an insert device. These systems measure test signals with and without an insert in the opening, the difference in intensity level being described as attenuation. Such methods measure insertion loss of the material but omit the numerous factors present when an earplug is in a human external ear canal. The values measured with these systems are usually very high and exceed those measured by non-physical methods. There is very little correlation between these measurements and those obtained by standard REAT methods. Although a few pilot efforts have been accomplished, there is no systematic effort underway to develop a physical method for inserts that is known to the author.

Performance Against Impulsive Sounds

The performance of hearing protectors against impulsive sounds has been measured and estimated by several investigators. Measured attenuation has usually been accomplished using the temporary threshold shift and miniature microphone methods described above. Miniature microphone measurements have been made both on human subjects as well as "dummy" head systems.

Estimations of protector effectiveness are generally based on extrapolations of data collected using current standard methods. The TTS methods can be used to identify the effectiveness of a particular protector against a particular impulsive noise, however, such tests must be repeated for each significant variation in the impulsive noise exposure. Also, estimations of attenuation based on measurements with non-impulsive sounds are not entirely satisfactory. The number of impulsive sounds in both the occupational and nonoccupational environment is quite large. In order for hearing conservation programs to effectively combat these signals, reliable measures of the protection provided to individuals is essential. The need for a standard procedure for evaluating the effectiveness of protectors against impulsive sounds has been expressed with increasing urgency by all sectors of the community dealing with hearing conservation and noise control.

Non-Linear Ear Protector Evaluation
Non-linear hearing protectors include two general classes of devices, one that usually contains a hole or orifice to aid face-to-face communication and perception of other signals in low level noise and one designed to provide different amounts of protection in different levels of sound. Present standard measurement methods are not appropriate for evaluating either type of protector. It is likely that the real ear attenuation at threshold measurements may underestimate the protection received in noise fields which is an advantage for users but a disadvantage for manufacturers. The requirement exists for uniform means of accurately describing the performance of both classes of these protectors. It is possible that a separate method will be required to evaluate each type.

Active Hearing Protectors
Active hearing protectors contain electronic systems that affect the sound under the device in some manner. For example, a muff type protector might be designed to amplify low level sounds in relative quiet

and to "cancel" sound under the earcup at high levels. Theoretically, the noise level at the ear could never reach high levels because it would be cancelled under the cup. In practice, the principle of cancellation is not 100% functional with noise signals. Nevertheless, this type of electronically augmented hearing protector must also be evaluated by uniform test procedures which have yet to be established.

Correlation Between Physical and Real Ear Methods

Physical measurements of hearing protector performance are essential for research, development, product improvement and quality control because they are quick and relatively inexpensive. The importance is obvious when the many changes and required measurements associated with these activities are considered. Results obtained with current standard subjective methods do not correlate well across test frequencies with results obtained with standard physical measurements. This lack of comparability between data leaves an unknown for the designer and manufacturer. Performance changes reflected in physical measurements due to product modification may not always indicate the same change in subjective results. Additional work is required to improve the correlation between the two types of measurement so one may be used to predict the other. However, it has been reported on various occasions that enough is not yet known about the physics of the human head to allow the desired correlation to be built into a physical measurement method.

Detection of Warning and Communication Signals

Hearing protection users are frequently in noise environments in which face-to-face voice communication and the perception of other auditory cues are essential. The noise reduction value of a protector provides no information regarding the perception of meaningful auditory cues when the device is worn. The need exists for some means of assessing and describing this property for hearing protectors. A uniform procedure that would identify this property and allow it to be compared among hearing protectors would be rather complex. Factors including the spectrum of the noise, the frequency and intensity of the auditory cues, the attenuation curve of the protector and even the hearing ability of the user are expected to influence such a procedure. In spite of the complexity of the problem, knowledge of the ability to perceive desired acoustic information with hearing protectors in noise would be very useful in many situations.

Laboratory Vs Field Performance

The performance of hearing protectors measured under laboratory conditions may differ from that measured in the field. The amount of difference in performance between the two situations varies with factors such as class of hearing protector, type of hearing protector within the class, condition of protector, extent of proper size, degree of accurate fit, discomfort and more indirectly with education about noise and hearing protectors, monitoring and follow-up of the organization and the motivation of the individual users.

This situation has been recognized for decades, but until recent times attention was directed to other principles of hearing protection. Laboratory evaluations are conducted under ideal conditions that differ from those in the field. Hearing protectors with the fewest opportunities for variance in size and fit, such as custom fit helmets and earmuffs, tend to show the best agreement. Those with more chance for variability tend to show less agreement. Only a small number of different devices have been measured under both conditions. Certain earplugs have shown different degrees of agreement, always with poorer performance in the field. However, it seems clear that these differences are not caused by a change in the performance of the protector in the field. They are a result of the kind of hearing conservation and protection program in effect at the time. There is questionable merit in identifying a hearing protector as poor just because it is part of a program that could benefit from improvements. Some protectors have less problem with factors like size and fit, and these will tend to show better agreement among the evaluation and use data. It is highly improbable that a set of guidelines could be established to treat this problem adequately; however, it is real and standardization groups have been asked to consider it.

Total Protector Evaluation

Interest has been expressed for a uniform procedure for evaluating the total hearing protector. Total protector is intended to represent all characteristics relevant to effective aural protection, which likely includes the items described in the several preceding paragraphs. A first step would involve the definition of "total" protector and of a comprehensive program that includes wearability, durability, performance, selection, care and use. Our understanding of hearing protection principles and technology is not sufficient at the present time to evaluate adequately the concept of the total protector

CONCLUSIONS

Substantial new knowledge is required to respond to identified needs for hearing protection standards. This knowledge must come from research and development activities. However, there are few investigators engaged in the work necessary to develop the needed technology. Lack of resources is most often cited as the reason that the investigative work is not initiated. Little change is expected in the amount of funds committed to hearing protection research. Consequently, the prospect for significant advances or breakthroughs in this technical area or of developing needed standards in the near term is not encouraging.

The role of standardization is vital to the total hearing protection community. Present standards represent the best procedures, by consensus, for accomplishing the specified tasks. Standardization groups continue to monitor, review and update established standards in accordance with the state-of-the-art. Experience and data acquired over the years demonstrate that the standardization process works effectively for hearing protection.

6. THE CANADIAN STANDARDS ASSOCIATION CLASSIFICATION OF HEARING PROTECTORS: HISTORY AND PRACTICAL PROBLEMS

Edgar A. G. Shaw

INTRODUCTION

Since industrial noise levels vary from place to place and hearing protectors differ in their performance characteristics, reliable ways of matching the protector to the noise are clearly needed. Quantitative methods of accomplishing this objective have, in fact, existed for two decades but, as we are painfully aware, all have fallen short of perfection. To appreciate the Canadian efforts in this field we need to be aware of parallel and complementary actions elsewhere (See Appendix I).

A HISTORICAL REVIEW

In 1957 the American Standards Association approved and issued "Z24.22-1957 Method for the Measurement of the Real-Ear Attenuation of Ear Protectors at Threshold" prepared under the sponsorship of the Acoustical Society of America[1]. Eight years later the Canadian Standards Association approved a standard of a very different kind "Z94.2-1965 Hearing Protectors"[2]. This standard defined "the performance requirements for devices for personal hearing protection" and, incidentally, included as an appendix "an outline of the needs for hearing protectors and various damage risk and protection criteria".

The writers of this concise Canadian document recognized that hearing protectors should be sufficiently robust to withstand the rough usage and varied environmental conditions encountered in Canadian industry. They also knew that the document would have little meaning if it failed to deal with the question of acoustical performance. In view of the qualitative difference between earmuffs and earplugs with respect to the shape of the attenuation curve[3,4], the members of the CSA Committee defined separate standards of performance for these two forms of hearing protector taking advantage of documentary material which may have come from a U.S. Military Specification issued in 1964[5]. The result was a table of sound attenuation requirements embodying the concept of "minimum group attenuation". For example, all earmuffs were required to provide mean values of attenuation at 0.5, 1, 2, 3 and 4 kHz totalling not less than 180 decibels whereas earplugs were to provide 135 decibels total. In effect the Committee members defined, or thought they had defined, a minimum standard of acoustical performance for earmuffs and a parallel minimum standard for earplugs.

Four years later, the American National Standards Institute set up a new Standards Committee for Hearing Protection (Z137), sponsored by the National Safety Council, to wrestle with the problems not covered by its other Committee, problems which had become more urgent with the passage of the U.S. Construction Safety Act of 1969 which extended the Walsh-Healey noise regulations to Federal construction contracts. This Committee quickly assimilated the Canadian experience and in 1971 circulated a working draft including a table of sound attenuation requirements. There were, however, important differences. In particular, Z137.1 made no mention of the form of the hearing protector but simply defined three Classes of acoustical performance A, B and C[6]. Nevertheless, the attenuation figures for Classes A and B, though not always identical with the corresponding figures in the Canadian document, were sufficiently similar to suggest that Classes A and B were at least related to the Canadian Muff and the Canadian Plug. It is probable that these Classes were inspired by a U.S. Military Specification issued in 1971[5] updating the 1964 document referred to earlier.

In the meantime, a new ANSI Working Group S3-52, sponsored by the Acoustical Society of America, had undertaken a critical review of Z24.22-1957 with a view to improving the accuracy and reliability of sound attenuation measurements. They quickly came to the conclusion that third-octave bands of noise and a quasi-diffuse sound field should be used and set in train the actions which eventually led to the approval of a new measurement standard, ANSI S3.19-1974[7]. That same year a British

Standard requiring third-octave band of noise and a quasi-diffuse field (BS15108:1974) also appeared, to be followed only one year later by an ISO document (ISO/DP4865:1975) with similar concepts[4].

By the time the first draft of the performance standard, Z137.1, went out for ballot there were indications that the new method of measurement might produce somewhat smaller attenuation figures than the old. For this and other reasons, Table 1, with its three Classes of protector defined in terms of attenuation, disappeared and was replaced by a Rating Factor K. In essence, the K-factor was defined as the reduction in A-weighted sound level calculated from the mean values of attenuation assuming that the protector was exposed to "pink" noise (equal energy per octave)[8]. Despite this and other changes consensus could not be obtained and in 1974 work on the standard was discontinued.

As it happened, the Canadian Standard was at that time under revision. When it emerged as CSA Standard Z94.2-1974[9] it was apparent that material similar to that deleted from the Z137.1 document had been incorporated in the new Canadian Standard. In particular, a table of sound attenuation requirements for Classes A, B and C (See Appendix 2) had replaced the sound attenuation requirements for Earmuffs and Earplugs approved in 1957. A footnote to the table made it clear that the classification of hearing protectors was based solely on the mean values of attenuation obtained in measurements made in accordance with American Standard Z24.22-1957. This footnote also discussed the variability of the attenuation and the factors which determine the magnitude of the standard deviation.

By 1979, most laboratories engaged in real-ear attenuation measurements in North America and elsewhere were working to ANSI S3.19-1974 and its counterparts. When the Canadian Committee met again in 1979 it recognized that change was imperative if the only North American Standard on hearing protector performance was to remain alive. Clause 6.2-Sound Attenuation was therefore amended to make measurements according to ANSI Z24.22 and ANSI S3.19 equally acceptable[10]. This simple pragmatic action has given the Canadian Standard a new lease of life and offered us the breathing space we need if we are to find better ways of handling hearing protector performance.

LABORATORY MEASUREMENTS AND FIELD PERFORMANCE

The factors which make it so difficult to control and determine the amount of acoustical protection received by the individual worker include the following:

1. Differences in measurement method (e.g. the use of pure tones as opposed to bands of noise);
2. Inherent errors in real-ear measurements (e.g. statistical errors);
3. Local differences in measurement technique (e.g. differences in the populations from which the subjects are drawn and differences in threshold tracking methods);
4. Production variations and inadvertent design changes (e.g. changes in material);
5. Physical differences between individuals using the protectors (e.g. tissue structure, amount of hair, etc.)
6. Incorrect use (e.g. incompatibility with other safety equipment, unsuitable eyeglasses, poor fit);
7. Deterioration with use and age (e.g. loss of cushion resilience, frame distortion, etc.).

It is worth noting that CSA Z24.22-1974 specifically mentions several of these factors. For example, Appendix A devotes several clauses to the field assembly of hearing protectors giving consideration to "soft suspension" hearing protectors, the use of spectacles, hearing protector components mounted on safety headgear, etc. In general the user is warned that the attenuation values provided for a given protector do not apply if a change affecting the attenuation is made in any part of the system. However, to place this Appendix and the Canadian Standard as a whole in perspective, we must take note of the lack of a certification procedure for hearing protectors in Canada. As a consequence there are no CSA-approved hearing protectors. In effect it is left to the supplier to provide the user with evidence that his protector satisfies the Standard. This situation is unlikely to change in the foreseeable future.

DISCUSSION

As we survey the history of hearing protector standards in the light of the practical problems which remain, it is natural to ask what has been accomplished with measurement and performance standards and what can reasonably be expected in the future. First, I suggest that the various Committees have not been mistaken in the view, implicit in the idea of standardization, that each type of hearing protector has a characteristic level of acoustical performance which is available to the user under controlled conditions of use. Second, I suggest that, despite the problems which remain, measurement standards such as ANSI S3.19-1974 have served to quantify this characteristic level of performance reasonably well. Third, I suggest that performance standards such as CSA Z24.22-1974 have focussed attention on several important aspects of performance thereby fostering the development of a hearing protector manufacturing industry which is able to respond to the rising demand for high quality products.

There is, however, one aspect of acoustical performance which we may have neglected. I am thinking of the vulnerability to acoustical degradation. Common sense would suggest that hearing protectors which are much superior to others under laboratory conditions would retain that lead in performance under poor conditions of use. Unfortunately, in this instance as we have seen,[3] common sense leads us astray for the hearing protectors which have the highest characteristic performance are often the most vulnerable to degradation". Since this vulnerability is unlikely to be properly reflected in the magnitude of the standard deviation found in laboratory measurement, no simple prescription such as the "mean minus " and "mean minus 2 " rules can be expected to yield reliable estimates of day-to-day performance. Perhaps, in the last analysis, this is why the concept of acoustical performance as a standard attribute seems for the moment to have lost some of its lustre and perhaps, if progress is to be made, we need to search for new concepts in hearing protector design and new approaches to performance measurement.

REFERENCES

1. American Standards Association Inc., Z24.22-57 American Standard Method for the Measurement of the Real-Ear Attenuation of Ear Protectors at Threshold (Sponsor: Acoustical Society of America) New York City, 1957.

2. Canadian Standards Association, Z94.2-1965 Hearing Protectors. Ottawa, April 1965.

3. Shaw, E.A.G., Hearing Protector design concepts and performance limitations. This Conference, 1980.

4. Shaw, E.A.G., Hearing Protector attenuation: A perspective view. Applied Acoustics 12, 139-157, 1979.

5. Nixon, C.W., Private Communication, 1980.

6. American National Standards Institute, Z137.1 Proposed first draft, American National Standard for Occupational and Educational Personal Hearing Protective Devices (Sponsor: National Safety Council). New York City, October 1971.

7. ANSI, S3.19-1974 Acoustical Society of America Standard Method for the Measurement of Real-Ear Protection of Hearing Protectors and Physical Attenuation of Earmuffs. New York City, 1975.

8. ANSI, Z137.1 Draft 3 American National Standard for Personal Hearing Protective Devices for Use in Noise Environments (Sponsor: National Safety Council). New York City, November 1973.

9. Canadian Standards Association, Z94.2-1974 Hearing Protectors. Rexdale, Ontario, 1974.

10. Canadian Standards Association, Amendment to Z94.2-1974 Hearing Protectors. Rexdale, Ontario, 1979.

Appendix I

Chronology of Actions in the U.S.A. and Canada Pertaining to Hearing Protector Attenuation Measurement and Hearing Protector Performance

Date	Organization	Action	Notes
1957	Am.Stds. Assoc. Sponsor: Acoustic. Soc. Amer.	Am.Std.Z24.22-1957-Method for the Measurement of the Real-Ear Attenuation of	Method requires free sound field with frontal incidence and pure tones.

		Ear Protectors at Threshold. - Approved.	
April 1905	Can. Stds.Assoc.	CSA Std.Z94.2-1965 -Hearing Protectors. - Approved	Covers performance requirements. Table I shows separate sound attenuation requirements for muffs and plugs.
Oct. 1967	CSA	Revisions to CSA Std.Z94.2-1965 - Approved	Sound attenuation defined by referencing Am.Std. Z24.22-1957. Mechanical specifications clarified and revised.
Oct. 1969	Am.Nat.Stds.Inst. Sponsor: Nat.Safety Council	Z137 Standards Committee for Hearing Protection - Inaugural meeting	
Nov. 1969	ANSI/ Acoust.Soc.Amer.	ANSI Working Group S3-52 - Inaugural meeting	Task: critical review of Am.Std. Z24.22-1957
Oct. 1971	ANSI/NSC	Z137.1-Proposed Am. Std. for Occupational and Educational Personal Hearing Protective Devices-Working Draft. - Circulated	Strongly influenced by CSA Z94.2-1965. Table I shows sound attenuation requirements for Classes A,B and C. Class A similar to CSA-plugs but <u>less</u> stringent at 125/250 Hz and 6000/8000 Hz.
May-June 1973	ANSI/NSC	Z137.1-Proposed Standard-2nd draft. - Letter ballot	Table of Classes now replace by "Rating Factor K" based on pink noise and A- weighted level at eardrum. - Not approved.

Date	Organization	Standard	Notes
Nov.-1973-Jan. 1974	ANSI/NSC	Z137.1-Proposed Standard-3rd draft. - Letter ballot	Changes in language. - Not approved, work discontinued.
Aug. 1974	ANSI Sponsor: Acoust.Soc.Amer.	ANSI S3.19-1974 ASA STD 1-1975 Method for the Measurement of Real-Ear Protection of Hearing Protectors and Physical Attenuation of Earmuffs. - Approved.	Real-ear method now requires quasi-random incidence sound field and 1/3-oct bands of noise. Supplemental physical method defines dummy head.
1974	CSA	CSA Std.Z94.2-1974 Hearing Protectors. - Approved.	Table of Classes revised: Classes A and B now identical with Z137.1 Proposal (see Working Draft); New Class C less stringent than Z137.1 Proposal except at 6000/8000 Hz. Many detailed revisions.
Aug. 1979	CSA	Amendments and errata to CSA Std. Z94.2-1974. - Approved	Sound attenuation clause revised to allow measurements in accordance with ANSI Z24.22-1957 or ANSI S3.19-1974
1980	ANSI Proposed sponsor: Am.Soc.Mech.Eng.	Z137.1-Proposed Standard - Further work recommended.	

Appendix II

Sound attenuation requirements for Classes A, B and C hearing protectors as specified in CSA Standard Z94.2-1974

Frequency Hz	Class A		Class B		Class C	
	Minimum Single Frequency Attenuation dB	Minimum Sum of Frequency Group Attenuations	Minimum Single Frequency Attenuation dB	Minimum Sum of Frequency Group Attenuations	Minimum Single Frequency Attenuation dB	Minimum Sum of Frequency Group Attenuations
125	None	25	None	18	None	6
250	None		None		None	
500	29		None		None	
1000	35		25		15	
2000	35	185	25	135	15	85
3000	35		25		15	
4000	35		25		15	
6000	None	60	None	50	None	40
8000	None		None		None	

A footnote to the table states that the sound attenuation requirements given in the standard "are based solely on mean sound attenuations ... It is equally important, however, to know the variability of the attenuation afforded by a protection device. This can be determined for a given percentage of the population from the standard deviation (σ) of the attenuation in dB, quoted at each test frequency ... The standard deviation includes the effects of variability in the threshold measurements of each person used to determine the attenuation of the device, day-to-day variation in the attenuation obtained for the same person (even though the device is fitted and worn correctly), and differences among attenuation values obtained with different wearers ....

Large values of standard deviation for one protector, compared to another, reflect primarily the relative difficulty in obtaining consistent attenuations with the device for ears and/or heads of various shapes and sizes."

7 A Test Facility for the Objective Measurement of Circumaural Hearing Protector Attenuation

J. A. Chillery

INTRODUCTION

Concurrent with the publication in 1974 of the British Standard method of measuring the attenuation of hearing protectors (BS 5108 1974) a need was expressed for a cheap, reliable and simple method of measuring this quantity which would be suitable for the quality control of quantity production and for monitoring the performance of protectors in use. It was acknowledged by the body responsible for BS 5108 1974 that the standard method was unsuitable for production testing and that further research was necessary before a suitable method, probably objective, would be recommended for this purpose.

As a consequence of these discussions Her Majesties Factory Inspectorate stated a requirement for research into the development of an 'artificial head' to be used for production testing with the additional goal that this device might, in the long term, be developed for the type testing of protectors. It was stated that the method of production testing should generate data of a quality that would facilitate decisions concerning the maintenance or removal of official approval of a particular protector. These requirements initiated a research programme, funded by the Health and Safety Executive, carried out at the Institute of Sound and Vibration Research of the University of Southampton. This paper constitutes a summary of that programme.

The first step in the programme was a review of the current literature[1]. Two separate, but naturally linked, areas of research were examined. Firstly, the design of hearing protectors and those physical parameters of the human head which influence their performance were studied and secondly, the principles underlying past and present methods of hearing protector attenuation measurement were investigated, particular attention being paid to objective methods.

The first part of the review identified important factors in the attenuation and measurement processes and this facilitated discussion of past and present methods of attenuation measurement. The conclusions of the review provided a firm basis for the development of an 'artificial head' although some of the points raised required further investigation. Accordingly a prototype 'head' was built and a short programme of research aimed at clarifying these points was undertaken.

This work was performed concurrently with an assessment of the practical problems associated with objective attenuation measurement which was accomplished using three contemporary 'artificial heads' on loan to ISVR.

The information derived from all the sources described above was then used to design a final version of an objective test facility. The characteristics of this device were studied and some preliminary attenuation measurements were performed. Comparison of these latter data with standard attenuation values encouraged the possibility of prediction of attenuation.

Literature Review

Introduction

Initial considerations, illustrated in Figure 1, led to the identification of nine parameters of the circumaural protector and of the head of a wearer with a possible influence on the attenuation measurement process. Several of these were found to be unimportant given that an insertion loss* technique was used. Other parameters were found to be important although the exact nature of their influence on an objective measurement process could not be ascertained.

---

* Insertion loss is defined as the difference between two values of sound pressure level measured at the same point in the vicinity of the ear, one measured with and the other without the protector in position.

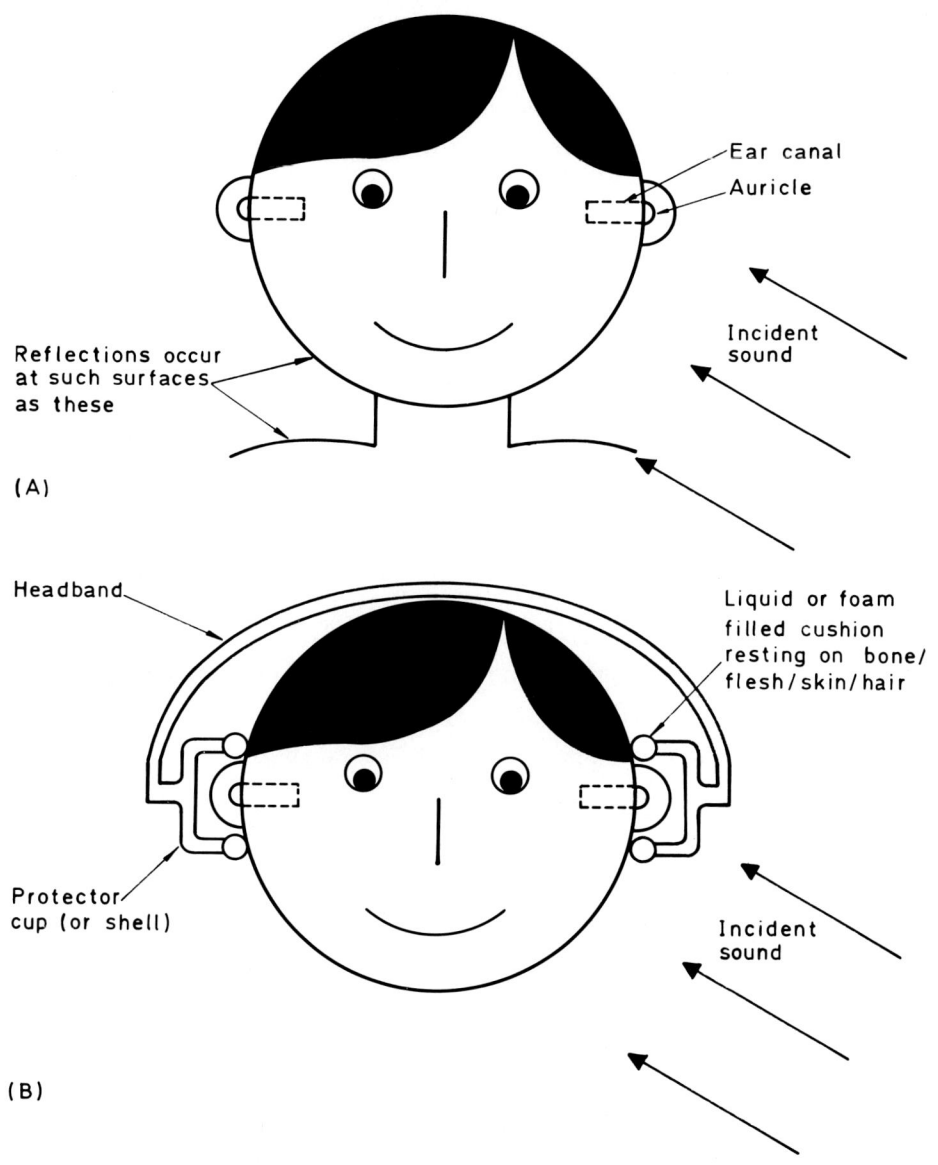

Figure 1. Illustrating important factors in the measurement of the attenuation of circumaural protectors.

A summary of the findings concerning these nine parameters is given below.

Head Geometry

The effect of the head, excluding the circumaural region, and upper torso were considered.[2-5] It was concluded that, given the use of an insertion loss type measurement, only a rough approximation to a head in size, shape and mounting arrangements would be satisfactory.

The contours of the circumaural region of the head were also considered and found to have a significant effect on the fit of the protector to the head[6-8]. Fit, or lack of it, is a component of the phenomenon known as 'leakage'. In order that the attenuation data generated by an objective method resemble that generated by REAT methods it would be necessary to model leakage in the objective method. One way to achieve this would be to model the circumaural contours.

Head Surface Covering

1. Hair: Although opinions differ in the literature as to the precise nature of the effect, it is generally agreed that hair has a deleterious effect on hearing protector attenuation[6-14] in that it diminishes the integrity of the seal between the protector and the side of the head. It can thus be regarded as a component of leakage and the same argument that has just been presented for cicumaural contours may be applied. That is, in order to simulate REAT data it may be necessary to represent the effect of hair.

To do this in a reproducible manner presents obvious difficulties. However, it may be possible to model leakage as a whole rather than model the individual components.

2. Skin and Flesh Layer: This parameter completes the description of the circumaural region. The action of the skin and flesh may be considered as being twofold. Firstly, it modifies the effect of the previous two parameters. For example, the leakage due to the notch formed at the junction of the jaw and neck may be modified as skin and

flesh in that region is squeezed into the gap between the protector and the head.

Secondly, the compliance of the skin and flesh layer interacts with that of the protector cushion and by so doing limits the attenuation. The literature was found to disagree about the exact nature of this interaction[7, 8, 14] but it is generally believed to be an essentially low frequency phenomenon.

It is clear from the above that a skin and flesh simulation would be a desirable component of an objective method intended to generate attenuation data similar to that produced by REAT methods. Attempts to model skin and flesh have been made in the design of previous objective methods. The most recent of these is the design contained in ASA STD-1-1975[15] which uses a layer of cast vinyl. However, there is little experimental evidence to support this particular choice of material.

3. Pinna and Concha: An objective measurement method in which the signal arriving at the observation point in the unoccluded state is important must have an ear replica capable of correctly modifying that signal. However, it was anticipated that the objective method developed here would utilise an insertion loss technique. This involved a subtraction process; that is, an occluded measurement would be subtracted from an unoccluded measurement.

In this case, as the literature indicated that the behaviour of the pinna and concha is not appreciably modified by occlusion,[17, 18] the effect of the pinna and concha would largely be eliminated during the subtraction[19].

4. Ear Canal: The argument used in the previous sections may be applied equally well to the case of the ear canal. However, the literature is not clear about the behaviour of an ear canal in the occluded state and thus it was felt that experimental evidence is required in this case.

The most convenient method of acquiring such evidence was considered to be to investigate the effect of changing the ear canal geometry on the attenuation values generated by an otherwise unchanged system.

Bone Conduction

The main conclusion from the literature dealing with bone or body conduction[12, 20, 25] is that the mechanisms of bone conduction are not yet fully understood, and that, even if they were, accurately modelling all the many conduction paths[26], would still present many problems.

A possible solution to this problem would be to utilise a correction curve. That is, to use one of the bone conduction threshold curves from the literature to set limits on the attenuation data produced by the objective method.

There are two drawbacks to this solution. Firstly, it is difficult to decide which of the bone or body conduction thresholds in the literature is the correct one in this case. Secondly, there exists the possibility that the circumaural protector influences the body conduction threshold[12] and that, therefore, different designs of protector produce different thresholds.

Given the above arguments it seemed wise to ignore, temporarily at least, bone conduction when designing an objective method.

Protector Characteristics

Four components of the circumaural protector were found to be significant with respect to attenuation mechanisms. These, the cushion, the cup mass, volume and the headband were examined from two points of view. Firstly, their relevance to the design of an artificial head was assessed and, secondly, their importance to the intended applications of the objective measurement method was considered.

From the first point of view these four parameters were found to be of importance only in that they form part of the mass-spring system of which the remaining component is the skin/flesh layer. This therefore stressed the importance of a skin/flesh simulation to an objective measurement intended to produce similar attenuation values to REAT methods.

From the second point of view, cup mass and volume were discarded as being irrelevant. Interest in these cases lay in the usage of the objective method; either for production testing or for monitoring the degradation of protectors with use. Although cup mass and volume are important components of the attenuation mechanism the literature showed that attenuation values are relatively insensitive to minor changes in these parameters[7, 27]. Therefore cup mass and volume were ignored when considering the calibration of the objective method.

This was clearly not the case with the protector cushion, which is the key component of a circumaural protector[8]. The literature was found to offer little information about the variation of attenuation with cushion characteristics. However, it can easily be appreciated that degradation of the cushion, for example a leak in a liquid-filled cushion, can cause appreciable loss of attenuation. In addition, it is not possible to estimate the variation in attenuation produced by fluctuations in production quality except to note that an objective method may be more sensitive to such variation especially in the absence of a skin/flesh simulation.

The last of these four parameters is protector headband force. The literature was found to contain information about the effect of this parameter on attenuation which indicated that, for a well designed and manufactured protector in a good state of repair, the attenuation would be insensitive to changes in headband force above a critical value[12]. However, in the absence of one or more of these conditions it may be that variations in attenuation with force could be quite large.

An objective measurement method would clearly show such variations but the cause would be unknown. In order to isolate the cause, an auxiliary method of measuring headband force would be required. As part of the experiments which followed the literature review a method to investigate the effect of headband force on attenuation was developed[28, 29].

Existing Artificial Heads

The information gained from the examination of the literature described above was used in an evaluation of 'artificial heads' described in the literature[9, 10, 30-35]. Eleven of these artificial heads all suffer from similar drawbacks and would not be suitable for standardisation. These drawbacks are:

1. In many cases the choice of design features of the head is not explained.
2. The effect of changes in the design is not explored.
3. Several of the designs are highly individual and would be difficult to standardise.

However, one head[35] was observed to fulfil many of the requirements of an objective test method. It was clearly designed as a standard and operation would appear to be quick and simple, probably producing repeatable data. Drawbacks with this device would seem to be minimal, however the design is somewhat inflexible in that the device is only suitable for the specified purpose and could not easily be adapted.

Conclusions

The literature review allowed the relative importance of nine parameters of a protector and the head of a wearer to be established and the information gained was of assistance in a critical analysis of previous objective measurement methods. This provided a sound basis for the development of an objective measurement method suitable for standardisation as a production testing tool and for further development. Areas requiring further investigation were isolated. These were as follows:

1. Investigation of the effect on attenuation values of different ear canal geometries.
2. Investigation of the possibility of simulating leakage in a simple, reproducible manner.

3. Investigation of the effect on attenuation values of different types of skin/flesh simulation.
4. Investigation of the effect on attenuation values of using different forms of ambient acoustic field.
5. Investigation of the effect on attenuation values of variations in headband force.

These five proposed areas of research were based on the assumptions that an insertion loss technique would be used and that the method might ultimately generate attenuation values similar to those produced by current REAT methods.

EXPERIMENTAL WORK
Introduction
Of the five areas pointed out by the literature review as requiring further investigation, three (I), (2) and (3) were considered to have an immediate bearing on the design of an objective test facility. The remaining two, (4) and (5), which could influence the method of using the test facility, could be investigated later. Accordingly a series of experiments were performed in order to assess the relative importance of skin/flesh and leakage simulations and of the ear canal geometry. The majority of this work was performed using a prototype objective test facility of flexible design. However, certain experiments were also performed using three contemporary 'artificial heads'. These were: -the Knowles Electronic Manikin for Acoustic Research, KEMAR[5]; a 'head' known as KOJAK[10]; a 'head' built to the design contained in ASA STD-I 1975[36].

The text below contains a brief account of this work. Unless otherwise specified experiments were performed in a near-diffuse field using the equipment shown in Figure 2[29].

Ear Canal Geometry
The effect on attenuation spectra of ear canal geometry was investigated in two ways. Firstly, by measuring the attenuation spectrum of a protector several times using different ear-like couplers and secondly, by

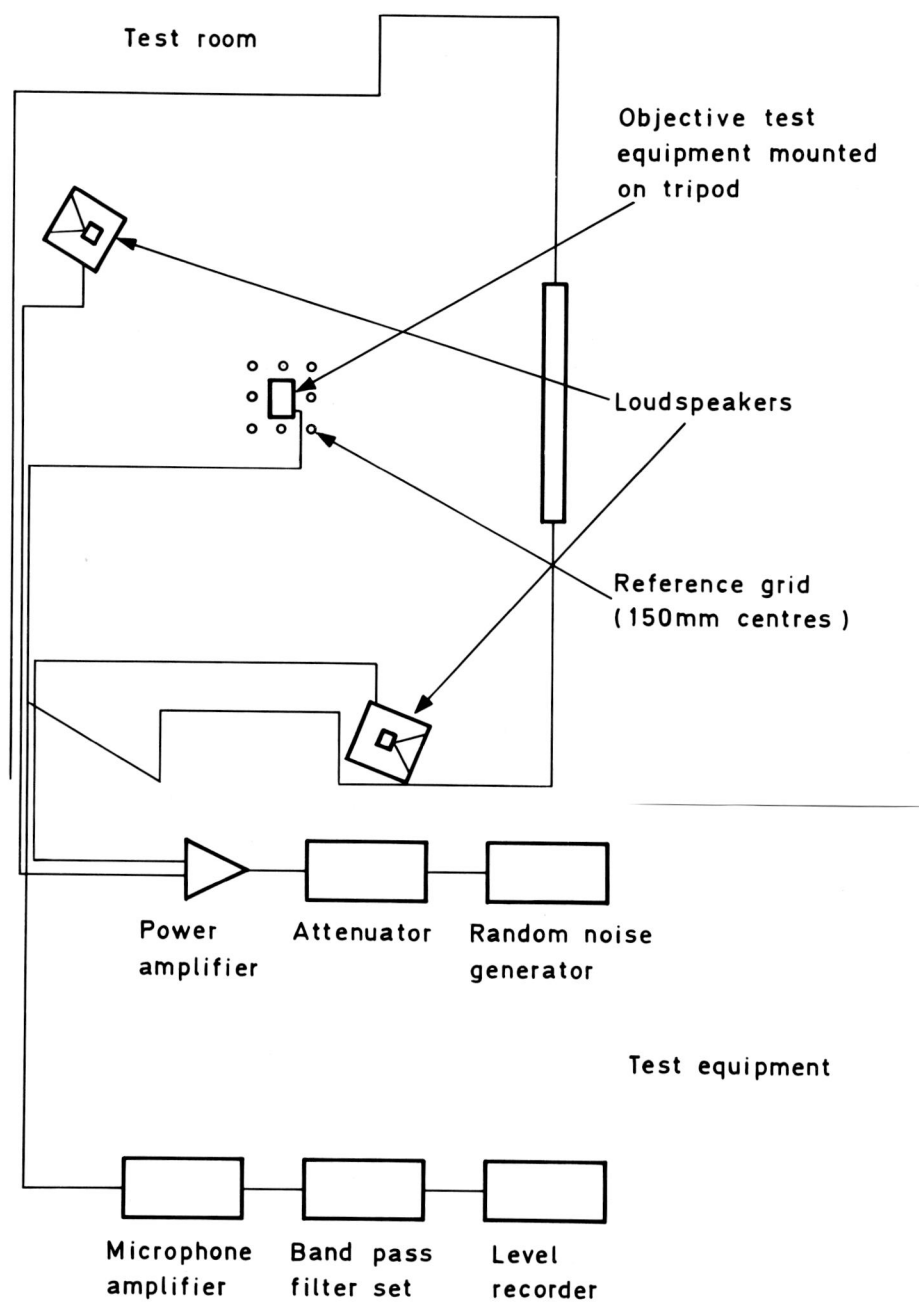

Figure 2. Showing experimental layout used for objective tests.

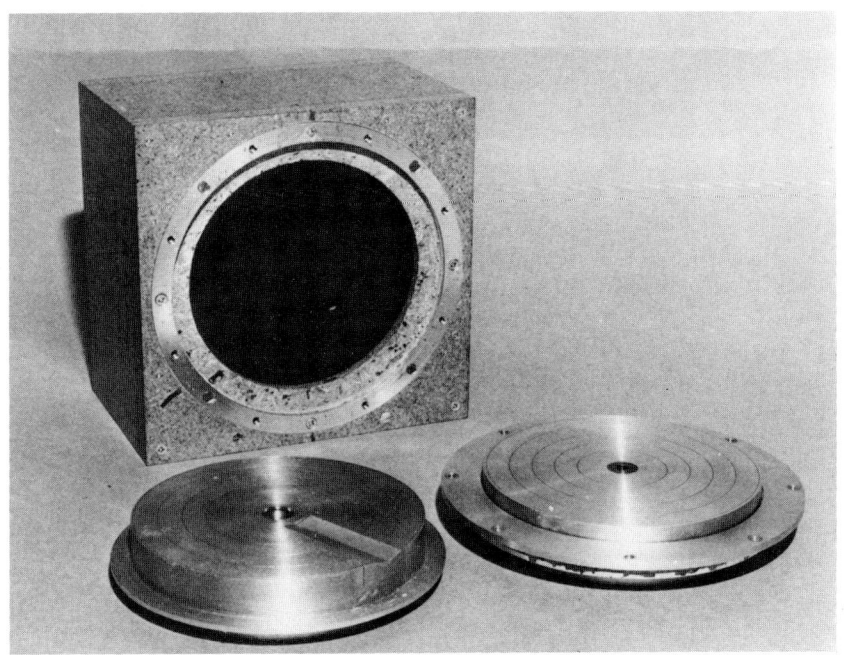
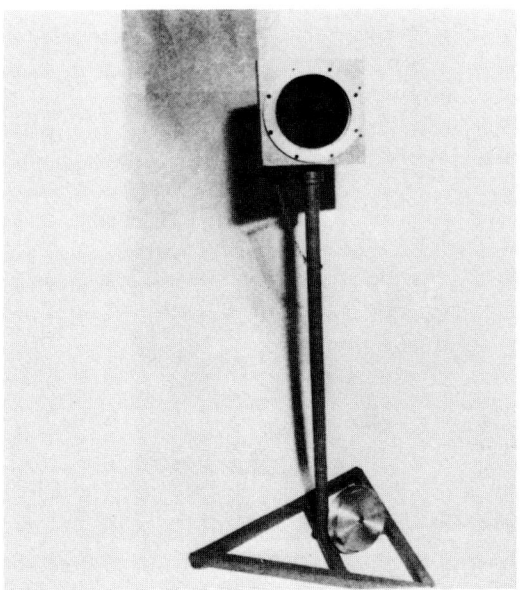

Figure 3. The ISVR prototype objective test facility.

studying the behaviour of the acoustic resonances inside an ear canal replica.

In the first case experiments were performed using the prototype 'head' shown in Figure 3, into which could be fitted a variety of ear-like couplers[29]. These were: three simple cylindrical couplers of internal dimensions (length x diameter) ½" x ¼", 1" x ½" and 1" x ¼"; the Bruel and Kjaer Type 4153 Artificial Ear; the Zwislocki Artificial Ear. Typical results from this work are shown in Figures 4 and 5.

Figure 4 shows spectra derived from the three simple couplers using the same earmuff. Although the high frequency differences are statistically significant in many cases it is clear that, in terms of practical attenuation measurement, the differences are unimportant.

The evidence from Figure 5 is less clear although similar trends may be observed. The marked differences at frequencies about 2000 Hz between the Zwislocki Artificial Ear and the remaining devices are ascribed to difficulties found when fitting protectors to the raised centre portion of this ear. The low frequency differences amongst the curves are judged to be a result of inadequate values of low frequency acoustic isolation of the Zwislocki and the Type 4153 which probably arose because the circumaural surface plates of both 'ears' are only one-quarter-inch thick.

Studies of ear canal resonance behaviour were made using KEMAR[5] and probe tube techniques developed at ISVR[37]. This well documented artificial head was developed primarily for studies of hearing aid response and contains a complete artificial ear including detachable pinna, ear canal and ear-like coupler. Using different lengths of small probe tube attached to a miniature microphone the sound pressure levels at different points along the ear canal axis were measured with and without occlusion of the ear by an earmuff of normal volume for single frequencies in the range 250-7000 Hz. This work was performed in a semi-anechoic room with low values of background noise.

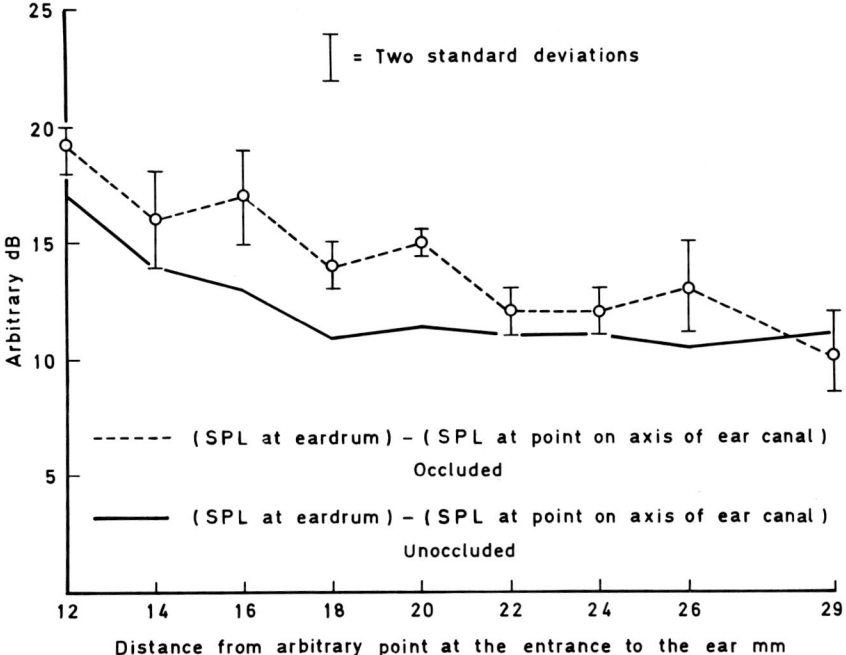

Figure 6.   Showing difference in the resonance pattern in Kemar's ear canal between the occluded and unoccluded states.

that, within broad limits, practical insertion loss measurements are independent of the method of acoustically coupling the measurement microphone of a test facility to the volume contained by the earmuff under test.

Circumaural Contours and Skin/Flesh Simulation

A brief study was made of the effect on attenuation of an idealised circumaural contour and a skin/flesh simulation both separately and in conjunction. Experiments were performed using the prototype test facility shown in Figure 3. An idealisation of the leakage produced by the circumaural contours was produced by cutting a radial groove of triangular cross-section (approximately 2.5 cm wide and 1.0 cm deep) into the surface of the test facility. Skin/flesh simulation was provided by a novel material known as LCS or SORBOTHANE manufactured by PERMALI

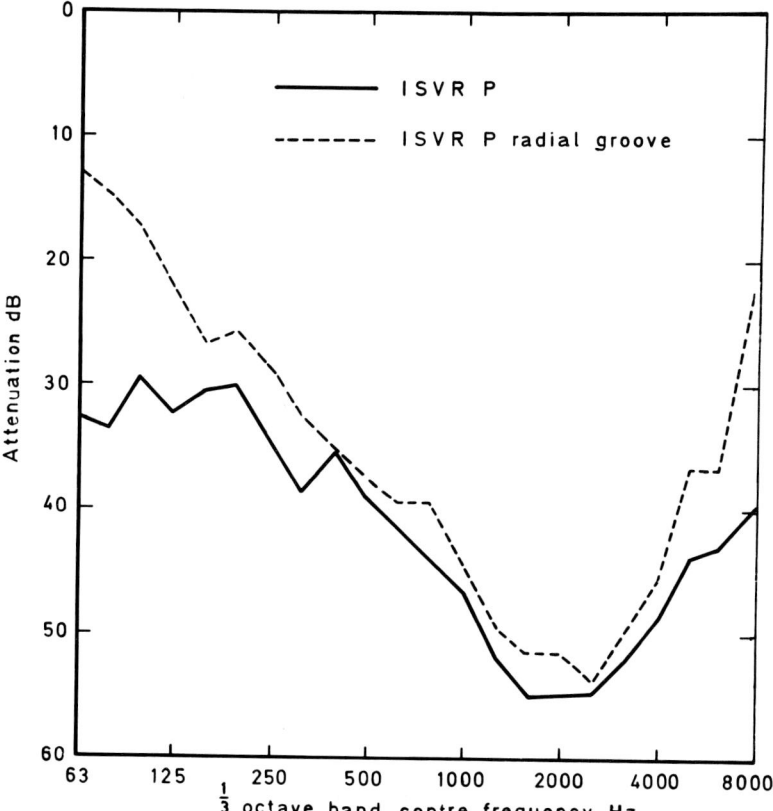

Figure 7. Variation in attenuation produced by radial groove.

GLOUCESTER LTD.

This material has unusual characteristics which give it a particularly flesh-like quality. Although a soft solid it exhibits some of the properties of a liquid of very high viscosity. It has a density of 1.34 gm/cm^3 coupled with a low flexural rigidity and a Shore value of 40 (00 scale), at room temperature. Two thicknesses, 2 mm and 6 mm, were used in these experiments, each sample being in the form of a disc which completely covered the active surface of the test facility, except for the 'ear canal' entrance.

Two earmuffs were used. One with liquid-filled cushions (A) and the other with foam-filled cushions (B).

In the first set of measurements the effect on attenuation values of the two thicknesses of LCS was measured using the normal non-grooved surface of the test facility. Neither earmuff responded in an important way to the changes in the surface beneath the cushion. Secondly, the effect of the circumaural contour was measured using the grooved surface. Here, although some minor high frequency decrease in attenuation was observed, earmuff B was again largely unaffected. Earmuff A however suffered considerable low and high frequency decreased in attenuation as shown in Figure 7.

Finally, the effect of the skin/flesh simulant LCS on attenuation values, measured using the grooved surface, was studied. As expected earmuff B was only slightly affected but the attenuation spectrum of earmuff A was raised at the low and high frequencies as shown in Figure 8.

The 2 mm layer restored the attenuation almost to the values observed for the non-grooved surface. The restoration was continued at the low and high frequencies when the 6 mm sample was used. However, a decrease, as yet unexplained, was observed over the mid-frequency range.

From these experiments it was concluded that there was no advantage to be gained at this time by the inclusion of either or both of circumaural contours and skin/flesh simulations in an objective test facility intended for production tests. Even if a suitable skin/flesh simulant could be manufactured reliably to a standard and did not 'age' significantly it is still clear that a much better understanding of the interaction betweean different surfaces and cushions is necessary.

Similarly the marked difference between the reaction of the two protectors to the different surfaces requires explanation before such contours could meaningfully be incorporated in the design of an objective test facility.

Existing Artificial Heads
In order to assess the practical problems of objective attenuation,

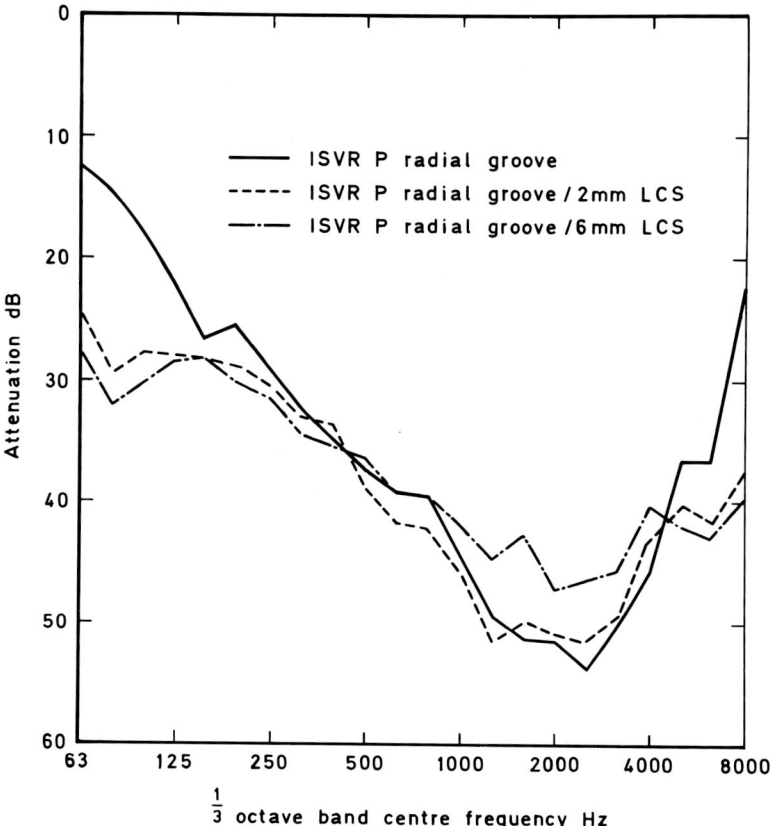

Figure 8. Effect of skin simulant on attenuation.

measurement experiments were performed using three existing 'heads' loaned to ISVR.

One of these, the ASA STD-1 1975 'head'[15], was designed specifically for the quality control of quantity production and another, KOJAK[10], was designed for the measurement of protector attenuation measurement. All three were found to be unsuitable, to a greater or lesser extent, for the quality control of protector attenuation.

Criticism of the ASA STD-1 1975 'head' arose from the failure of two separately constructed versions of this 'head'[29, 38] to achieve the acoustic isolation spectrum (60 dB at all test frequencies) specified by the standard. It was considered unlikely that the quality of engineering at the two establishments where these 'heads' were constructed would be exceeded by other potential users and that the fault lies with the design of the ASA STD-1 1975[36] 'head' which possibly does not pay sufficient attention to the elimination of leaks.

A second, minor criticism of the ASA STD-1 1975[36] 'head' was that the effects produced by the angle of the 'head' and the cast vinyl surface layer do not justify their inclusion in the design. The attenuation spectra produced by this 'head' differed little from equivalent spectra produced by the prototype ISVR 'head'. The effect of these two features has also been investigated by other workers[38] who also concluded that there was little to be gained, for a quality control tool, by the addition of these features.

Also, the artificial skin was found here to lengthen the experimental period as it was more difficult to clean and replacement required great care.

The main criticism of the head 'KOJAK'[10] was that although the data produced offers useful information about the behaviour of earmuffs on artificial heads the device is of too complex a construction to be suitable for quality control work. In addition, the acoustic isolation of the device is unknown and also, a lengthy test period is necessary.

It was found that severe practical problems arose when using a simulation such as KEMAR[5]. The presence of a flexible pinna which must remain undistorted and the lack of suitable reference points made it extremely difficult to reproduce the placement of the protector on the head. It was found that changes of position indiscernible to the eye produced changes in attenuation of up to 15 dB.

From the experiments with these three 'heads' it became clear that only the most simple device would be suitable for the measurement of earmuff attenuation for the purposes of quality control. None of the devices examined were found to offer any advantages over a simple mounting for a microphone with provision for attachment of the headband.

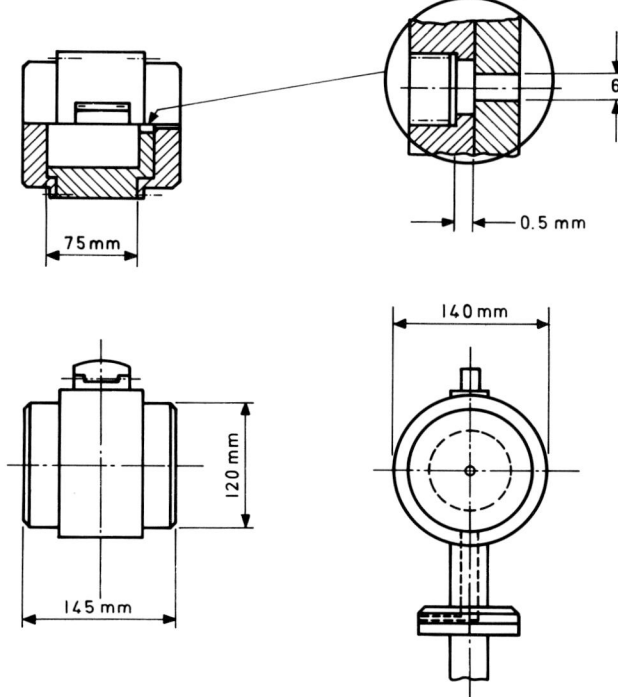

Scale 1:4

Figure 9. Details of the ISVR objective test facility.

THE OBJECTIVE TEST FACILITY

Introduction

The conclusions from the literature review and the results of the experimental programme were combined in the design of a final version of the objective test facility or 'artificial head'.

A sketch of the 'head' showing details of the design is shown in Figure 9.

Figure 10 shows the 'head' when assembled and also the brass cup, used for acoustic isolation measurements.

The fundamental intention of the design was to produce a simple device for quality control work with very high acoustic isolation whilst at the same time incorporating a capacity for changing the geometry. This flexibility was envisaged as allowing changes in the basic dimensions of

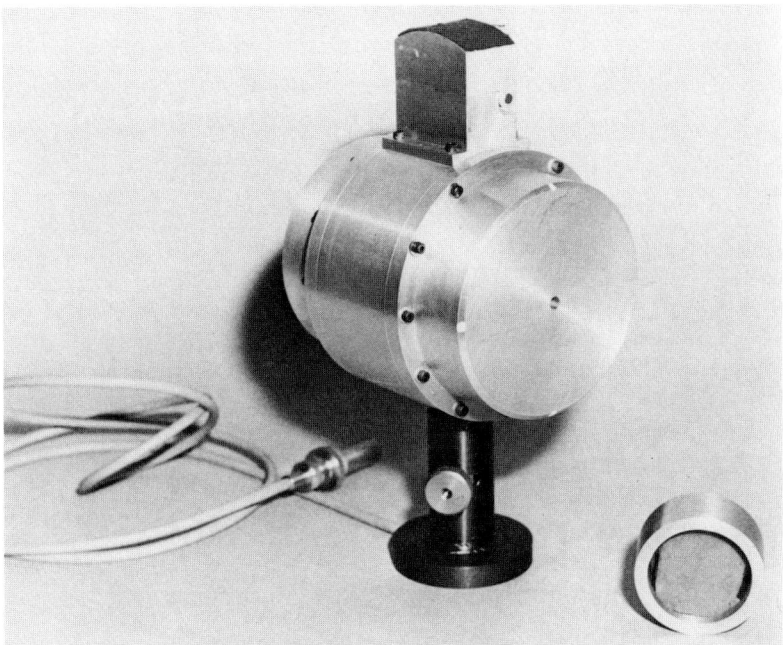

Figure 10.   The ISVR objective test facility.

the 'head' and changes in the nature of the surface in contact with the protector under test which would facilitate both the development of improved protectors and further development of the 'head' itself.

These considerations led to the concept of a central mainframe, containing the microphone and with high acoustic isolation, to which could be attached accessories to interface the device to the protector in the manner desired. That is, the accessories would not be essential to the acoustic seal which would only be disturbed to replace defective components and therefore comparisons amongst attenuation spectra measured using the same protector under different conditions could be performed quickly and easily.

The 'head' mainframe and accessories were constructed from Duralumin to the dimensions shown in Figure 9. These dimensions may be adjusted at will be choosing different accessories. The values chosen approximate those of the median human head[38, 39].

The 'head' is supported by a pillar constructed from mild steel. Earlier success, in terms of acoustic isolation, of the ISVR prototype head had been attributed in part to the housing of the microphone emitter follower inside the body of the device. Here, the volume inside the mainframe was insufficient for this purpose and an alternative method was required. By choosing heavy gauge tubing for the support pillar it was found possible to mount the emitter follower inside the support pillar. The internal diameter of the pillar was such that the emitter follower was a push-fit and it was clamped in position using screwed collar arrangement. The emitter follower cable exit was via a shallow groove machined into the underside of the baseplate brazed onto the support pillar. This baseplate was of such dimensions that it mated with the support platform of the vibration isolated tripod.

When the baseplate and the tripod were securely clamped together the emitter follower cable was compressed between the two in the groove and a good acoustic seal was achieved. Sealing between the mainframe and the support pillar was easily achieved by screwing the pillar, with a taper thread, into the base of the mainframe. In this condition the acoustic isolation was shown to be in excess of 65 dB at all frequencies except 6300 Hz and 8000 Hz where it was 61 dB and 63 dB respectively.

Mainframe

Details of the mainframe are shown in Figure 9. The design shown represents a slight modification of the original concept in that a screw-in plug to seal what is shown as an open end was dispensed with as being unnecessary for these experiments but could be added to the system at a later date.

The mainframe is a right cylinder with three features of interest, the first of these is a hole, let into the centre of the endface, which is machined such that a Bruel and Kjaer Type 4166 microphone cartridge with the protective grid removed can be screwed firmly into it. When the microphone is fully inserted the diaphragm plane lies just below the plane of the outer surface of the endface. This is necessary so that when an accessory is fixed onto the endface the fragile diaphragm of the microphone is not damaged.

Clearly, mounting the microphone in the mainframe meant that it was displaced from the sound field inside the protector to be measured by a distance equal to the thickness of the accessory. This was regarded as an advantage for several reasons:

1. It was essential to the concept of a mainframe to which could be attached accessories without disturbing the acoustic seal.
2. It placed the delicate microphone cartridge at a point where it would not be easily damaged.
3. It obviated any problems with summation of the sound field[35] in that the microphone operates under the same conditions independently of whether the orifice is occluded or not.

Displacing the microphone from the contact surface in this way was justified by the work described earlier where it was shown that there were only slight variations amongst the data gathered from the ISVR prototype 'head' using a variety of couplers. That is, the attenuation spectra generated using an insertion loss method of measurement were largely independent of the microphone placement and the nature of the path between the microphone and the protector sound field.

The second feature of interest is the hole let into the curved surface of the mainframe. This was tapped to accept the support pillar which, containing the Bruel and Kjaer Type 2619 emitter follower, is inserted into the mainframe such that the end of the Type 2619 protrudes slightly above the interior surface of the mainframe. This allows contact to be made between the Type 2619 and the Type 4166 using a Bruel and Kjaer Type UA0023 flexible adaptor. The practical minimum radius of curvature of the flexible adaptor formed a convenient lower limit on the internal dimensions of the mainframe.

The third interesting feature of the mainframe is the provision made for the attachment of a headband contact surface analogous to the top of the human head. The influence of this on the test data was unknown and therefore the headband contact surface was hinged so that it could be swung away after protector adjustment, and measurements could then be made both with and without contact between the headband and the test facility.

Accessories

The two endplates used were identical except that one had a ¼" diameter coaxial hole. Both were machined to be a push-fit onto the mainframe and were firmly attached using allan screws. As may be appreciated the endplates are easy to manufacture and a range of these with different thicknesses (to change head width), angles, contours and surface treatments could easily be produced. The flexibility introduced into the system by these possible accessories is one of the main features of the design. However, initial interest in the device lay in its usefulness as a quality control tool and therefore only simple endplates were manufactured.

ATTENUATION MEASUREMENT USING THE ISVR OBJECTIVE TEST FACILITY

Introduction

The characteristics of the test facility were examined. The effects of different types of test sound field, test field sound pressure levels and degrees of contact between the headband of a protector and the top of the test facility on attenuation spectra were studied. The knowledge thus gained was combined with information derived from earlier experiments with the prototype and other 'artificial heads' to produce the equipment specifications and test procedure described below.

Following this some preliminary measurements of the attenuation of protectors previously tested using the British Standard method[40] were made. The coefficients of the regression line of subjective on objective attenuation were calculated.

Equipment

The instrumentation and test environment were similar to those used in earlier experiments and shown in Figure 2. A 'pink' noise signal was used to power two loudspeakers placed asymmetrically in a normal hard-walled room. The sound field produced was diffuse almost to within the specifications of the British Standard for the subjective measurement of protector attenuation[40]. Signal analysis was performed using standard analogue instruments although the broad band nature of the test sound field clearly argues for the future use of digital analysis techniques which would decrease the experimental period considerably.

Procedure

The experimental procedure finally decided upon was as follows. The protector to be tested was removed from storage and fitted to the test facility with headband contact. This entailed ensuring that the headband was adjusted to the correct width and that the protector cups were symmetrically placed on the headband and on the test facility surfaces. If the headband was of more than one piece this was also adjusted to be symmetrical. The protector fitted tightly to the test facility. The positions of the cups were then marked (with a dab of paint) and the protector carefully removed and returned to storage. Any additional protectors were then adjusted in the same way.

After measurement of the unoccluded spectrum at the test facility when placed in the test field, the test facility surfaces were cleaned and the protector to be tested was then placed on the facility in such a way that the previous adjustments were not disturbed, the headband was firmly in contact with the 'head' top and the protector cups were symmetrically placed on the appropriate surfaces. A light horizontal momentary force was then applied to both cups along the axis of the test facility. The occluded spectrum was then measured and the protector carefully removed and returned to storage. Other protectors to be tested were then treated in the same manner. This process was repeated five times and the unoccluded spectrum measured again.

The mean value, at each test frequency, of the five occluded values was then subtracted from the corresponding mean value of the two unoccluded values provided that the latter had not changed by more than 1 dB. Otherwise the sound generation system was checked for malfunction.

Protector attenuation measurement using the ISVR objective test facility
The attenuation spectra of four protectors were measured using the ISVR test facility and the method described in the previous section. The purpose of this work was firstly to check that the method was viable for protectors in general and secondly to produce comparisons between data derived from this objective technique and that produced by current standard subjective methods. Although the primary purpose of the ISVR test facility was as a quality control tool it has also been developed to be a flexible base from which either a type test or a tool for the investigation of protector characteristics may be developed. Also, before this device can be used for quality control, measurements of many samples of many types of protectors must be performed in order to allow the setting of standards.

Table 1: Linear Regression of subjective on objective attenuation for four protectors

Frequency	r^2 Correlation Coefficient	Slope	Intercept
63	0.82	0.63	4.7
125	0.05	0.13	7.6
250	0.97	0.61	0.61
500	0.23	0.34	12.1
1000	0.66	0.59	5.6
2000	0.35	0.32	15.9
3150	0.51	0.52	11.8
4000	0.80	0.43	14.6
6300	0.72	0.62	5.1
8000	0.94	0.34	16.0

The following measurements represent a first step towards the accomplishment of these objectives. The protectors tested all had foam-filled cushions and plastic headbands. Subjective data were available.

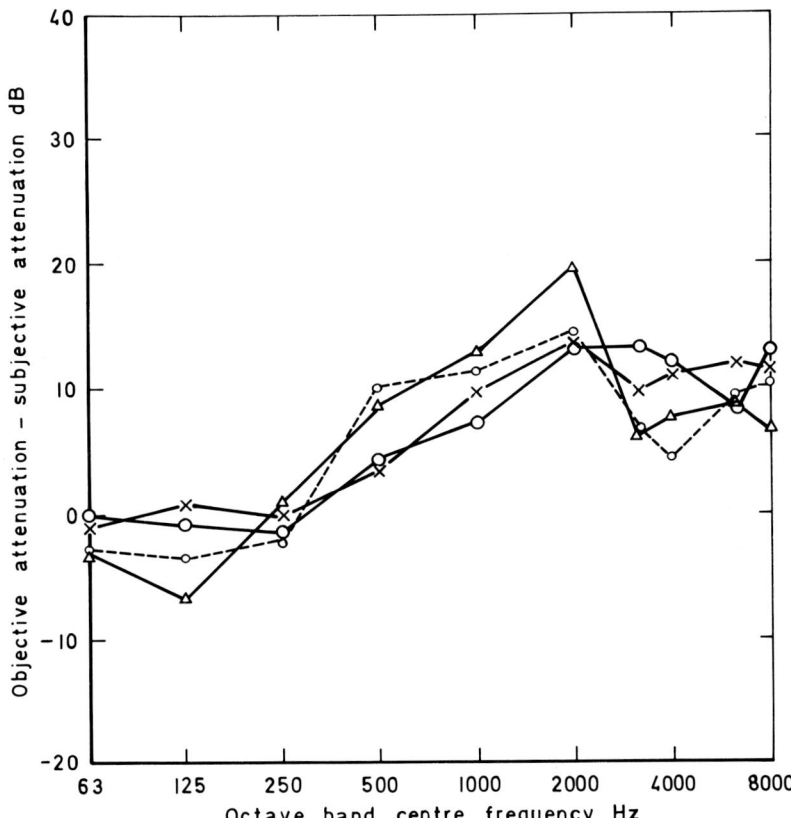

Figure 11. Spectrum of difference between objective and subjective attenuation measurements for earmuffs with foam filled cushions.

Differences between the subjective and objective data at standard[40] subjective test frequencies were calculated and the results are shown in Figure 11. The coefficients of the regression line of subjective attenuation on objective attenuation are shown in Table I.

It may be seen that the curves in Figure 11 all follow a similar pattern. The differences are at a low minimum at frequencies below 250 Hz and then rise steadily to a maximum value at 2000 Hz. A second minimum occurs at around 4000-6300 Hz and a second maximum at 8000 Hz. Similar trends may be observed in the results of other workers[7].

Although not ideal, the values of correlation coefficient are sufficient to encourage the collection of more data. Further work in which the attenuation spectra of many samples of many types of protector would be measured both subjectively and objectively is required. Suitable analysis of these data might allow the following:

1. Prediction of subjective values of attenuation from measured objective values with appropriate confidence intervals.
2. Calculation of objective and subjective inter-protector sample variances which would allow quality control limits to be set.

CONCLUSIONS

Stages in the design of an objective test facility primarily intended for the quality control of quantity production have been described. Important features of the design are high acoustic isolation (greater than 60 dB at all test frequencies between 63 Hz and 8000 Hz) and simplicity of use. Additional features have been incorporated, without affecting the primary design goals, which extend the possible use of the device.

The performance of the device using various test sound fields and procedures was examined. It was found that reliable data were generated using a simply obtained diffuse field and a simple test procedure.

Use of this device for quality control would require criteria to be established. Further work in which attenuation spectra of many samples of many types of protector would be measured both subjectively and objectively in order to provide a basis for such criteria has been suggested. It was also proposed that a different analysis of such data might lead to the production of a method of predicting subjective values from measured objective values.

Shortage of time precluded the performance of all but a pilot study of one sample of four protectors. These data cannot be used as a basis for quality control criteria but do encourage the possibility of prediction of attenuation values.

ACKNOWLEDGEMENTS

The author thanks the Health and Safety Executive for their financial support, through the Medical Research Council (Grant Number A850/149.11), of this project and Professor R.R.A. Coles for his assistance in the production of this paper.

REFERENCES

1. Chillery, J.A., Attenuation properties of circumaural hearing protectors: A review of the factors involved in their objective measurement. Institute of Sound and Vibration Research Memo No. 576, The University of Southampton, 1978

2. Abbagnaro, L.A., Bauer, B.B., Torick, E.L., Measurements of diffraction and interaural delay of a progressive sound wave caused by the human head. J. Acoust. Soc. Amer., 58, 693-700, 1976

3. Kasten, R., Lotterman, S.H., Azimuth effects with ear level hearing aids. Bull. of Prosth. Res., 10-7, 50-61, 1967

4. Shaw, E.A.G., Transformation from the free field to the ear drum in the horizontal plane. J. Acoust. Soc. Amer., 58, 1848-1860, 1974

5. Burkhard, M.D., Sachs, R.M., Anthropometric manikin for acoustic research. J. Acoust. Soc. Amer., 58, 214-222, 1975

6. Webster, J.C., Ear defenders: Measurement methods and comparative results. Noise Control 1, 34-42, 1955

7. Zwislocki, J.J., Factors determining the sound attenuation produced by earphone sockets. J. Acoust. Soc. Amer., 27, 146-155, 1955

8. Shaw, E.A.G., Thiessen, G.J., Improved cushion for ear defenders. J. Acoust. Soc. Amer., 30, 24-36, 1958

9. Joyce, P.G., Determination of the attenuation characteristics of circumaural hearing protectors for impulse noise. Development Branch Notes DN 50 Reference YS/150/050, Quality Assurance Directorate (Weapons), Development Branch, Woolwich, 1973

10. Russell, M.F., May, S.P., Objective tests for earmuffs. J. Sound. Vib., 44, 545-562, 1976

11. Soilleux, P.J., The design of more effective acoustic ear protectors. SRDE (RSRE) Memo No T21/78 BR 724-24, Christchurch, 1973

12. Gorman, A.G., Factors affecting the design of circumaural hearing protectors. Paper presented at a Symposium at the National Physical Laboratory, Teddington, Middlesex, England 1976

13. Whitham, E.M., Martin, A.M., An investigation of an artificial ear

technique for the evaluation of hearing protectors. Tech Memo 513, Institute of Sound and Vibration Research, The University, Southampton, 1976

14. Zwislocki, J.J., Ear protectors, in Handbook of Noise Control by Harris, C.M., McGraw Hill Book Co. New York, 1957

15. AMERICAN STANDARDS ASSOCIATION, Method for the Measurement of Real-Ear Attenuation of Ear Protectors at Threshold. ASA Z24-22, 1957

16. Brinkmann, K., Broksch, K-H, Sound attenuation provided by ear defenders Parts I and II. Uber die Schalldammung von Gehorschutzern, Z Hor-Ak/J. Audiol. Tech., $\underline{9}$, 178-193, 1970 and $\underline{10}$, 10-28, 1971

17. Shaw, E.A.G., Ear canal pressure generated by circumaural and supra-aural earphones. J. Acoust. Soc. Amer., $\underline{39}$, 471-479, 1966

18. Shaw, E.A.G., Thiessen, G.J., Acoustics of circumaural earphones. J. Acoust. Soc. Amer., $\underline{34}$, 1233-1246, 1962

19. Rood, G., Towards a semi-objective method for the measurement of the acoustic attenuation of flying helmets. Paper presented at a Symposium at the National Physical Laboratory, Teddington, Middlesex, 1976

20. Barany, E., A contribution to the physiology of bone-conduction. Acta-Otolaryngol Suppl XXVI, 1938

21. Bekesy, G., Vibration of the head in a sound field and its role in hearing by bone conduction. J. Acoust. Soc. Amer., $\underline{20}$, 749-760, 1948

22. Tonndorf, J., Bone-conduction. Chapter 5, in TOBIAS (1972) pp 195-235; Academic Press, New York and London, 1972

23. Khanna, S.M., Tonndorf, J., Queller, J.E., Mechanical parameters of hearing by bone conduction. J. Acoust. Soc. Amer., $\underline{60}$, 139-148, 1976

24. Zwislocki, J.J., In search of the bone conduction threshold in a free sound field. J. Acoust. Soc. Amer., $\underline{29}$, 795-804, 1957

25. Nixon, C.W., Gierke, H.E., Experiments on the bone conduction theshold in a free sound field. J. Acoust. Soc. Amer., $\underline{31}$, 1121-1125, 1959

26. Tonndorf, J., Bone-conduction. Chapter 5, in TOBIAS (1972) pp 195-235; Academic Press, New York and London, 1972

27. Zwislocki, J.J., An investigation of certain means of sound attenuation at the ear. AD 257039, Armed Services Technical Information Agency, Arlington Hall Station, Arlington, Virginia, USA 1961

28. Cox, J.P., An apparatus for the measurement of hearing protector headband force. BSc Final year project, Dept of Mechanical Engineering, The University, Southampton, 1978

29. Chillery, J.A., Objective measurement of the attenuation of circumaural hearing protectors. Institute of Sound and Vibration Research Memo No 602, The University, Southampton, 1980

30. Forstall, J.R., Manikin measurements of the noise attenuation provided by flight helmets. AD 676 885, Naval Aerospace Medical Institute, Pensecola, Florida, Aug 1968

31. House, M.E., Martin, A.M., Howell, K., Cockpit noise -flight helmet attenuation. A contract progress report 1499 for the Ministry of Defence, Sept 1972. Institute of Sound and Vibration Research, The University of Southampton

32. Unsworth, G.W., Acoustic attenuation of the Mk II flying helmet. BSc final year project, Faculty of Engineering and Applied Science, The University, Southampton, 1972

33. Schiller, E., Rosenfeld, J.B., Development of objective technique for ear protector attenuation measurement. Reports 1, 2 and 3, Project 920-46, US Naval Applied Science Lab, Brooklyn, New York, 1967, 1968, 1969

34. Michael, P.L., Bolka, D.F., An objective method for evaluating ear protectors. Final report, Dept of Health, Education and Welfare Grant 1 RO1 OH 00341-01, Environmental Acoustics Laboratory, 3 Psychology Building, Pennsylvania State University, USA, 1972

35. Gorman, A.G., Objective measurement of hearing protector performance. Proposals presented to ISO/TC 43/SC 1/WG 17 meeting June 1977 by A.G. Gorman, Technical Director, Racal-Amplivox Ltd, Wembley, Middlesex, England

36. ACOUSTICAL SOCIETY OF AMERICA, Method for the Measurement of Real-Ear Protection of Hearing Protectors and Physical Attenuation of Earmuffs. ASA STD-1, 1975

37. Lower, M., Institute of Sound and Vibration Research, The University, Southampton Private communication, 1976

38. Whittle, L.S., Sutton, G.J., Robinson, D.W., The objective measurement of hearing protectors of the circumaural type. National Physical Laboratory Acoustics Report Ac 87, 1978

39. Bolton, C.B., Kenward, M., Simpson, R.E., Turner, G.M., An Anthropometric survey of 2000 Royal Air Force Aircrew 1970/71. RAE Tech Report 73083, Procurement Executive, Ministry of Defence, Farnborough, Hants, 1973

40. BRITISH STANDARDS INSTITUTION, Method of measurement of attenuation of hearing protectors at threshold. BS 5108: 1974

Personal Hearing Protection in Industry, edited by P. W. Alberti, Raven Press, New York ©

8 Acoustical and Mechanical Properties of Earmuff Type Hearing Protectors and Their Testing

K. Brinkmann and M. R. Serra

INTRODUCTION

In the Federal Republic of Germany, as in many other industrial countries, noise-induced hearing loss has, in recent years become the most frequently recognized occupational disease. This has led to increased efforts to improve hearing protectors which, in the absence of appropriate noise control, must still be used in many workplaces as the last resort to prevent hearing impairment. Hearing protectors should not only produce adequate noise reduction but also be sufficiently comfortable so that they can be used for a full work shift.

In order to prevent the use of inadequate products, a German standard[1] has recently been promulgated, which includes requirements for various acoustical and non-acoustical characteristics of hearing protectors, together with corresponding test procedures. Only models which have been approved and classified according to this standard may be offered for industrial application in future. It is the aim of the standard to ensure that an approved hearing protector model has a sound attenuation sufficient for many practical noise situations and an acceptable degree of comfort in wear, both properties being equal for all protectors of the same model within reasonable tolerances and being essentially stable over a long period of use. The requirements are of particular importance for hearing protectors of the earmuff type which, generally, are made of many individual parts and which are subject to numerous strains in practical use.

Details of the requirements and test procedures of the standard are described and discussed, and then the concepts for future testing are presented.

REQUIREMENTS, TEST PROCEDURES AND MEASUREMENT RESULTS
Measurement of Sound Attenuation
Subjective Procedure

One of the most important properties of a hearing protector is its sound attenuation. In many countries it is determined according to the so-called threshold shift method which has been laid down, for instance, in the German standard DIN 45 611[2]. In principle, this procedure consists of two determinations of the threshold of hearing with a number of otologically normal test subjects tested first with open ears and then with ears occluded by the hearing protector. In the Physikalisch-Technische Bundesanstalt (PTB) this procedure has been applied for many years. At the moment the measurements are still carried out in a large, anechoic room with sinusoidal sound signals in the frequency range from 63 Hz to 8000 Hz. It is planned, however, to change to a quasi diffuse sound field and to carry out the measurements with third octave band noise, as stipulated in the present American standard[3] and in a new international standard[4] in order to be closer to actual practice.

At the time of writing, about 160 different models of hearing protectors have been tested in the PTB by the threshold shift method. Figure 1 gives a summary of the results. It contains about 80% of the data available. Each plotted value represents the mean of the individual attenuations obtained by one hearing protector on 10 test subjects. Different symbols characterize different kinds of protectors. Additionally, the limiting curves of sound attenuation caused by bone conduction[5,6] are given. The diagram gives an idea of the characteristic performance of different kinds of protectors and the large variety of the amount of attenuation within each group (for details see ref. 7).

The selection of hearing protectors on the basis of sound attenuation curves is a difficult problem in practical noise situations, because in general the necessary, detailed knowledge of the noise spectrum does not exist. For this reason several different approximation procedures have

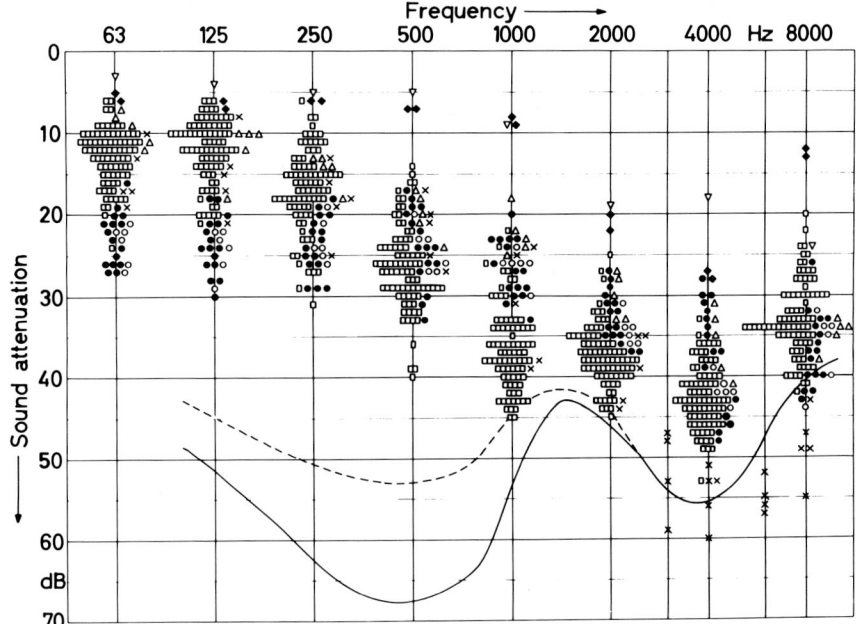

Figure 1. Results of sound attenuation measurements
■ earmuffs   ● prefabricated resilient earplugs
○ malleable earplugs   △ protective downs
▽ dry surgical cotton   × sound protecting helmets
◆ individually molded permanent earpieces

been suggested which require only one figure to characterize the attenuation performance of the hearing protector and which enable selection to be made on the basis of the total sound level of the noise measured by means of the frequency weighting curves C and/or A of a sound level meter[8].

Another unsolved problem is what proportion of the total population of users should really be protected? It is well known that the individual performance of a hearing protector may display considerable variation among users due to physiological and anatomical factors and because of the fitting procedure. If only the mean values are taken into account when calculating the noise reduction afforded by a device, as given in Fig. 1 for example, about 50% of the population in question is insufficiently protected. It is necessary, therefore, to reduce the mean attenuation by some safety margin, which will be a compromise between under-protecting a minority and over-protecting a majority of users in most environments.

The procedure laid down in the German standard[1] follows the idea of Waugh[9]. The so-called "characteristic sound attenuation" is calculated in a way similar to that of "Noise Reduction Rating"[10] apart from the fact that instead of two standard deviations, only one standard deviation and an additional safety factor of 2 dB are subtracted from the mean attenuation figures and no additional allowance is made for possible variations of hearing protector performance in different noise environments. Waugh's thesis that a noise-related safety factor is unnecessary because any uncertainty due to spectral differences disappears in the large spread of individual attenuations was proved with our own data[11]. An example of the characteristic sound attenuation calculation is given in Table 1. It is expected that with this method, about 95% of users will be adequately protected.

A minimum value of the characteristic sound attenuation of 7dB, below which no approved type of hearing protector may fall, has been specified in the standard. This minimum value has been so laid down that protective downs made of glass fibres, which are largely established as hearing protectors and which have proved good in practical use at numerous places of work, just meet the requirements. The characteristic sound attenuations of the great majority of hearing protectors available on the market are well above this limit as can be seen from the histogram in Figure 2. Any additional classification was not felt necessary.

Objective Procedure
The threshold shift method described so far is a time-consuming and metrologically difficult method which is not suitable for routine measurements on greater numbers of hearing protectors, e.g. within the framework of production control. For this purpose and for a simple determination of whether the sound attenuation of a hearing protector has changed after mechanical or thermal strains, an objective measuring

Table 1: Example for the calculation of the characteristic sound attenuation Z of a hearing protector

Octave-band Frequency in Hz	A-Weighted Octave-band Sound Pressure Levels of a Hypothetical Noise (Pink Noise) L_{A_i} in dB	Sound Attenuation of the Hearing Protector		Person-Related Safety Factor S_p in dB	Effective A-weighted Octave-band Sound Pressure Levels of the Hypothetical Noise When the Hearing Protector is Worn $L'_{A_i} = L_{A_i} - (d_i - s_i - S_p)$ in dB
		Mean Values d_i in dB	Standard Deviation s_i in dB		
63	65.3	7.4	3.3	2	63.2
125	75.4	10.0	3.6	2	71.0
250	82.9	14.4	3.6	2	74.1
500	88.3	19.6	4.6	2	75.3
1000	91.5	22.8	4.0	2	74.7
2000	92.7	29.6	6.2	2	71.3
4000	92.5	38.8	7.4	2	63.1
8000	90.4	34.1	5.2	2	63.5

The effective overall A-weighted sound pressure level L'_A when the hearing protector is worn is the logarithmic sum of the 8 octave-band levels of the last column: L'_A = 80.8 dB.

The characteristic sound attenuation (Z) is: $Z = L_C - L'_A$

where L_C = 100 dB is the overall C-weighted sound pressure level of the hypothetical noise from column 2.

Thus Z = 100 dB - 80.8 dB = 19.2 dB follows.

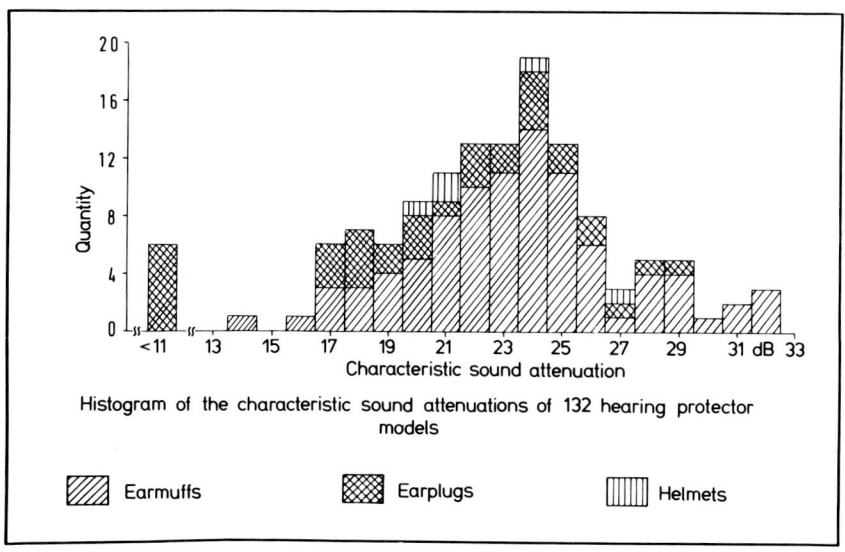

Figure 2. Histogram of the characteristic sound attenuations of 132 hearing protectors

procedure is a prerequisite.

Dummy heads for carrying out such measurements on hearing protectors of the earmuff type have been in use in the PTB for a long period[12]. Even though it is not currently possible to reproduce all relevant physiological and anatomic properties of the human head (e.g. its mechanical impedance, bone conduction) in an "artificial head", i.e. the subjective procedure cannot yet be replaced by an objective one, objective insertion loss measurements represent a very useful complement to the threshold shift method.

A very simple acoustic test fixture which will receive an international standard[13] (Fig. 3), has proved to be suitable for the intended application[14]. Compared with the dummy head specified in the American standard[3], the ISO test fixture provides similar critical dimensions and a slightly higher internal acoustic isolation. No attempt was made to simulate human flesh, resulting in somewhat higher insertion loss data at low frequencies, especially with earmuffs with liquid-filled cushions, but

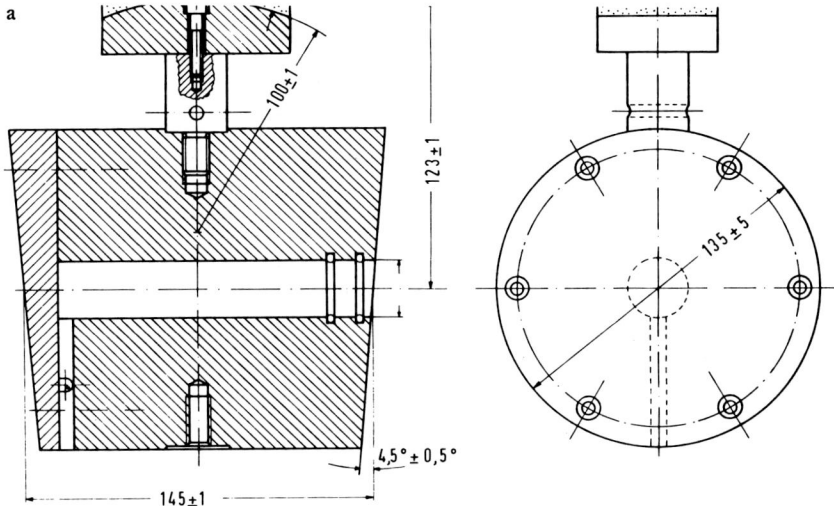

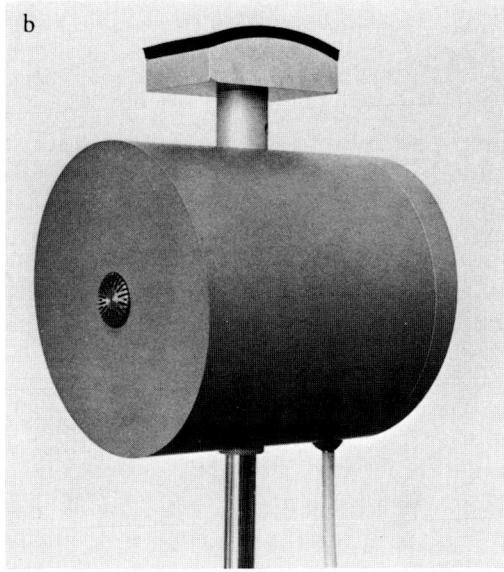

Figure 3 a,b. ISO acoustic test fixture for objective insertion loss measurements on hearing protectors of the earmuff type.

presumably being of advantage with respect to the long-term stability and the comparability of test results. Insertion loss measurements are to be carried out with third octave band noise either in a free sound field or in a diffuse one. The test of 10 earcups of every type is provided for in the

German standard[1], some of the earcups being new and others having been previously subjected to certain mechanical and climatic strains (see Sections on Mechanical Tests and Climatic Tests). The total spread of the insertion loss data must not exceed a given maximum value, which is 12 dB in the total frequency range from 63 Hz to 8000 Hz in the case of hearing protectors with foam-filled cushions and 16 dB or 12 dB for hearing protectors with liquid-filled cushions in the range from 63 Hz to 200 Hz and 250 Hz to 8000 Hz, respectively. Measurement results are shown in Figures 4 and 5 indicating that good quality protectors just meet the requirements.

Mechanical Tests
Construction

The construction test of a hearing protector of the earmuff type serves to ascertain whether the headband can be adequately adjusted and the fastening of the earmuff sufficiently moved in order to guarantee a good fit of the hearing protector, even in the case of very different sizes and shapes of head. For this purpose simple dummy heads of varying heights and widths are used[1]. A test of these set-ups with numerous hearing protectors of different types resulted in some problems particularly for hearing protectors mounted on a safety helmet and in the case of hearing protectors with moveable headbands, if the band is worn at the neck. In these cases improvements of the hearing protector construction seem necessary.

Application Force, Application Pressure

A sufficient application force is the prerequisite for a close fit of a hearing protector and thus for its sound attenuation. On the other hand, comfort in wear can be noticeably reduced with an increase of the application force. For this reason the measurement and control of the application force is of particular importance. In the PTB, the measurement is carried out by means of an appropriately converted commercial scale (Figure 6). An alternative is already specified in the American standard[3]. As the measuring value depends considerably on the setting of the headband, its careful adjustment to given dimensions, i.e. 145 mm

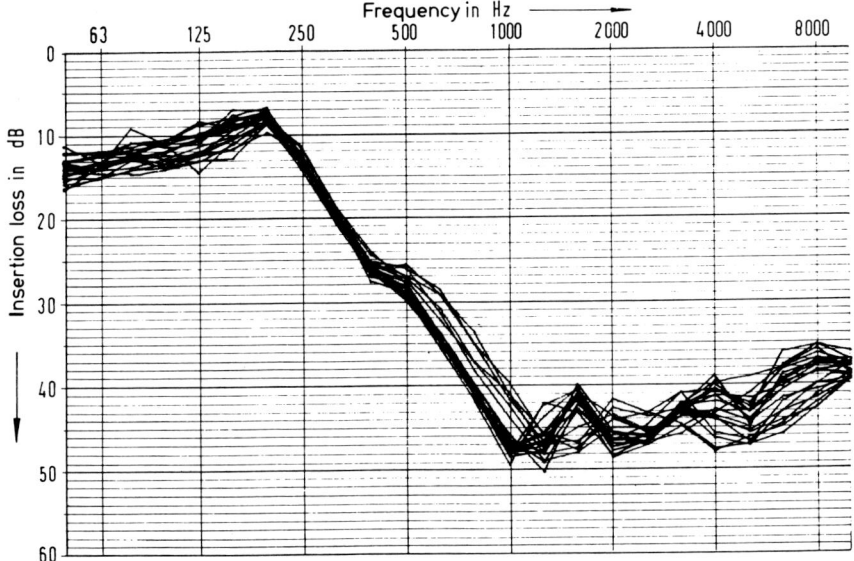

Figure 4. Insertion loss of 20 identical new earmuffs (foam cushion) at the test fixture of fig. 3, measured with third octave band noise in a diffuse sound field.

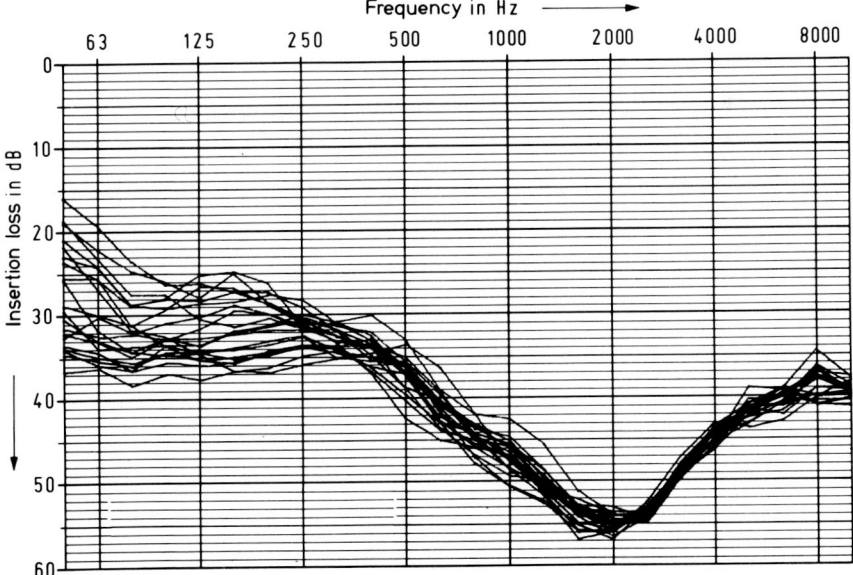

Figure 5. Insertion loss of 20 identical new earmuffs (liquid cushion) at the test fixture of fig. 3, measured with third octave band noise in a diffuse sound field.

between the two cups and 129 mm between the centre of the headband and the centre line between the cups is of great significance. Attention has also to be paid to the primary treatment of the headband in order to obtain reproducible results[12]. An uncertainty of measurement of about 2% to 4% resulted from recent comparative measurements.

In the German standard it has been laid down that the application forces of different hearing protectors of identical type must not deviate from the mean value by more than $\pm$ 1 N. This requirement is not met by all hearing protectors available at the moment[12]. Even the permissible maximum value of the application force of 12 N (mean value) is exceeded by numerous types, as shown in a survey of measurements carried out on different types (Figure 7).

However, it is not the application force alone that is decisive for comfort in wear[15]. This applies in particular to hearing protectors with broad cushion seals where the force is distributed over a larger area. For this reason the standard stipulates that in the case of hearing protectors with application forces above 12 N, the application pressure has to be additionally determined. If this pressure does not exceed the value of 4000 N/m^2, the hearing protector can be approved.

In order to determine the application pressure, the sealing cushions are dyed with stamp ink and, the headband of the hearing protector being expanded to a given span, prints are made of both sealing cushions. In Figure 8 an example is shown for two different hearing protectors. The areas are measured by means of a planimeter.

Strain of the Headband Due to Bending
In use, the headband of a hearing protector is exposed to a considerable strain due to expansion. Assuming that a hearing protector is put on and taken off about ten times during a working-day, more than 2000 headband expansions to values above the usual head width are obtained in one year. It must be a requirement that this strain does not cause any significant alteration of the application force, for this might have an effect on the

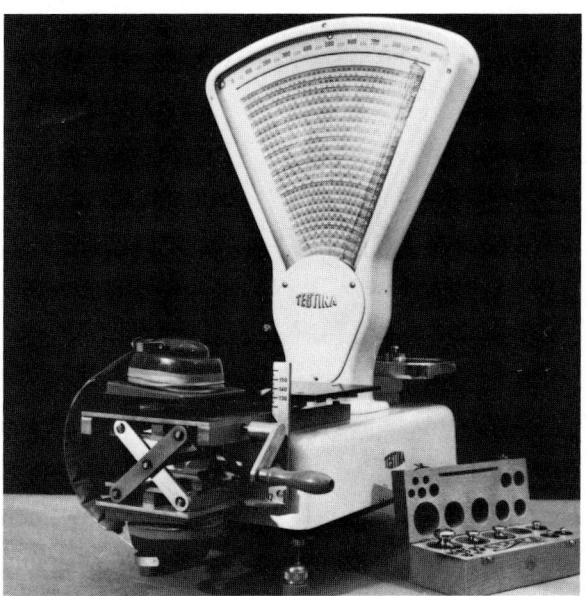

Figure 6. Device for measuring the application force of hearing protectors.

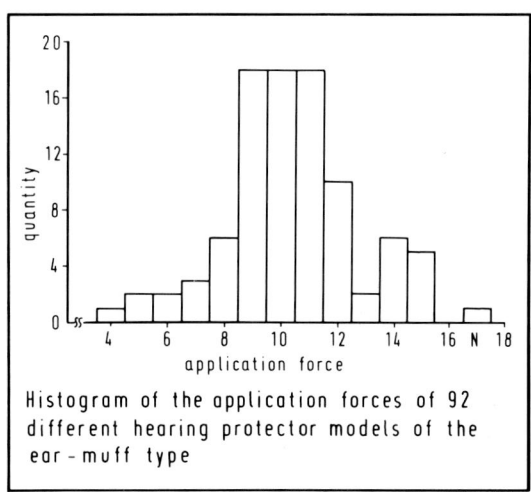

Histogram of the application forces of 92 different hearing protector models of the ear-muff type

Figure 7. Histogram of the application forces of 92 different hearing protector models of the earmuff type (the force figures refer to a separation span of the earcups of 140 mm, formerly used. Increasing this span to 145 mm would result in about 10% increase of force on the average).

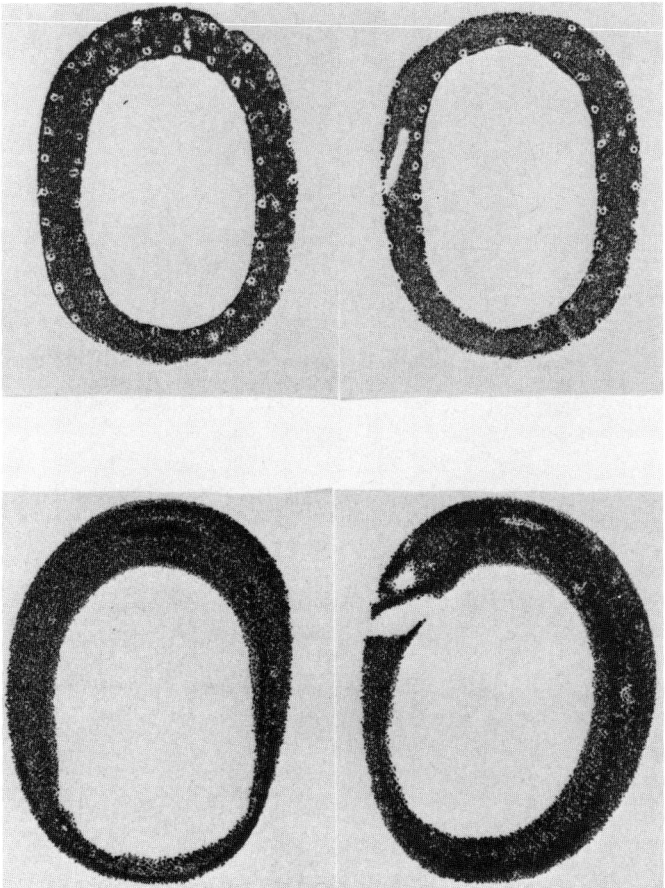

Figure 8. Prints of the sealing cushions of two different hearing protector models.

wearing properties and the sound attenuation.

For the performance of the corresponding test the apparatus represented in Figure 9 was developed in the PTB. By means of this apparatus it is possible to bend 3 hearing protectors at the same time to the intended span of 180 mm in an approximately sine-shaped movement. The frequency is about 0.2 Hz; the number of expansions can be preset (3000 are specified). The application force is determined before and after the expansion.

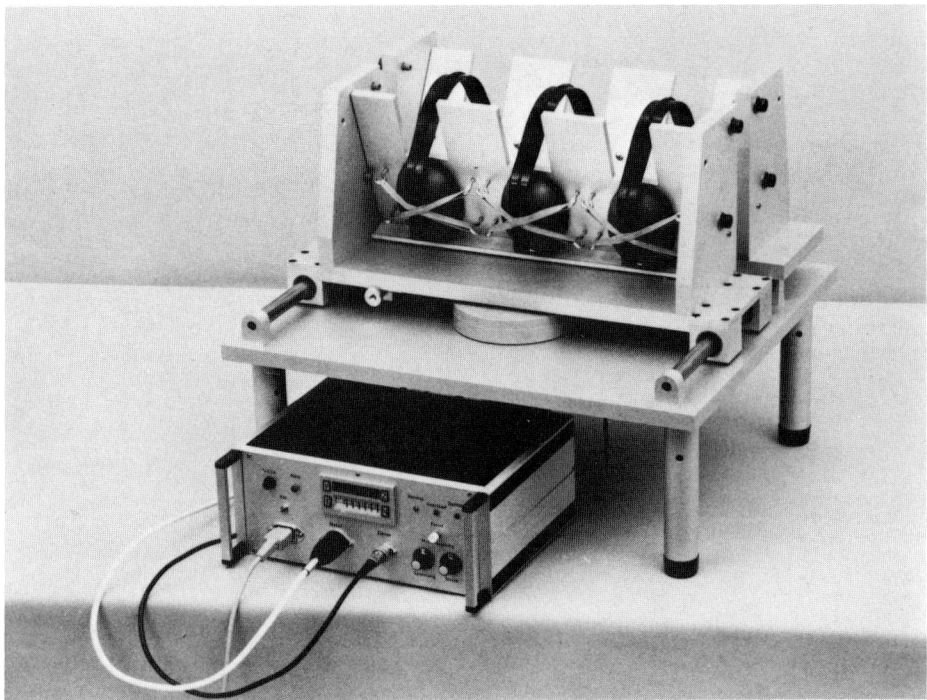

Figure 9.   Apparatus for the expansion of headbands.

Initial tests have shown that with plastic headbands the application force tends to be reduced (in the case of the hearing protectors tested so far, up to about 20%), whereas the application force tends to show a slight increase in the case of metal headbands.

Strain Due to Dropping

For this test the hearing protector is first stored for 4h at a temperature of $0°C$. It is then dropped six times on a horizontal floor of smooth concrete from a height of 1.5 m. As a consequence of this, the hearing protector must not tear or break. Damage to the sealing elements is permissible. The purpose of this test is to exclude damage which might lead to an unnoticed reduction of the sound attenuation. Splitting of the sealing cushions, is not considered a safety hazard, because in this case they can be exchanged or a new hearing protector be used.

Previous tests have shown, however, that weak points are to be found in the headband fastenings of the earmuffs. It is true that even in this case, breaking does not lead to a safety hazard, because further use of the hearing protector is precluded, but it does represent a negative quality feature.

Climatic Tests
Humidity Effects
In earlier investigations[12] it had been noticed that the application force of some hearing protectors was already reduced by storing them for some time under normal climatic conditions. This behaviour could be explained by a humidity absorption of the plastic material used and led to the simulation of this long-term humidity effect in a short test. For this purpose the hearing protectors are stored in a water bath at a temperature of $50°C$ for 24h. The application force is measured before and after storage.

Corresponding investigations were recently carried out with 15 different hearing protector models of the earmuff type by means of the apparatus shown in Figure 10. Two groups are clearly distinguishable: in the case of the hearing protectors with metal headbands and some of the hearing protectors with plastic headbands the application force changed only slightly or not at all (-11% at the most). In the case of 7 out of 12 hearing protectors with plastic headbands, however, the application force decreased by 22% to 28%.

Influence of High and Low Temperature
Here additional requirements are concerned which have to be met only by specially marked hearing protectors. The behaviour at high temperatures is determined by the measurement of the application force before and after a 4-hour storage at a temperature of $60°C$. The behaviour at low temperatures is first determined by the drop test (see Strain due to Dropping) after a 4-hour storage at $-20°C$. Here, no tearing or breaking must occur. The alteration in the application force is then determined.

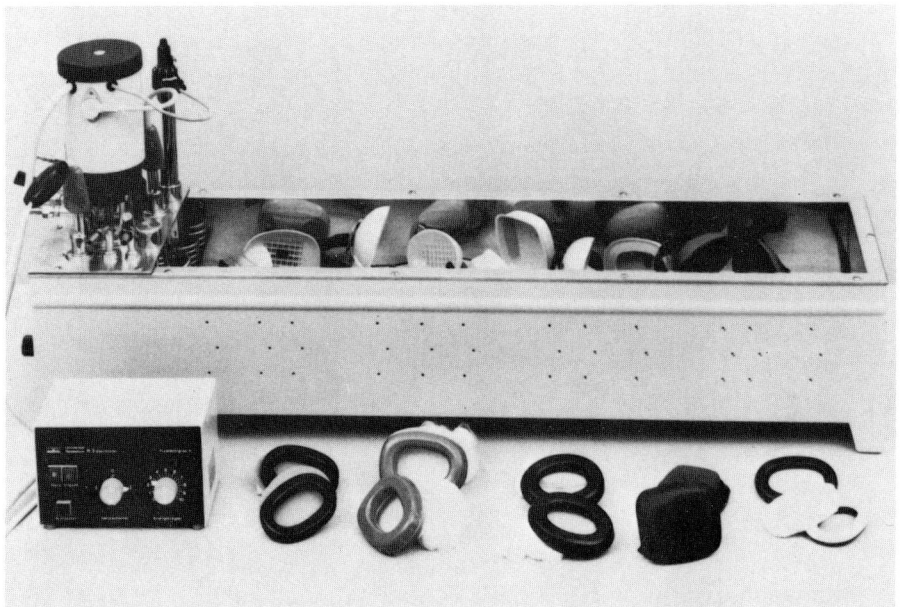

Figure 10. Tempered water bath for testing humidity effects.

TYPE APPROVAL TESTS

Future type approval tests of hearing protectors of the earmuff type will be performed according to the test scheme shown in Figure 11. Five specimens of each model have to be submitted. Three of them are first tested with respect to their construction and application force, and the humidity, mechanical and temperature tests are performed later. During this procedure the application force must not change altogether by more than 20%. In the case of a positive result the six cups tested previously are compared with 4 brand new ones on the acoustic test fixture for the insertion loss afforded. If the spread of data is not too great the final subjective determination of the sound attenuation is performed using the three original specimens.

When preparing the standard, several other additional requirements such

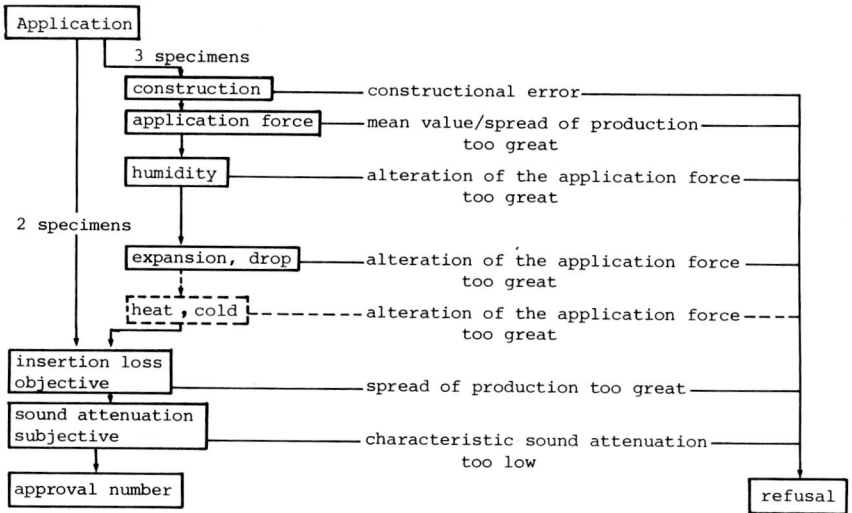

Figure 11. Functional scheme for the type test of a hearing protector of the ear-muff type according to DIN 32 760.

as inflammability and vibration strain were discussed. But, finally, the decision was made to confine the standard to the most important characteristics in order to keep testing time and testing costs within tolerable limits. Nevertheless, it is expected that due to this test procedure, unsuitable hearing protectors will be discovered and thus a contribution made towards a general improvement of quality.

REFERENCES

1. DIN 32760. Gehörschützer; Begriffe, Sicherheitstechnische Anforderungen, Prüfung. 1980.

2. DIN 45611. Messung der Schalldämmung von Gehörschutzern nach der Hörschwellenmethode. Oktober 1965.

3. ANSI S 3.19-1974. Method for the measurement of real-ear protection of hearing protectors and physical attenuation of earmuffs.

4. ISO/DIS 4869. Acoustics - Measurement of sound attenuation of hearing protectors - Subjective method.

5. Zwislocki, J. In search of the bone-conduction threshold in a free sound field. J. Acoust. Soc. Amer. $\underline{29}$, 795-804, 1957.

6. Nixon, C.W.; V. Gierke, H.E. Experiments on the bone-conduction

threshold in a free sound field. J. Acoust. Soc. Amer. 31, 1121-1125, 1959.

7. Brinkmann, K. Noise reduction provided by hearing protectors. Proc. 9th Int. Cong. Acoust. - Sevilla Symposium on Hearing and Industrial Noise Environments 61-70, 1977.

8. A summary table of proposed single number measures of hearing protectors noise reduction. Available upon request from E-A-R Corporation, Indianapolis, USA.

9. Waugh, R. Calculated in-ear A-weighted sound levels resulting from two methods of hearing protector selection. Ann occup. Hyg. 19, 193-202, 1976.

10. Berger, E. Single number measures of hearing protector noise reduction. EAR Log 2 (1979). Available upon request from E-A-R Corporation, Indianapolis, USA.

11. Brinkmann, K. Unpublished data.

12. Brinkmann, K.; Brocksch, K. -H. Zur Anwendung objektiver Meßverfahren bei der Prüfung von Kapselgehörschützern. PTB-Ak-12, März 1977.

13. ISO/DP 6290. Acoustics - Simplified method for a measurement of insertion loss of hearing protectors of earmuff type for quality control purposes.

14. Brinkmann, K.; Serra, M.R. Objektive Schalldämmungs-messungen an Kapselgehörschutzern im freien und im diffusen Schallfeld. PTB-Bericht PTB-Ak-15, Oktober 1978.

15. Acton, W.I.; Lee, G.L.; Smith, D.J. Effect of head band forces and pressure on comfort of earmuffs. Ann. occup. Hyg. 19, 357, 1976.

9

EVALUATION OF THE COMFORT OF PERSONAL HEARING PROTECTORS

André Damongeot, Michel Tisserand, Ghislain Krawsky, Jean-Pierre Grosdemange, and Daniel Lievin

INTRODUCTION

The wearing of individual hearing protector is always uncomfortable. Among the most frequently recorded comments are: a modification of perceived sounds, a pressure over the temples, a congestion of the ears, sweaty ears, an irritation of the auditory duct, a sensation of isolation. Though acoustic efficiency has to remain paramount, there should be a search for the slightest discomfort. Examination of available devices shows that maximum efficiency is not always reached because of comfort. For example, ear-plugs which can be more easily tolerated in some ambiances, or worn continuously, may be as efficient as less comfortable earmuffs; in the same way, earmuffs with liquid filled seals are both more efficient and more comfortable than some sponge seals, because of a better tightness linked to a better distribution of the application force. Such considerations led us to perform subjective evaluations of the comfort of the devices together with acoustic attenuation measurements. In the case of the earmuffs, we then looked for a relationship between the comfort and some physical characteristics of the devices, such as mass, application force, frame tightness, the hardness of the pad . . . in order to determine which ones of these factors were the most important.

SUBJECTIVE EVALUATION OF COMFORT

Subjective measurements of comfort have been performed on 24 models of earmuffs. Two types of investigations have been performed: an evaluation of global comfort, and a questionnaire on the criteria of comfort.

Global Comfort

The earmuffs were evaluated by 10 subjects - students - who performed 10 tests for each device, i.e. a total of 2400 measures.

The method used was that of "absolute judgements" described by Woodworth[1]: each element of the series is presented separately, by means of a drawing of lots; the individual has to evaluate his sensation: he expresses it with an acceptance or a refusal (positive or negative answer). In practice each test takes 10 to 30 seconds. A rest of 10 to 15 minutes is given at the end of every series. Preliminary training acquaints the subjects with the experiment and defines their judgement. The subject is asked to appreciate the global comfort of the device and its retention on the head even during movement.

The results of these tests are presented on figure 1. On the Y-axis there is the proportion of positive answers relatively to all the answers, for each device. On the X-axis there are, by classes of increasing comfort, the code numbers of the earmuffs. The dispersion of the results is measured with the average variation ($\bar{E}$):

$$\bar{E} = \frac{1}{N} \sum_{i=1}^{i=N} \left| x_i - \bar{x} \right|$$

with N = number of subjects;
x_i = grade given by each subject to each earmuff (number of positive answers);
$\bar{x}$ = average of the grades given to each earmuff for the whole tests.

The proportions of positive answers are between 0.03 and 0.92. There are differences between the devices, but the dispersion of the grades between subjects for a single earmuff shows that the discrimination is

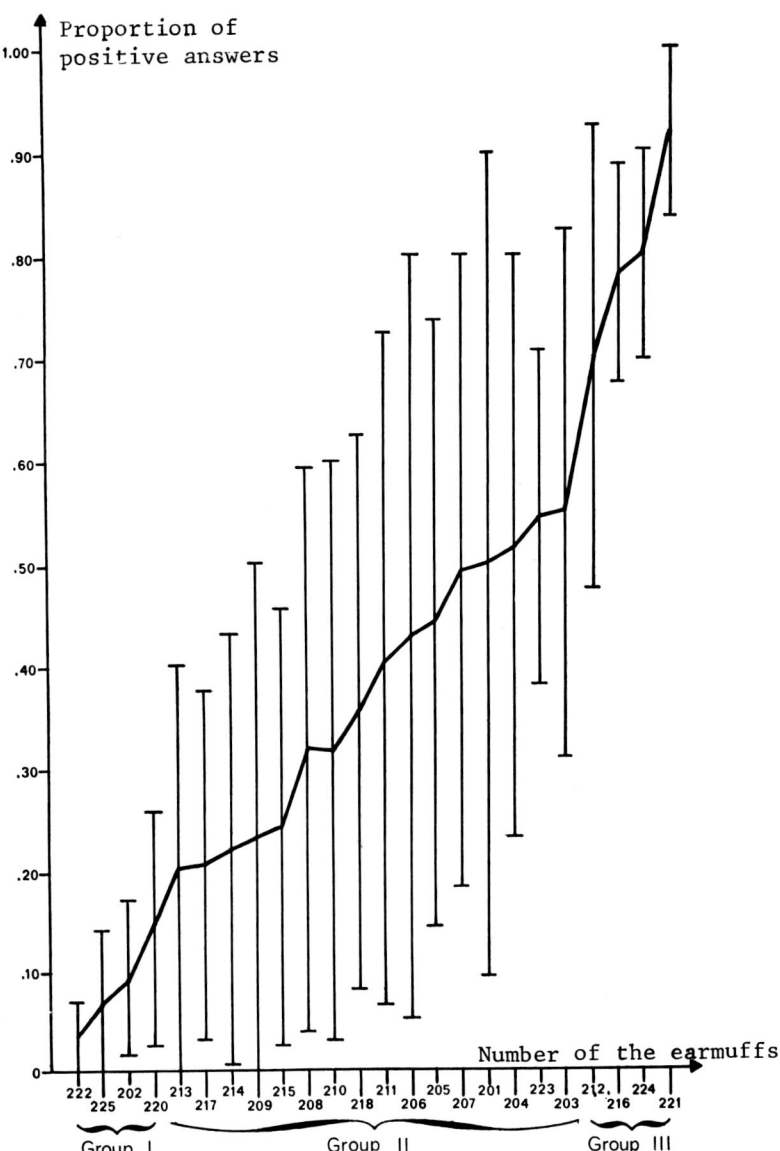

Figure I. Classification of the earmuffs according to the global comfort.

weak between devices with adjoining classifications. The separation into three groups has been made where there were noticeable gradient changes. There is in both of the extreme groups: group I (the worst ones) and group 3 (the most comfortable ones) a certain convergence, of the quality of appreciation, shown as a smaller average variation.

Questionnaires on the Comfort Criteria

Two other subjective studies, by means of questionnaires, have been carried out:

- one aimed at checking, for a longer period (1 hour) the results of the global comfort classification;
- the other enabled the subjects to express the specific deficiencies of each earmuff. The most frequent complaints were: compression by the pad, insufficient inner dimensions of the cup, unpleasant contact of the frame. Details are given by Tisserand and Krawsky[2].

EVALUATION OF THE PHYSICAL CHARACTERISTICS OF THE PROTECTORS

The mass of the device and the application force of the cups may be elements of discomfort. The average application pressure measured between the pad and the skin, is obtained from the ratio between the application force of the cups and the surface of contact.

The overpressures at the prominent parts of the skull come from the incapacity of the pad to diffuse the pressure over its whole surface and then to adapt exactly to the anatomic relief. The necessary pressure to a determined deformation is the parameter expressing this lack: it will be called "necessary pressure to the adaptation to a local contour".

When the application force of the cups is optimum (compromise between comfort and acoustic efficiency), it should not change for the different widths of heads. As a matter of fact, though a setting of the length of the spring usually allows a modification of this application force, the user has no precise criteria to perform such a setting. The earmuff has therefore to tolerate slight variations in force. Then, one may suppose that the tightness of the spring is minimum.

A complaint which is often recorded from the users of these earmuffs is heat discomfort in a warm environment (Brouha[3], Wisner[4]). Temperatures measurements have been made from subjects under exposure to a radiant source. Even though thermic discomfort caused by the protectors has clearly been identified, such measurements did not allow discrimination between the protectors.

Measurement of Mass
The mass of the earmuffs was between 148 and 375 g, i.e. 3 and 8% of the average mass of the human head.

Measurement of the Application Force of the Cups on the Head
These measurements have been done with three widths of head: 120, 148, and 168 mm. The results are presented in figure 2 (on the X-axis there are the code numbers of the earmuffs; on the Y-axis, there are the forces, given in Newtons). The earmuffs have been classified according to the increasing values of the holding force at average width. We see that the differences between holding force at maximum width and force at minimum width vary largely according to the earmuffs. The springs making up the frames have therefore different tightnesses.

Tightness of the Spring

Let F be the application force
l = width in between cups
The average tightness of the spring is: $\frac{\Delta F}{\Delta l}$

This had been calculated for each earmuff and is between 48 and 270 newtons per meter.

Average Pressure
The measurement of the application surface from a model of the head allows the calculation of the average pressure

$= \frac{force}{surface}$

This calculation has been done only for an average width of head (148 mm). The values are between 1900 and 9100 Pa (newtons per sq. meter).

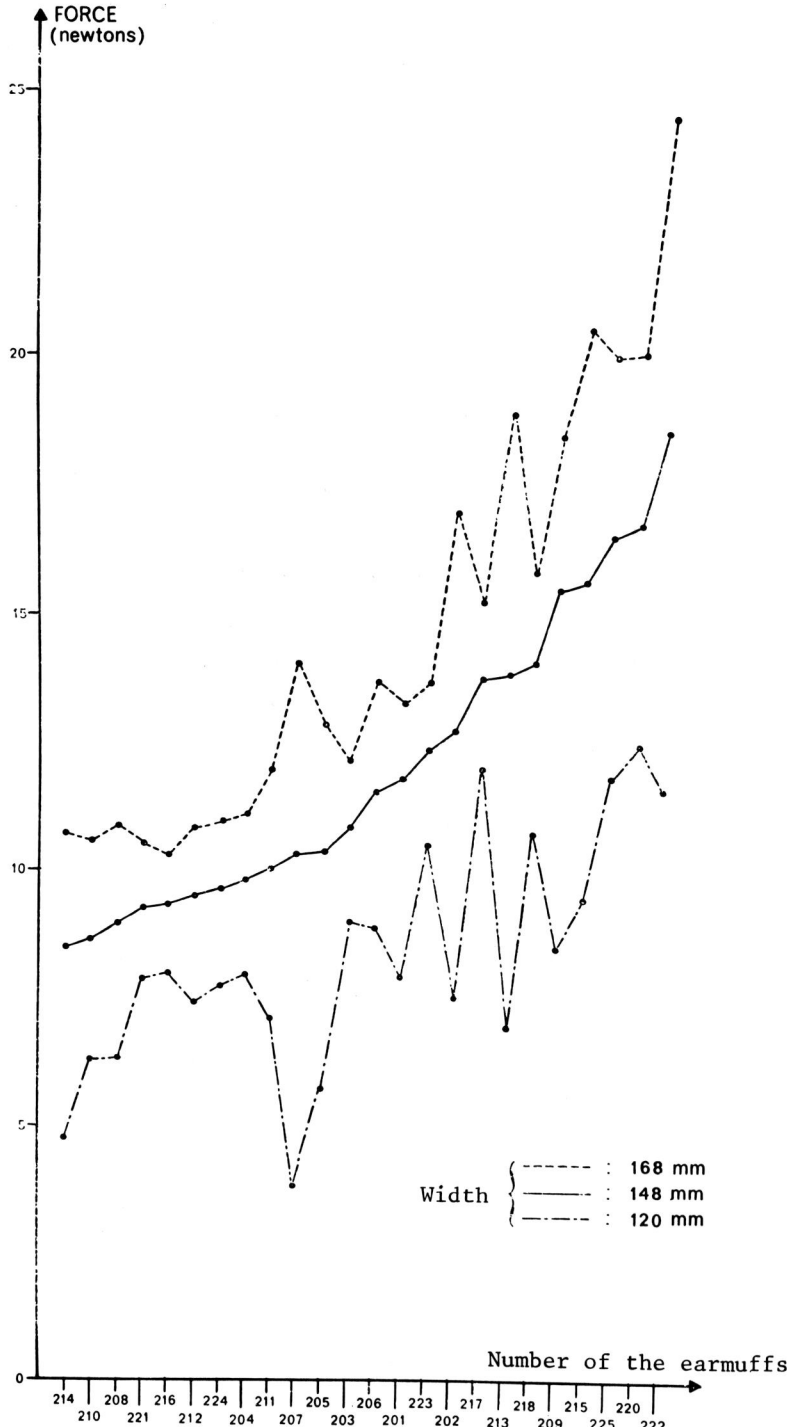

Figure 2.   Application force of the cups on the head.

Necessary Pressure for Adaptation to a Local Contour

The testing device was a cylinder of 3 mm in radius presented from its right section extremity which created a 2 mm depression. The pressures recorded in these conditions were similar to the local overpressures existing between the pad and the skull at prominent places.

The adaptation pressure for 23 earmuffs was between 45 and 395 . 10^2 Pa. One earmuff was completely out of this range with an adaptation pressure of 1380 . 10^2 Pa.

CORRELATION BETWEEN THE GLOBAL GRADE OF COMFORT AND THE PHYSICAL CHARACTERISTICS OF THE PROTECTOR

The non parametric correlation test p of Spierman, appropriate for small samples was used

$$p = 1 - \frac{6 \Sigma d_i^2}{N(N^2-1)}$$

with
- N = size of sample
- d_i = ranks difference between homologous elements of both distributions;
- p varies from -1 to +1 (negative or positive correlation); the value 0 indicates absence of correlation.

The following correlation coefficients were obtained:

The Mass: $p = + 0.10$ (fig. 3)

Contrary to common belief, this criterion is without influence on global comfort. However such a result is logical: on the one hand, the force due to weight (1.5 to 3.7 N depending on the earmuff) creates a small sensation compared to the sensation caused by the application force which is between 8 and 18 N; on the other hand, the mass of the earmuffs (0.15 to 0.37 kg) is small compared to the one of the head (an average of 4.6 kg).

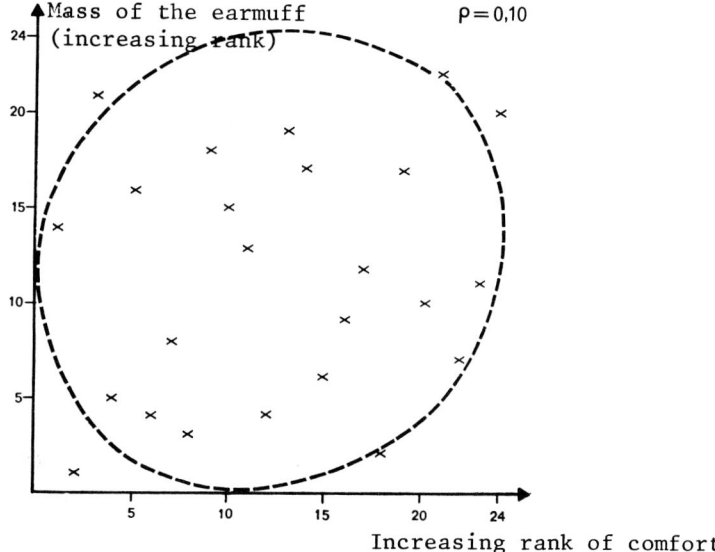

Figure 3. Rank correlation between global comfort and mass of the earmuff.

Also the very small horizontal distance separating the atlanto-axial pivot joint from the axis joining the two cups of the earmuff causes the moment of inertia, relative to the pivot, to be small and less influential on the muscles of the neck. It has to be clearly said that this result is only valid for the range of the masses measured in this sample. The complaints commonly made about the excessive weight are not justified for this sort of protectors. If they still exist, they probably have as an origin, other mechanical effects (application force, pressure).

The Application Force of the Cups: $P = -0.61$.
The correlation coefficient indicates a modest connection, the application force seems rather to be influenced by another characteristic which is related to it: the tightness of the spring.

The Tightness of the Spring $P = -0.76$ (fig. 4)
This criterion seem to be the determinant for global comfort. This result is similar to that obtained by Von Lupke[5] for whom tightness is the main element of discomfort of an earmuff against noise. In theory, it is possible to obtain similar application forces with springs having very

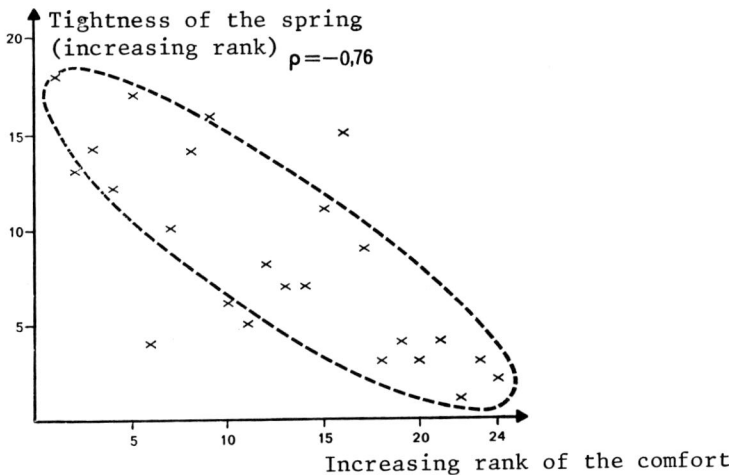

Figure 4. Rank correlation between global comfort and tightness of the spring.

different tightnesses. But in practice, as for the frames of the earmuffs under study, high application forces mainly appear when tightness is rather strong.

Consequently, it is possible that a good correlation between comfort and tightness partly expresses the correlation between comfort and application force. There are other reasons for the importance of tightness in global comfort:
- for an earmuff without an adjustable spring band, a small tightness is necessary to give an identical force for all the widths of head;
- for an earmuff with an adjustable frame, when there is a small variation in width, there is an important force variation, and therefore a difficult setting when tightness is high;
- the setting used for the band is a compromise between acoustic insulation (a high application force is wished), comfort (small force) and size requirements (width and height of the head).

Our experience in these settings showed that it was difficult to give a sufficient emphasis to the application force in such a compromise. Therefore, tightness has to be low in order to have an application force independent of the settings of the frame.

Average Application Pressure of the Flap: P = - 0.63
The importance of this criterion is moderate. Its interpretation is obvious.

Adaptation Pressure to a Local Contour: P = - 0.74
This index is very important to global comfort. It mainly expresses the equalization of the pressure at the different contact points between the flap and the skull. The different results are grouped in the following table:

Physical criteria	Mass	Application force	Tightness of the frame	Average application pressure	Adaptation pressure to a relief
Correlation coefficient with the global comfort	0.10	- 0.61	- 0.76	- 0.63	- 0.74

CONCLUSION

The results correlating the comfort and physical parameters of the earmuffs, show that, contrary to common opinion, the mass of the protector does not have an important influence on its comfort, at least in the range of the considered masses. However, the tightness of the head band and "the adaptation pressure of the pad to a contour" (in fact its stiffness) have a very important unfavorable influence. Just below these parameters in importance are, the application force and the average application pressure.

Independantly of these results about the earmuffs, we can also comment on the problem of comfort of individual protectors against noise on a more general basis. The experience obtained by the INRS, during the last ten years, concerning tests in laboratory as well observations from the working environment, allow the following additional generalizations to be made:

- It is unnecessary and even inappropriate to choose a device giving an acoustic attenuation much superior to the one necessary to protect a worker from the dangers of noise: the sensation of isolation is much more.
- Helmets providing complete head enclosure are the most efficient protection against noise, but they are also the most uncomfortable and should only be used for extremely high noise levels. Their typical application is in military or aviational fields.
- Earmuffs should be preferred to ear-plugs for casual use because it is easy to take them off and to put them on again; however continuous use is difficult. They can also incorporate radio or low frequency induction receivers, and this allows both speech communication, and the provision of musical programs, which helps stimulate their use.
- Ear-plugs, on the other hand are more acceptable during a continuous use, especially in warm or humid environments. They are also less noticeable and this may get rid of reserves caused by some "fear of being ridiculous". Single-use plugs should be preferred when strict conditions of hygiene are impossible.

Ultimately, the best appreciation of comfort, or of discomfort, is still done by the user himself. It seems to be important, if only for psychological reasons, to give him a choice between several devices.

REFERENCES
1. Woodworth, R.S., Psychologie expérimentale, tome II, P.U.F. - PARIS, 1949

2. Tisserand, M., Krawsky, G., Grosdemange, J.P., Lievin, D., Protecteurs individuels contre le bruit - Méthode d'évaluation du confort. Les cahiers de notes documentaires, n° 73, 4e trimestre, 443-452, 1973.

3. Brouha, L., Physiologie et industrie. Gauthier-Villars -PARIS, 1963

4. Wisner, A., Physiologie du travail et ergonomie. Conservatoire National des Arts et Métiers - PARIS - 8 fascicules, 1970

5.   Lupke, A., Gehörschützer II. Ergebnisse von Messungen und Trageversuchen. Arbeitsschutz, n° 12, 395-402, 1964.

Personal Hearing Protection in
Industry, edited by P. W. Alberti,
Raven Press, New York ©

10 Measurers' Choices in Standard and Nonstandard Testing of Hearing-Protector Effectiveness

Jerry V. Tobias

One might expect, in a discussion of "Protector Evaluation" only to hear presentations about standards for the measurement of hearing-protector effectiveness. However, we find that, although the published standards went through a long and careful analysis by large numbers of interested people in order that the final product would be uniformly acceptable, many of the researchers, engineers, physicians, audiologists, physicists, psychologists, scientists and technicians who use and apply the standards modify recommended techniques, interpret them in ways that were not originally intended, or ignore them completely. When this process of modifying, interpreting and ignoring is applied knowledgeably, it serves as one of the major ways in which we prevent our standards from growing old and outdated. However, the process isn't always based in wisdom, and too often, the mutations that we hear about lead to poor rather than to improved data-gathering techniques.

This paper discusses some of the ways in which techniques are shaped by the people who do the testing and about some of the consequences --good and bad -- of that shaping. In order to protect the naive, and because the sorts of problems discussed arise repeatedly in many places, specific sources will not be cited except in one or two extreme cases.

Let us start by looking at the special situation that arises when a standard test will not measure something that a manufacturer claims for his protector. The case that most of us are familiar with involves one of the kinds of earplugs for which the manufacturers claim nonlinear performance. That is, a plug is advertised as letting low-intensity sounds through but as attenuating high-intensity sounds. The ones I know about are perforated devices either with or without a mechanical closer inside the perforation. When these kinds of plugs are tested according to the American standard[1], they behave like earplugs with holes in them: they let the sound into the wearer's ear canal. Yet one manufacturer who markets a custom-molded perforated plug has sent out literature that claims that ". . . above 85 dB, the noise is attenuated to 85 dB. The higher the noise the more efficient the attenuation. Thus noises of 140 to 150 dB are attenuated to 85 dB . . .". How can you test to see if that plug actually can do such a thing? Several techniques come to mind, and none of them is standard. One might ask listeners to match loudnesses between an isolated plugged ear's percept and an isolated unplugged ear's percept. Or one might measure temporary threshold shift after noise stimulation of a naked ear and compare that to the shift in the same ear with the plug. Or, rather than make a psychological measurement, one might make a physical measurement by putting a sound source in one room, a microphone in an adjacent room, and filling the only hole in the wall with the earplug. Intuitively, this physical measurement may seem reasonable, but of course walls in acoustic fields behave differently than human heads in similar fields, so the results won't tell you much that you can use. The writer's reaction to all of this is tempered considerably by comparing the claim just quoted with the theoretical limit on earplug attenuation[2] and seeing that the claim is well beyond what is possible.

However, before leaving this issue, it should be noted that such perforated earplugs do indeed have the potential for nonlinear performance[3]. Constructed properly, they give only a few decibels of attenuation for external sounds up to 110 dB sound pressure level, then increase to about 15 dB of attenuation as the external level rises from 110 to 140 dB. And finally, above 140 dB SPL, the attenuation increases by 1 dB for each 2 dB increase in the sound. That results can hardly be squared with the claim of perfect compression above 85 dB, but it shows that, in situations in which the primary exposure is to high-level _impulse_ noise, the plugs might help. Of course one must be confident that the wearer will only use them in impulse noises before they are recommended.

By the way, the person who determined how much attenuation perforated plugs actually give elected yet another measuring technique, and it's one that is quite different from anything mentioned so far. He ran physical attenuation tests in cadaver ears.

Let's get back to the testing of standard types of hearing protectors. A highly visible example of a measurer's influence on test results turned up in 1975 when Consumer Reports magazine[4] printed an article about hearing protectors and their efficacy. More people are likely to have read -- and believed -- that essay than are likely ever to see the lab reports and hearing-protector studies that any of us have done or will do. The results they reported were based on a short set of tests done using the ears of one person. Apparently, Consumer Reports was satisfied that the attenuations found by stuffing up the external auditory canals of their experimental subject would be universally applicable to all their readers. Several of us wrote to them at the time to say that a standard for making such tests existed, to explain why standard testing is desireable, useful, and important, and to suggest that one gets very little information about population variability from tests run on a single subject. To the best of the writer's knowledge, all that wisdom about standard versus nonstandard testing received was a standard letter of acknowledgement.

A form letter was not what we wanted. What we really hoped for was a publication in Consumer Reports of results derived from standard tests. Let me speculate for a moment about why they used the kind of test that they did. Perhaps they had seen the 1957 American standard[5], which was then current, and decided not to use it. What reasons might they have for such a decision? That standard calls for the use of an anechoic chamber for testing, and anechoic chambers are not in the armamentarium of most general-purpose engineering laboratories. In fact, the best light that I can put on the case is that they saw the requirement for a free-field testing space and therefore set aside the entire standard. (The 1975 standard[1] that calls for a simpler-to-create space was not yet in general circulation at the time they were doing their work.) But setting aside the standard, excusable as it might be on the grounds of the special acoustic environment, is still not excusable when one considers the ways in which the article ignores what was already known about the importance of condensing attenuation data into single numbers that permit rational comparisons of various hearing protectors, in which it ignores what was already known about the effect of the specific noise in which the device is to be used on the amount of attenuation the protector can give, in which it ignores the variability in effectiveness of hearing protectors between one wearing and the next as a function of how they were put on, and in which it ignores the fact that, for earplugs, one person's ear canals are not like anyone else's nor even quite the same today as they were yesterday. (One likely reason that custom-molded earplugs don't work quite as well as some of the moldable or premolded, over-the-counter types is that the tissues of the auditory canal change character with time as a result of such things as outside temperature, water retention in the tissues, wax accumulation and so on.) So I have to conclude that even if the tests had to be done somewhere other than an anechoic chamber, too many other problems prevented that popular publication from saying anything very useful about what sort of device might offer the most protection.

The problems in that instance are clear. In some other cases, the results are a lot more difficult to interpret either fairly or correctly. A long succession of workers has been trying to find ways to test hearing protectors in order to meet some special requirement of the protector or of the available testing environment or of a client with an unusual need. I look with a bit of extra skepticism at the results of modified or of nonstandard tests. I am skeptical, in fact, even when I read or hear about something that was done in exact accord with an accepted standard. Yet I don't want to throw away some useful procedures just because they have not reached consensual acceptance. For example, when I'm feeling especially negative about a test technique, I stop to remind myself that I would have reacted in just that same way ten years ago if someone had recommended determining the attenuation characteristics of a pair of acoustic earmuffs by using a sort of flat-plate coupler instead of a listener's head. Today, such a coupling method, bypassing the use of listeners, is a part of the current American standard.

One group consistently dashes my hopes. That group is composed of the optimistic people who say that they have found a reasonable and inexpensive way to test insert hearing protectors in the ears of the actual users by bringing factory workers into the hearing conservation area and running tests on them under an audiometer's headset. For the more naive tester, the belief that this kind of measurement leads to meaningful results seems to stem from the idea that an audiometer is, after all, a standard and calibrated sound source and that the numbers on its attenuator dial are accurate enough for measuring hearing thresholds and so must be accurate enough for measuring thresholds under earplugs. The more thoughtful -- but still naive -- tester considers that hearing-protector attenuations are not derived from any absolute measure of sound pressure, but rather are a relative measure that compares a nonattenuated hearing threshold with an attenuated one in the same ear. The people all conclude that such tests leads to accurate results.

Let us ignore the likelihood that the usual audiometric test booth behaves like an acoustic sieve at low frequencies, and let us also ignore the instrumentation problems that are associated with using an audiometer as a sound source -- for example, its attenuator commonly has a step size no smaller than 5 dB and calibration errors are permitted that can modify that step size randomly; its output is limited at some frequencies by an amount that may prevent any useful measurement at all when a worker is tested with an earplug and some hearing loss. Ignoring all that, one still must face the ultimate problem with testing under a headset: geometry. That problem is nearly as important with a circumaural set as with the kind more commonly used. The baseline values are found while the ear is open, and the test values are found while the canal is stuffed full of something. The size of the cavity into which the earphone is working is changed and the result is not necessarily two comparable thresholds. And since one cannot judge if they are comparable, one cannot be sure that subtracting one from the other will give you a useful, precise number. One cannot be confident that the number expresses a relative change in <u>attenuation</u>. Even if the step sizes were small enough to tell one just how well the earplug worked, one would still be measuring not only the attenuation characteristics of the device in the ear, but the effects of all the architectural changes that the device creates in the test environment. It modifies the volume under the earphone. The smaller the volume, of course, the greater the effects are likely to be, and the volume is not just a function of having a plugged ear canal, but of having an earplug handle that fills space outside the canal.

The results of an audiometer-headset test and the results of a standard test can be expected to be similar at some frequencies and dissimilar at others. The variations themselves will vary from one set of ears to another. Therefore, even when someone furnishes a correlation coefficient to demonstrate similarity of results between an audiometer test of some earplugs and a standard test, the correlation can come out spuriously high unless the data are presented frequency by frequency instead of lumped all together. Until many such correlations have been shown to be quite good, and until attenuators with smaller steps than 5 dB are used, I have to reject the results of that kind of test. It is too easy to visualize situations in which a worker gets convinced that a poor earplug is doing something useful for him. And it is too easy for the tester to come to believe that comparative ratings for several types of earplugs measured under his audiometer's headset are surely a function of the quality of the plugs rather than of the size of their handles.

Another result of naivete is apparent in the advice one hears given by measurers who may have tested one type of earmuff, one type of premolded earplug, and one type of custom-molded plug and who then generalize from that small sample. They may say (as two of them did in print) that custom-molded plugs are better than premolded plugs. Had they performed standard tests or had they tried to, had they limited their conclusions to comparisons of the brands that they tested, or had they used more than two or three subjects, I might feel more generously inclined toward their work. But as it is, such bad testing coupled with such broad generalizing coupled with a recommendation that can be interpreted as self-serving (because they seem to be in a business in which selling custom-made earplugs will make them more money than selling off-the-shelf earplugs will), leads me to conclude that these people are not just naive; they are either stupid or they are consciously misleading their clients. Either way, the variations in standard procedure that they use are potentially dangerous and expensive.

Let me use myself as a bad example before mentioning some good ones. When I first tested a series of earplugs about ten years ago, I followed the standard, but I learned quite soon that the standard didn't help me in making direct comparisons. In fact, at that time, researchers were only starting to devise procedures that would permit direct comparisons between hearing protectors. No satisfactory technique was yet developed to account for the fact that the hearing protection one might expect from a given device has to be a function of the noise in which the device is worn, and certainly no one had yet found a reasonable way to describe an earplug's or an earmuff's performance without reference to the specific noise environment in which it would be worn. Not until Botsford[6] and Johnson and Nixon[7] looked at ways to simplify the noise spectrum used in attenuation calculations were we able to set aside that problem with a clear conscience. So lacking a method ten years ago, I invented one. It was dreadful. I measured the area under the high-frequency part of the attenuation curve for each protector and assigned a number proportional to that area. It seemed reasonable at the time because high frequencies contribute more to potential hearing damage; but in retrospect, it was a poor -- or at least an inadequate --guess. I try to remember that when I see some of the poor guesses that turn up in print today. (I also comfort myself that, when I learned better, I contributed a little[8,9] to the understanding of the mathematics underlying comparative ratings of hearing protectors and that I then published an appropriate set of comparative earplug ratings[10].)

Let me give you some evidence that the people who do the testing can improve the results that are reported as well as spoil them. If one uses numbers that have been collected according to either the old or the new American standard, one discovers that direct comparisons between devices are nearly impossible. The data are required to be reported in means and standard deviations at each tested frequency, but how can one compare such a table full of numbers with a similar table for another protector? The standard doesn't say. So, some thoughtful users of the standard considered new ways to handle the data. I already mentioned that a composite or a typical or a representative noise spectrum had to be developed for use in calculating how much noise would get past a given protector. Users also needed to do something that would give them a prediction of the potential damage of the noise that gets through to the tympanum. Most wound up including A-weighting[11] (or something like it) in their calculations in order to resolve that question. Still another calculation is needed before one can make maximum use of hearing-protector ratings: one had to know how well the device being tested would work on people who are not among the best users of that device; i.e., it was necessary to look at the effectiveness of each protector for people who get less-than-optimum attenuation with it. The American standard simplifies this best. If data is collected according to the standard, one already has the numbers that will permit estimation of the effectiveness of a tested protector on poor users. The standard deviations at the several frequencies[+] can be considered as estimates of the population's variability at each frequency, and if one then elects to calculate the single-number, composite attenuation value for that device (in the representative noise spectrum and weighted for the prediction of potential hearing damage) not from the mean attenuation that was measured, but from the attenuation one or even two standard deviations below the mean, one can estimate not just how well the protector will work on an <u>average</u>, fiftieth-percentile user, but how well it will work on somebody in the sixteenth percentile or the second percentile. And that, in fact, is the reason that the United States Environmental Protection

---

[+] As a sidelight, the American standard gives instructions for the calculation of the standard deviations that are not quite appropriate. It would be proper to calculate the variability based on a mean score from each tested subject. The standard calls for a calculation based on all scores from all subjects. The effect is that the reported standard deviations tend to be somewhat smaller than they ought to be.

Agency's hearing-protector labelling procedure[12] calls for calculations made two standard deviations below the mean. They wish to protect the person for whom the device doesn't work quite as well as it does for the average user.

The calculation of the E.P.A. Noise Reduction Rating includes a whole family of positive contributions by measurers of hearing protectors. One additional kind of computation has been suggested[10] but it is not part of that rating system. On the grounds that decibel numbers are hard for people to understand, that they may give a false sense of precision, and that they may lead to buyers selecting one protector over another because of a difference of a nonsignificant decibel or two, I once recommended that published ratings be in the form of naming the class of performance rather than specifying an attenuation value. In my example, I used the digits 1 through 6, with 1 being best -- first class. E.P.A. said that if they accepted that approach, manufacturers whose products were on a borderline between classes would have a good reason to complain. I pointed out that agricultural products, among others, are categorized into classes without that problem, and I pointed out that the Noise Reduction Rating has the potential for placing every product on a borderline, but E.P.A. disagreed. I am still not sure if they made the best choice, but it is certainly a good one.

Neither the American standard nor the E.P.A. computational procedure says anything substantive about how to select the human subjects for testing or about how to fit the hearing protectors to the subjects' ears. Again, measurers are making choices. Some choose their subjects more or less randomly, from the belief that only with that sort of selection can the variability values give a reasonable approximation to the ways in which the protector will work away from the laboratory. Others, suggesting that the increased variability one gets with a heterogeneous group of subjects leads to unreliable results -- that is, the results are not precisely repeatable -- began to collect experienced listeners for their tests of hearing protectors.

A similar difference of opinion exists about how the hearing protector that is to be tested should be fitted to the subject. Some say that, in this regard, the test needs to imitate the actual-use situation, so they give their subjects the manufacturer's printed instructions and have them apply the protectors based on that information. Others, again concerned about decreasing the variability of the results, use only subjects for whom the device under test is particularly good and place the hearing protector on or in their ears in the way that leads to maximum attenuation.

Manufacturers, who are paying laboratories to run these tests for them, clearly should prefer measurers who come out with the best results --the better the measured attenuation two standard deviations below the mean, the better their hearing protector's Noise Reduction Rating. Anything that improves the mean, such as selecting only the best subjects and making the best possible fittings of the protectors, and anything that decreases the size of the standard deviation, such as homogenizing the population of test subjects, will lead to good scores. Manufacturers should be pleased. But the ultimate users probably should not. Those scores no longer serve the purpose that the Environmental Protection Agency must have intended. When variability is artificially decreased, one no longer has a reasonable basis for judging how well a given device will work on the person at the second percentile among wearers of that device. These labs are doing everything strictly according to the standard. They are not cheating. They are not changing the rules. Yet when they publish data, they show ratings at the mean that are often very close to the ratings one or two standard deviations below the mean. By compressing the range of normal variations, they give attenuation values that say nearly nothing about real-world variability. As a result, one begins to believe that their data are no more informative than if they had been collected on a single subject. With regard to letting one estimate population variances, the results are almost like the ones that were published in <u>Consumer Reports.</u>

Measurers of hearing protectors need to continue to evaluate and re-evaluate test procedures, to modify them, to interpret them, and to ignore them at the proper times. The influence of those procedures and their variations on economics, on safety, and on health are potentially enormous.

REFERENCES

1. Acoustical Society of America Standard Method for the Measurement of Real-Ear Protection of Hearing Protectors and Physical Attenuation of Earmuffs, ASA STD 1-1975, 1975.

2. Zwislocki, J., In Search of the Bone-Conduction Threshold in a Free Sound Field. J. Acoust. Soc. Amer., 29, 795-804, 1957.

3. Forrest, M.R., Ear Protection and Hearing in High-Intensity Impulsive Noise. In D.W. Robinson, ed.), Occupational Hearing Loss, Academic Press, New York 1971.

4. Consumers Union, Hearing Protectors. Consumer Reports 40, 618-621, 1975.

5. American Standards Association, American Standard Method for the Measurement of the Real-Ear Attenuation of Ear Protectors at Threshold. American National Standards Institute Z24.22, 1957.

6. Botsford, J.H., How to Estimate dB(A) Reduction of Ear Protective Devices for Use in Noise Environments, Sound and Vibration 7, 32-33, November, 1973.

7. Johnson D.L., Nixon, C.W., Simplified Methods for Estimating Hearing Protector Performance. Sound and Vibration 8, 20-27, June, 1974.

8. Tobias, J.V., Simple Rating of Hearing-Protector Effectiveness. J. Acoust. Soc. Amer., 57, S 73, 1975.

9. Tobias, J.V., Johnson, D.L., The Typical Noise: First Step in the Development of a Short Procedure for Estimating Performance of Hearing Protectors. J. Acoust. Soc. Amer., 63, 207-210, 1978.

10. Tobias, J.V., Earplug Rankings Based on the Protector-Attenuation Rating, P-AR). Federal Aviation Administration, OAM Report AM-75-11, 1975.

11. American National Standards Institute, Specification for Sound-Level Meters, American National Standards Institute S1.4, 1971.

12. Environmental Protection Agency, Noise Labelling Requirements for Hearing Protectors. Federal Register 42, 56139-56147, 1979.

11 THE *IN-SITU* MEASUREMENT OF THE ATTENUATION OF HEARING PROTECTORS BY THE USE OF MINIATURE MICROPHONES

G. M. Rood

INTRODUCTION

Standardised methods of measuring the acoustic attenuation of hearing protectors, either by the British Method (BS 5108: 1974)[1] or the equivalent American Method (ASA STD-1: 1975),[2] use a subjective processing task in asking the subjects involved in testing to provide estimates of occluded and unoccluded threshold, with and without some form of hearing protector. The difference in dB between these thresholds is classified as the acoustic attenuation of the protecting device. Previous methods (ASA Z2422-1957)[3] had used a pure tone signal to provide the sound field and single frequencies of 125, 250, 500, 1000, 2000, 3000, 4000, 6000, 8000 Hz were used. The current standards use a refinement of this technique, and 10 one-third octave bands of random noise are used in place of the pure tone signals. This change of signal and a better noise field has provided a test with fewer error variances.[4]

Whilst widely accepted, this real ear at threshold (REAT) method has several disadvantages, namely:

i   The test bands are generally an octave apart, and so no attenuation information is obtained for frequencies between the bands. The lack of this information could lead to mistaken conclusions in cases where a seal, earshell or cavity resonance occurs and causes a significant decrease in attenuation at a frequency not in any test band.

ii It has been shown[5] that in using subjects to detect threshold values, masking of the lower frequency test signals occurs in the ear canal, thus providing an overestimate of hearing protection at low frequencies.

iii Subjective methods are both costly in capital equipment and time-consuming in testing, especially where type-testing or production testing is involved.

iv The REAT methods preclude the testing of hearing protectors either in high noise environments or in the type of noise field in which the protector is to be used. In addition, if a protector is tested by threshold methods, and is to be used in high noise environments, as is inevitably the case, the protector attenuation should be shown to be independent of noise level -which involves more testing and generally more assumptions.

Whilst these REAT methods provide valuable information and have been the mainstay of attenuation measurement over the last few decades, the methods have evolved historically from techniques that were possible at the time, [6,7] when no reliable alternative methods were available. The relatively recent evolution of reliable miniature microphones with acceptable bandwidths has allowed techniques to be developed which, while having some disadvantages, generally remove the constraints of threshold methods.

Development of a technique using direct measurement of the noise field at the ear by the use of miniature microphones has been pursued at RAE in an attempt to provide a method which overcomes the constraints of REAT methods and provides equally accurate results, but retains the virtues of simplicity and cheapness and significantly reduces testing times. The method described was developed from techniques used by RAE for in-flight recordings in strike and other high-speed aircraft, which previously had provided analysis of communication system performance in the air.

Very simply, the method makes use of miniature or sub-miniature microphones which are placed under the flying helmet or protector earshell, affixed either to the subject at the entrance of the ear canal or to the earmuff opposite the ear canal entrance. A direct analysis is then made of the measured noise in the bandwidth required.

This method of using the human in a passive role will be called 'semi-objective', the human being passive rather than active (i.e. using any form of intelligent processing) as in the REAT method, which will be called 'subjective'. At the other end of the scale, the removal of the human element by use of an artificial head, ear or ear model will be called 'objective'.

It is quite obvious that with all these types of testing, there will be some differences in the measured attenuation of a single protector caused by differences in method; for instance on most artificial ears or heads air leakage from inside the earshell is not a problem, whilst it is a significant problem when using a human for testing. Similarly in the subjective REAT method neural or physiological noise is a problem, whilst it is negligible in semi-objective and absent in objective testing.

To see how these factors affect results for hearing protectors, an experiment was set up to test a hearing protector by the different methods. All these methods were used, namely subjective (to BS 5108: 1974), semi-objective and objective (artificial ear), but only the initial analysis of the subjective and semi-objective results is shown here, since the results from the objective comparisons are still being processed and confirmatory experiments being carried out. However, the results indicate that a reliable and repeatable semi-objective method with all of its attendant advantages, may be used in place of REAT methods.

EQUIPMENT
The Hearing Protectors
In the pilot study, the protector was a standard, commercially available unit, with a single-piece headband providing a headband force of approximately 1 kgf. The cups were constructed of melamine, each cup having a volume of 175 ml and weighing 85.5 gm. The seal was of a low-

compliance liquid-filled type, with a stated compliance of 1.2×10^{-5} M/N at 125 Hz.

The three subsequent studies involved the use of two standard flying helmets, and one standard flying helmet with experimental earshells. The helmets comprised:

i   a standard in-service current RAF flying-helmet, the Mk 2/3 series helmet, which contains ear-muffs having seals of the low-compliance liquid-filled type.

ii   a standard Mk 4 flying-helmet, which is the service replacement helmet for the Mk 2/3 type. The helmet itself is of similar construction to the Mk 2/3, but the earshells are similar to those of the hearing protector and the seals are of the foam-filled, high-compliance type.

iii   a standard Mk 4 flying helmet as in (ii) above, but with an experimental earshell of different dimensions and constructed of DMC.

Measuring Microphone

The microphone type used throughout this series of semi-objective tests was the Knowles Electronics Ltd. miniature electret microphone Type BT 1759 which has dimensions of 8 mm x 5 mm x 2.25 mm. The free field response, shown in Fig. 1, is +2 dB from 100 Hz to 5 kHz and the circuitry used, Fig. 2, is such that levels may exceed 130 dB before noticeable distortion appears. Fig. 3 shows measured distortion levels against a high-quality standard half-inch microphone at 140 dB. The circuitry[8] was originally designed for use with a noise dosemeter to permit direct measurement of noise dose under the flying-helmet in flight.

Under laboratory conditions the microphone is placed on the subjects' ear at the entrance to the external auditory meatus, using a flat lead (0.25 mm thick) to provide a signal path, this lead allowing minimal extra

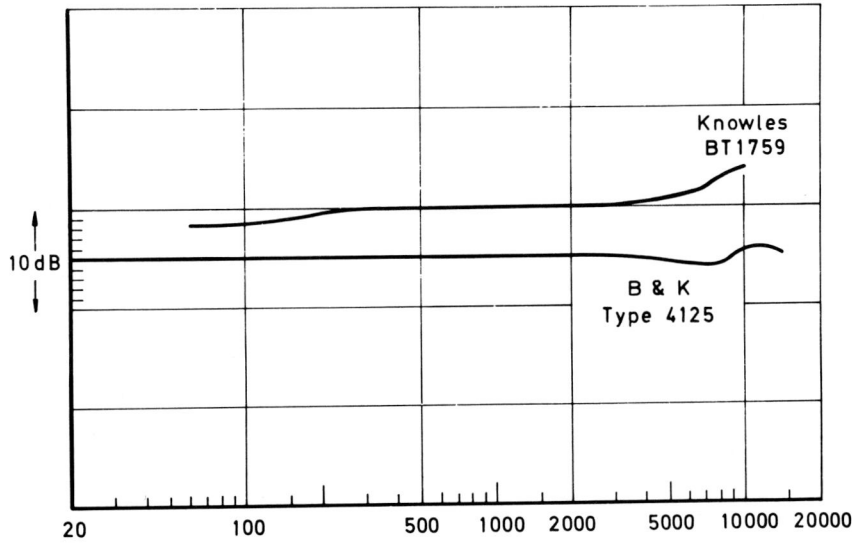

Figure 1a. Free Field Frequency Response of Knowles and B & K microphones.

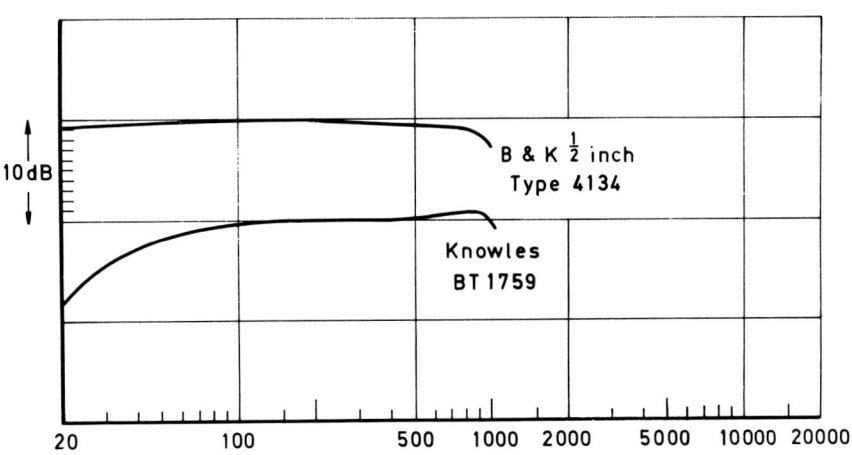

Figure 1b. Pressure Response of Knowles and B & K.

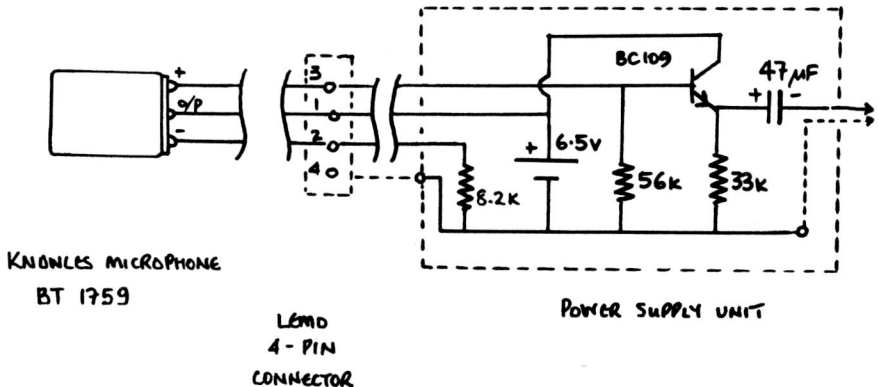

Figure 2.   Microphone Circuitry.

leakage past the helmet ear seals.

Noise-Generating and Measuring Equipment

The equipment was set up using the BS 5108 REAT rig at the Institute of Sound & Vibration Research (ISVR) at the University of Southampton.[9] This allowed the ten 1/3-octave bands of random noise required for BS 5108 REAT tests to be produced. Non-coherent broadband noise was produced from four random-noise generators feeding through suitable spectrum-shapers to the same rig.

Analysis was by Bruel and Kjaer one-third octave Real Time Analyser (Type 13347 and 2131). Bruel and Kjaer Type 2608 or 2609 Low Noise Amplifiers were used to amplify the microphone signals where necessary.

SUBJECTS

For the pilot study, the 15 subjects were chosen from staff and students at the ISVR and included both male and female subjects.

For the subsequent three helmet studies, a specific population resembling aircrew was required. 15 students from the University Air Squadron were used and were considered to be a random selection of a specific

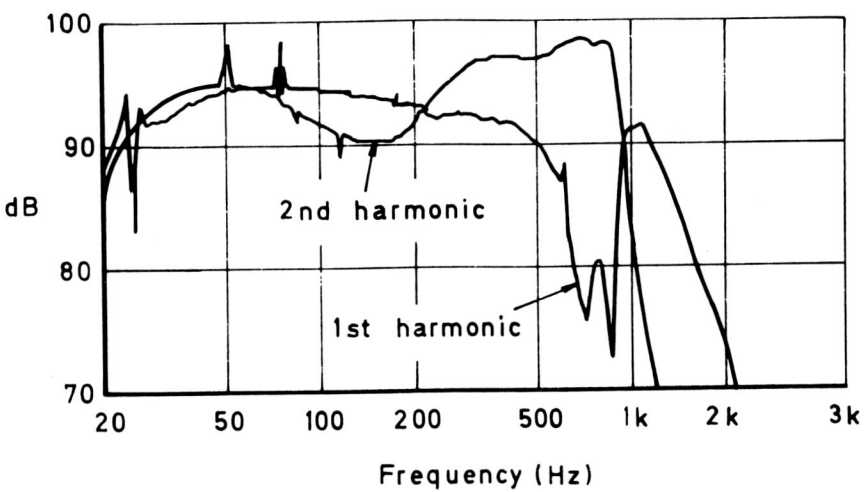

Figure 3a.   Knowles Type BT1759 Miniature Electret Microphone.

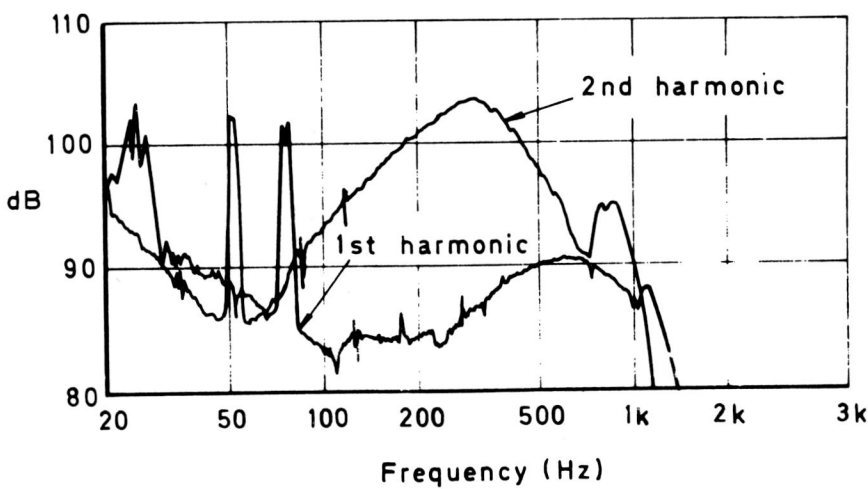

Figure 3b.   Band K Type 4134 ½ inch Condenser Microphone.

Figure 3a & b.   Distortion Levels for Fundamental of 140 dB.

population. This requirement was formulated since service aircrew generally have short hair and are clean shaven. By contrast many of the student population have long hair and/or beards which promote leakage past the ear shell seals, producing poor attenuation at low frequencies. All the Air Squadron students were currently in flight-training, or had flown regularly, and were used to wearing flying-helmets.

Anthropometric data in the form of head measurements were taken on all the flight-helmet subjects to allow a comparison with a wider ranging anthropometric study of aircrew.[10,11]

METHOD OF TEST

The methods described in this paper are the subjective real ear at threshold (REAT) method and the semi-objective method using miniature microphone.

The REAT method allows investigation of the insertion loss technique alone to estimate the acoustic attenuation of the protector whilst the use of miniature microphones allows both insertion loss and transmission loss to be measured. In this context insertion loss is where the unoccluded ear is exposed to the noise field or band of noise, and the threshold is determined or the noise level is measured; the ear is then occluded with the protector and the measurements are repeated. The difference between the two sets of measurements (in dB) is called the acoustic attenuation. Transmission loss is where the protector is fitted and the noise at the ear and the noise external to the ear shell are determined simultaneously, the difference in dB again being classified as the acoustic attenuation.

The sequence of tests for the subjective/semi-objective comparisons is listed below. It was arranged so as to provide a minimisation of error variance (e.g. the helmet was not refitted between insertion loss and transmission loss measurements).

    1.   Pre-test calibrations and helmet/protector fitting.
    2.   REAT Randomised procedure Occluded/unoccluded.

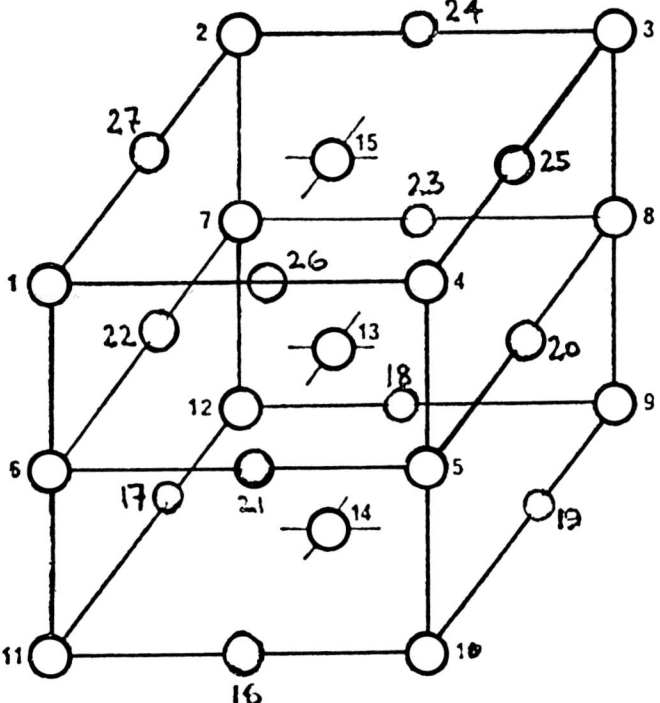

Figure 4.   Positions of measurements in cube.

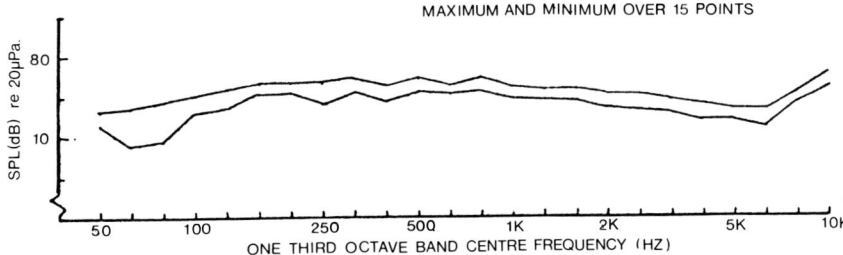

Figure 5.   Maximum and Minimum Levels of Noise Field.

3. Fit microphones to both ears.
4. Measure unoccluded 10 1/3-octave bands.
5. Measure unoccluded broad band spectrum.
6. Don helmet.
7. Measure occluded: broad band spectrum.
8. Measure occluded: 10 1/3-octave bands.

9. Fit outside microphone for transmission loss measurements.
10. Measure inside and outside microphones: 10 1/3-octave bands.
11. Measure inside and outside microphone: Broad band spectrum.
12. Completion of experiment. Post test calibrations.

Noise Field

The noise fields were either the ten one-third octave bands of random noise, or a broad-band approximation to pink noise over the range 50 Hz to 10 kHz. The diffusivity of the field was determined by measurement of the field at 28 points in a 300 mm cube, the centroid of the cube being that position where the head of the subject was placed during the tests. Both the measuring points and the levels of the field are shown in Figs. 4 and 5.

RESULTS AND DISCUSSION

The results presented here represent the initial analysis of the subjective versus semi-objective tests since these represent the primary objective of the series of experiments. Later analysis will compare these two methods with those objective methods also tested during the experiments (i.e. artificial ear results) to allow a three method comparison to be made, with the ultimate aim of providing a wholly objective test which provides the 'correct' attenuation characteristic of a hearing protector or flying helmet. The normal statistical studies have been carried out (though the details are not given here) on the experimental data - and it was found that the normality of distributions, and homogeneity of the data etc, would allow parametric analysis techniques to be utilised.

Insertion Loss Versus Transmission Loss (Semi-Objective Data)

The grand mean values (the mean of tests 1 and 2 and of both ears) for the Mk 4 helmet are plotted against each other in Fig. 6. In this particular case at frequency bands up to and including the 3.15 kHz band there are no statistically significant differences (p 0.01) except in the 1 kHz band -a difference of 2.8 dB. In the remaining 5 bands from 4 kHz upwards there

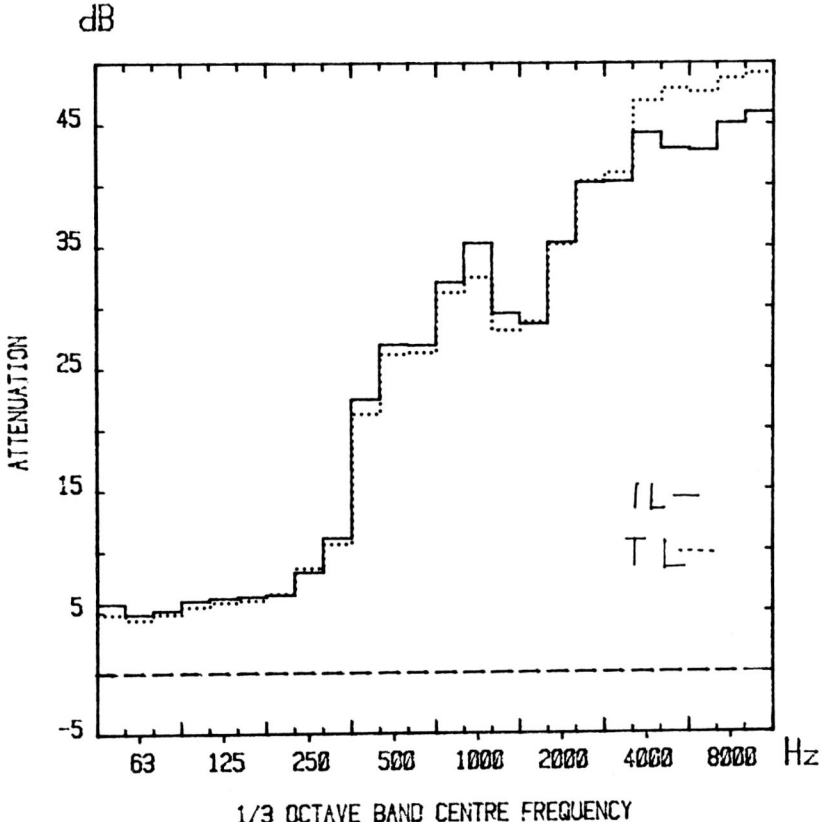

Figure 6.   Insertion v Transmission Loss: Mk 4.

is a significant difference in all bands. Similarly for the remaining two helmets, the trend is the same between the two techniques, but there are significant differences in some bands.

Since the differences at low frequencies are so small (effectively 1 dB up to 500 Hz) there is a possibility that the higher frequency effects are due to the short wavelengths and the precise placing of the microphones on the subjects' ear. It was believed that any systematic error variance from placing of the microphones would equate to zero, as with the random error variance. Perhaps this is not so, and experiments to investigate the field under the muff are now in progress. The most probable source of error, however, is a small but consistent systematic error variance that may occur in the relative calibration between the inner and outer microphones when using the transmission loss techniques. Calibration appears to be critical, as errors of up to 1 dB at medium frequencies and up to 3 dB in the four highest bands (5 kHz-10 kHz) may occur. These, although small in practical terms, tend towards the larger side for statistical purposes and are systematic errors which do not tend to zero. This possibly may be resolved by a study of the different calibration techniques now being carried out.

Whilst the differences are important and reasons for the discrepancies must be found, the problems of differences between statistically significant and significant practical differences arise. With semi-objective data, 60 data points are processed for each frequency and generally standard deviations fall below 5 dB -except at the highest frequency bands - so that the standard error is approaching 0.5 dB. With the lower freqency band standard deviation of less than 2 dB, the standard error approaches 0.35 dB. Thus differences between means of 1.5 dB can be statistically significant. Thus there is a discrepancy between a difference of _practical_ significance, say 2 dB or more, and the corresponding _statistically_ significant difference which may be 1 dB or less in some cases. In these cases it is felt that whilst the differences may be significant (should be further analysed to find an explanation), in practice it would be permissible to conclude that, apart from the higher frequency bands, both techniques provide the same answer. This is more clearly seen in Fig. 7 where the differences for all frequency bands is shown for all three helmets. Up to the 4 kHz band the differences between the two techniques is less than 3 dB, with 10 bands out of 20 having differences less than 1 dB for the Mk 2/3 and 16 out of 20 for the Mk 4 helmet. Above 4 kHz the differences become greater, rising to a maximum of 5.8 dB in one case in the 5 kHz band.

Generally it is felt, however, that either technique may be used, and the differences up to the 4 kHz band do not exclude either technique being compared with the other reasonable confidence, which will however, be

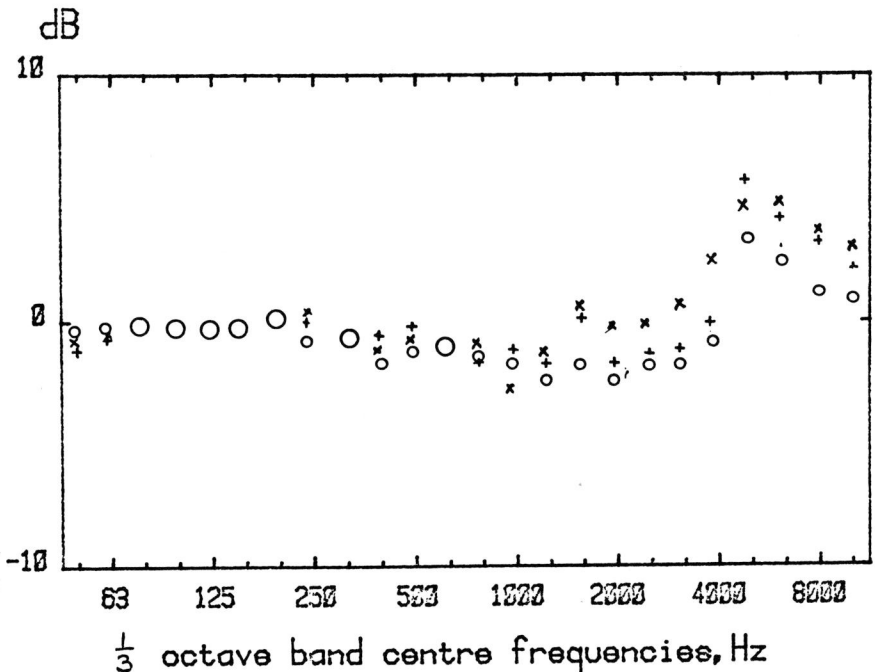

Figure 7. Summary of Differences Between Insertion Loss and Transmission Loss Techniques. Large circles are where all points are within 1 dB.

quantified as further research into the differences progresses.

Replications: Runs 1 and 2

REAT methods use a single replication since analysis of REAT data has shown that the intra-subject variance is small compared with inter-subject variance and thus more subjects are more important than more replications. The results obtained here support this statement since for the REAT data obtained for all three helmets, there is no significant difference in any of the 10 frequencies between replication. Similarly for the semi-objective tests, the results for the grand mean of left and right ear for the Mk 4 helmet by the Insertion Loss method and for the Mk 2/3 helmet for the Transmission show there is an insignificant difference

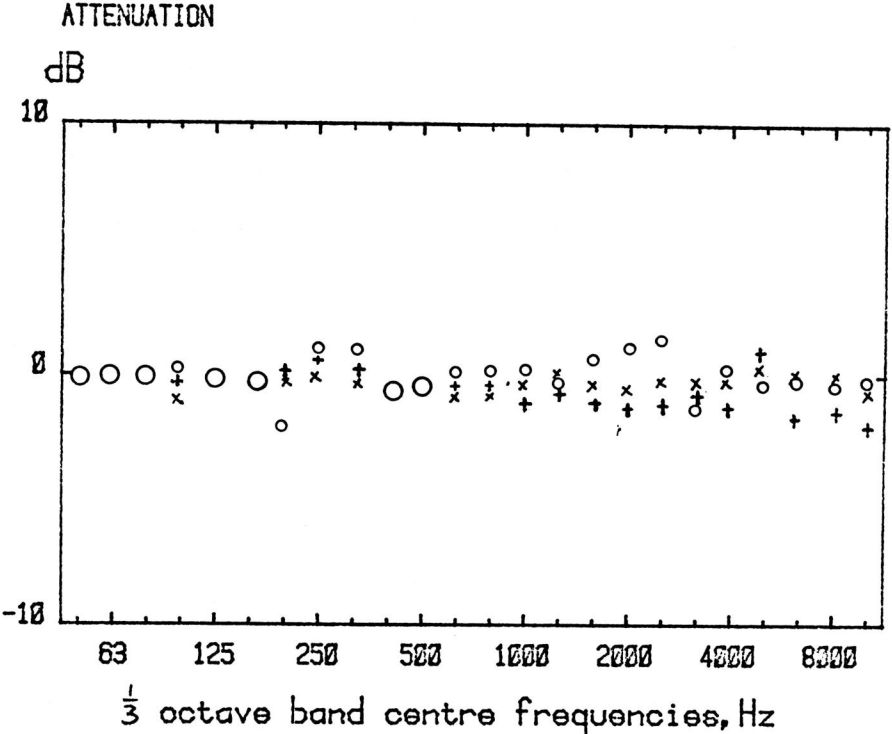

Figure 8. Summary of Run 1 versus Run 2 Data for all Helmets. Large circles are where points are within 1 dB.

between runs. For all three helmets there are only two bands where the significance of the differences between replications rises to 1%, in the Mk 4 alt helmet at 3.15 kHz for the insertion loss technique (0.76 dB), and for the same helmet in the 50 Hz band (0.85 dB) with the transmission loss technique.

The summary in Fig. 8 of the comparison between replications for the insertion loss technique for all three helmets shows clearly that for all practical purposes there is no difference between runs and that to perform only one run would entail no loss of accuracy.

Differences Between Left and Right Ears

With the use of miniature microphones, sound pressure levels in both ears

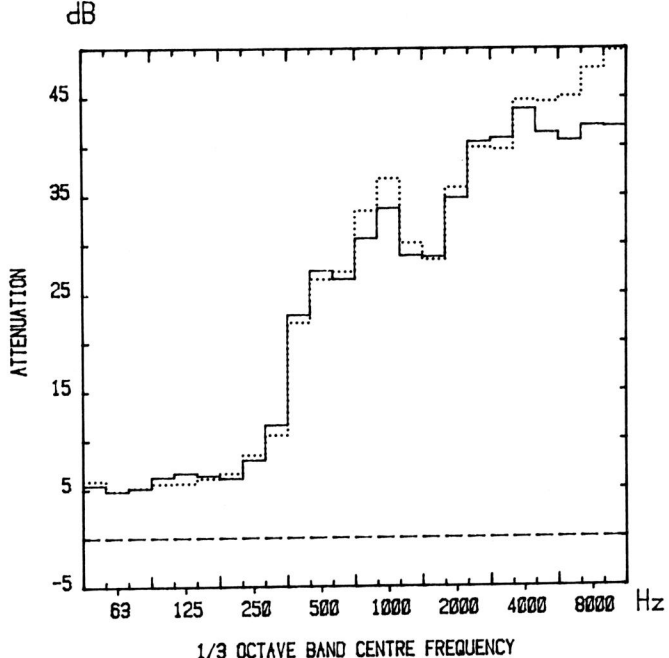

Figure 9.   Insertion Loss: Left v Right: Mk 4.

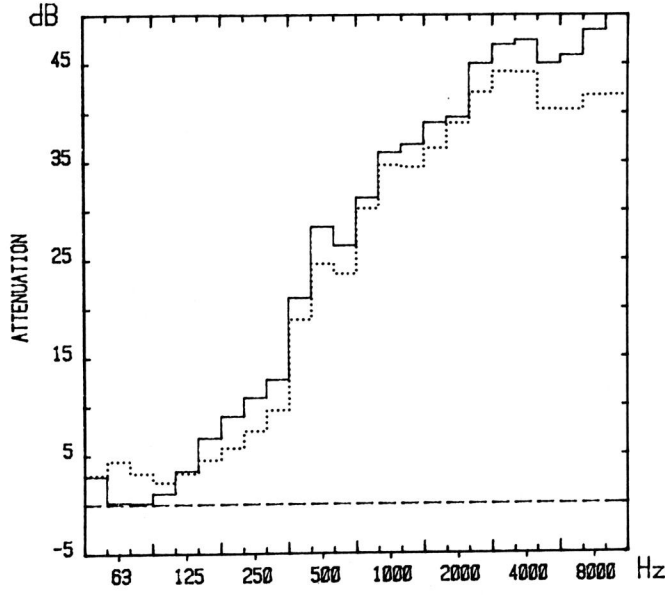

Figure 10.   Insertion Loss: Left v Right: Mk 4 alt.

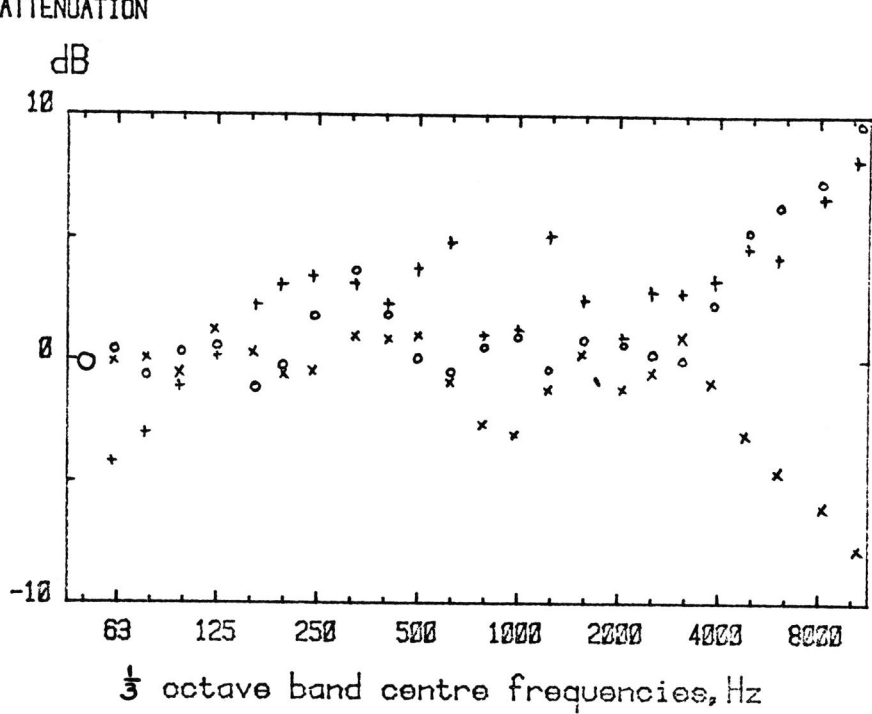

Figure 11. Summary of Left Ear and Right Ear Differences.

may be measured, and, unlike the REAT method, differences between ears may be shown. The mean values for left and right ears for both runs were combined. The plots in Figs. 8 and 9 show samples of the helmets and highlight the differences which occur between ears. For example in Fig. 9 whilst there are only significant differences (p 0.01) in the 1 kHz band, and all frequency bands above and including 5 kHz; in Fig. 10 differences of the same significance are apparent in no fewer than 16 of the 24 bands. The reasons for these differences are under investigation and no reasons are yet apparent, but it is interesting to note that when left and right ear data are combined to form a mean for separate runs, no significant differences occur. Thus until rational explanations are available for the differences, the mean of both ears should be used. These differences are highlighted in Fig. 11 which summarises data for all three helmets, for insertion loss, and clearly shows the scatter of the difference data.

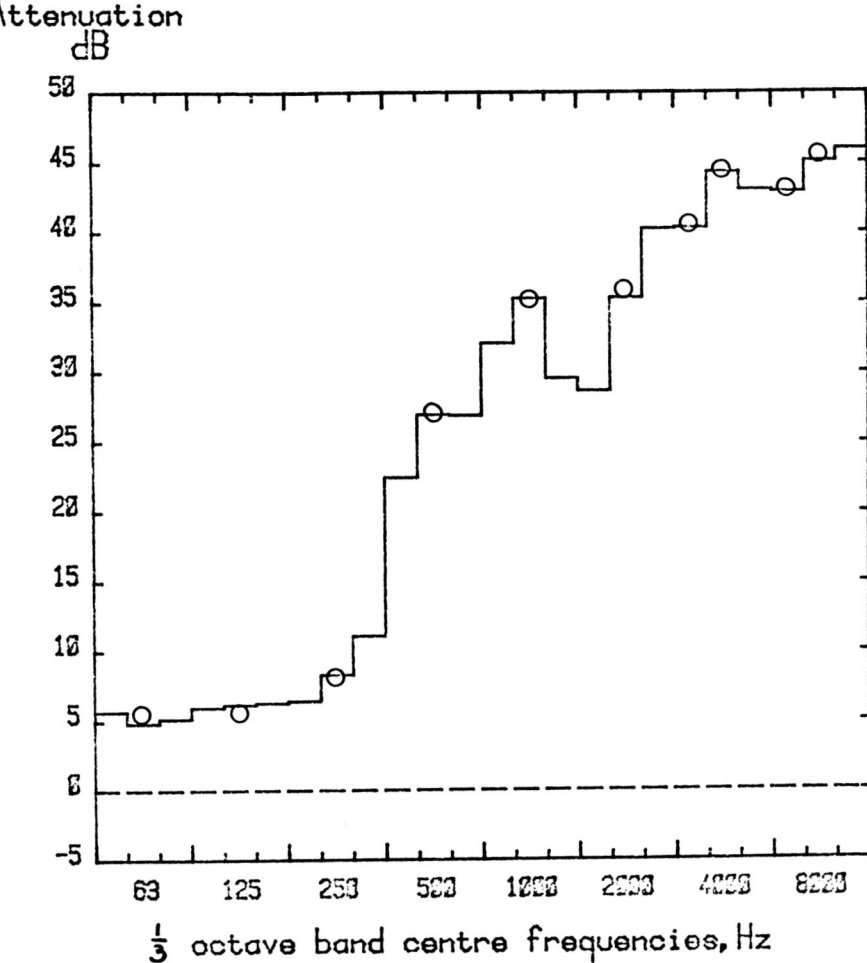

Figure 12. Comparison of Broad Band and One-Third Octave Band Attenuation Results: Insertion Loss: Mk 4 Helmet.

Differences Between Broad Band and Sequential Band Results

When REAT methods are utilised, data is only available for the ten one-third octave bands of noise used and information between these bands is lost. The use of broad band noise allows information over a wide band to be obtained.

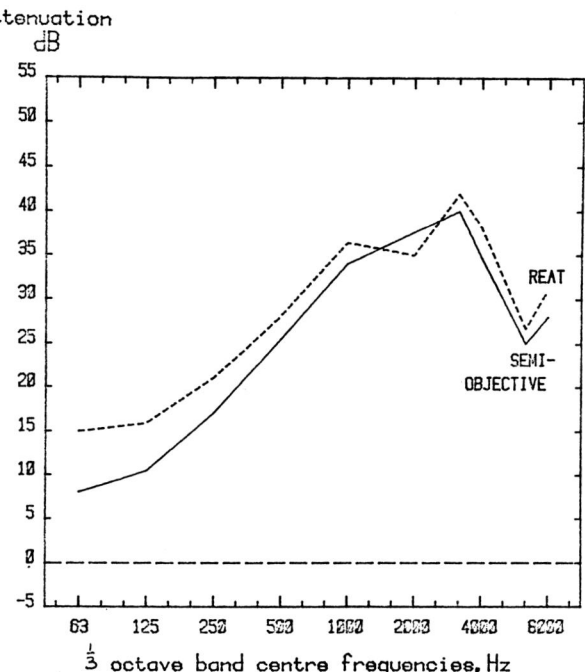

Figure 13. REAT Versus Semi-Objective Results: Hearing Protector.

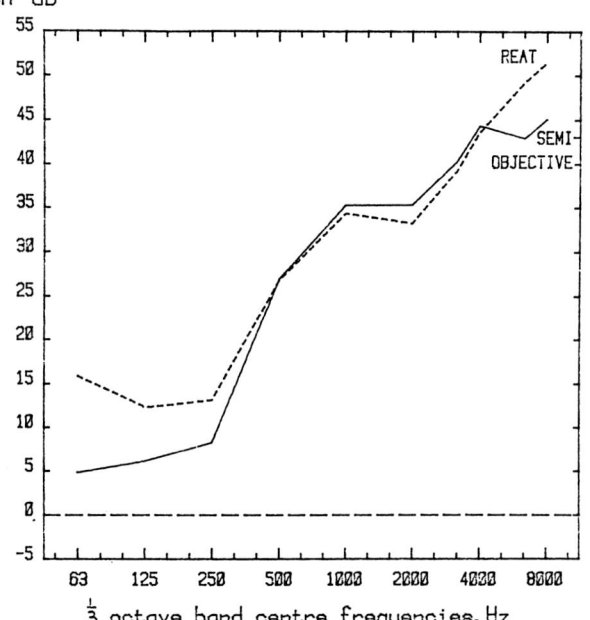

Figure 14. REAT Versus Semi-Objective Results: Mk 4 Helmet.

Fig. 12 shows the result of Insertion Loss Measurements on the Mk 4 helmet and compares the attenuation results using broad band noise and those obtained with the ten one-third octave bands under similar circumstances. The greatest difference for this helmet is less than 1 dB and for all helmets is less than 2 dB except for the Mk 2/3 helmet in the 8 kHz band where the difference is 2.6 dB. When summarised, the differences between attenuation measured from one-third octaves and those measured by broad band noise are insignificant, and thus broad band noise may be used and this permits considerably more data to be obtained rapidly.

Differences Between REAT and Semi-Objective Results

The final graphs, Figs. 13 and 14, exemplify comparisons between subjective (REAT) and semi-objective insertion loss tests for the hearing protector and the three flying helmets. Each protecting device was measured using the same subjects for each technique, and, as detailed previously, during the same session.

Inspection of the figures shows three noticeable trends which were apparent with all devices tested. At low frequencies, that is, in the 63, 125 and 250 Hz bands, the attenuation measured by the REAT method significantly exceeds that measured by the comparative semi-objective method. A two tailed 't' test shows significant differences (p 0.01) in the 63 Hz, 125 Hz and 250 Hz bands. At medium frequencies between the 500 Hz band and the 4 kHz bands there is a good agreement between the two methods, whilst above this frequency there is a divergence with significant differences, again with the REAT values exceeding the semi-objective values in all four cases.

Fig. 12 also shows an interesting dip in the REAT results on the 2 kHz band, suggesting perhaps a bone conduction threshold limit, which, of course, would not be shown by the microphone method. When these types of body/bone conduction thresholds are reached, one of the limitations of semi-objective methods becomes apparent, and research is needed to find reliable body/bone conduction thresholds to provide corrections for semi-objective methods. This dip does not show in the helmet results, probably because the outer shell of the helmet attenua- tes the higher frequency noise to below the possible bone conduction limit.

CONCLUSIONS

The results show that the use of a miniature-microphone semi-objective method may be used successfully in place of the standardised REAT methods. The standard deviations are not significantly different, and with the smaller standard errors of the mean and the amount of additional data available over the extended frequency range of testing, it is felt that the method provides an attractive, accurate and simpler alternative to REAT methods - methods which are perhaps anachronistic. It is clear that either the Insertion Loss or Transmission Loss technique may be used and the results using either agree well from the 50 Hz band to the 4 kHz band, (i.e. the mean attenuation values are all within a maximum of 3 dB of each other - in the majority of cases within 2 dB). In the 4 remaining bands above 4 kHz there is a divergence and differences up to 5 dB can occur. However, either insertion or transmission loss techniques may be used with confidence up to 4 kHz, and where frequencies above this are required, the insertion loss technique, with no danger of calibration errors, will provide reliable data. In general the insertion loss technique is used at RAE in the laboratory; but where high levels of noise are required (i.e. above an Leq of 75 dB(A) at the subjects' ear) or in-flight measurements are necessary, only the transmission loss technique is possible.

A further area requiring investigation is whether or not there are discrepancies between the attenuation of the left and right earshells. The scatter in Fig. 10, which summarises the difference between left and right ears, is clearly shown. However, when both ears are summed and the mean value taken and compared between the replications then no significant difference occurs. Thus, providing the data at both ears are used, no loss of accuracy will occur. As part of this particular exercise it is also shown that there is no difference between mean values for replications, and thus a single run is adequate, and as noted previously this is also true for all the REAT tests, where neither the means nor variances are significantly different.

The conclusions to be drawn from the comparison of the broad band noise data and that obtained from the one-third octave data is that the differences are insignificant and that, quite apart from the obvious advantages of obtaining the additional information contained in the bands between the one-third octave measurement bands, either method may be used to measure the attenuation characteristic. The further major advantages are that all 10 or 24 frequency bands may be measured simultaneously instead of sequentially, thus providing a considerable saving in testing time, and that the broad band spectrum may be analysed, if necessary, in frequency bands narrower or broader than the one-third octave bands, allowing a greater flexibility in analysis.

The final comparison, that of the REAT method against the Semi-objective method using miniature microphones poses a more fundamental question: that is which is the 'correct' method of attenuation determination? Obviously over the medium frequencies from 500 Hz to 4 kHz there is no significant difference, and at the higher frequencies the differences may, at least in the first analysis, be looked upon as academic from a practical viewpoint, since 6 or 7 dB difference on an attenuation of over 40 dB is negligible. Nevertheless it may be important and research is in progress to try to explain the differences. The major problem, at least in the aircraft industry, is at low frequencies where there is a great deal of noise, and there is difficulty in increasing the attenuation of flying helmets because of constraints of size and weight. One would wish to accept the markedly greater results obtained by the REAT method, but the research of Anderson and Whittle of the National Physical Laboratory,[5] convincingly suggests that these figures are due to masking by physiological noise in the auditory meatus. If this is the case, the attenuation measured by the miniature microphone is likely to be closer to the 'correct' value than the REAT figures.

It is considered that valid results can be obtained by semi-objective methods using the transmission loss technique with measurements at both ears of 15 subjects in a single run. The major advantage would be that the testing time - using computer analysis techniques - would be reduced by around 95%. The testing time for a single subject by REAT methods is approximately 1 hour for 2 runs, whilst with the proposed semi-objective method the testing time can be reduced to 1 minute, plus a further 2 minutes or so for fitting and removal of the microphones. Thus it should be possible to carry out a single comprehensive test on a flying helmet or hearing protector, which will give data as accurate as a probably more accurate than those from the corresponding REAT tests, and significantly reduce the overall testing period.

REFERENCES

1. British Standards Institution, British Standard Method for the measurement of real-ear attenuation at threshold of hearing protectors BS 5108, 1974

2. Acoustical Society of America Standard, Method for the measurement of real-ear protection of Hearing Protectors and Physical Attenuation of Earmuffs ASA STD 1-1975

3. American Standards Association, Measurement of the real ear attenuation of ear protectors at threshold ASA Z24.22, 1957

4. Whittle, L.S., Robinson, D.W., On the measurement of real-ear attenuation of hearing protectors by Standardised test methods. National Physical Laboratory Acoustics Report Ac 79, 1977

5. Anderson, C.M.B., Whittle, L.S., Physiological Noise and the Missing 6 dB. Acustica, $\underline{24}$ 261-272, 1971

6. Stevens, S.S., Griffin, D.R., Goffard, S.J., Volkman, J., The Acoustic Design of Earphone Sockets Helmets and Headsets. OSRD Report Contract No. 1366, 1942

7. Wilkie, D.R., The Acoustic Properties of Flying Helmets FPRC 732, 1950

8. Rood, G.M., Baines, D.C., A meter for the measurement of noise dose under circumaural hearing protectors. RAE Technical Memorandum FS 96, 1976

9. Whitham, E.M., Martin, A.M., The ISVR Facility for the Evaluation of hearing protectors following the British Standard procedure. ISVR Memorandum 558, 1975

10. Bolton, C.B., Kenward, M., Simpson, R.E., Turner, G.M., An

Anthropometric Survey of 2000 Royal Air Force Aircrew 1970/71 RAE Technical Report 73083, 1973

11.   Hobbs, P.C., An Anthropometric Survey of 500 Royal Air Force Aircrew Heads, 1972 RAE Technical Report 73137, 1973

12 Hearing Protector Attenuation in High Noise Levels

Larry E. Humes, Daniel F. Konkle, and Jay W. Sanders

INTRODUCTION

The current American standard for the assessment of hearing protector attenuation (ANSI S3.19-1974)[1] describes two methods of evaluation. In the primary method, hearing protector attenuation is determined for one-third octave bands of noise by establishing the difference in sound-field air-conduction thresholds for the protected and unprotected conditions. Sound-field threshold is determined first without the hearing protectors in place and then with the protectors placed appropriately, with the difference in these two threshold values comprising an estimate of the attenuation provided by the protector. Thus, the primary method of the current American standard is a real-ear method that makes use of threshold-level acoustic signals to evaluate the effectiveness of hearing protectors. Hearing protectors, however, are designed for use in high noise levels. An assumption underlying the use of the primary method to evaluate hearing protector attenuation is that the attenuation provided by the protector is constant regardless of noise level. That is, it is assumed that the attenuation determined at low noise levels is the same at high noise levels.

Perhaps in recognition of the possible weakness of this assumption, the American standard also describes a secondary method for the determination of hearing protector attenuation which incorporates high noise levels. In particular, this method utilizes a manikin to obtain physical estimates of the attenuation provided at noise levels in excess of 85 dB SPL (re: 20 Pa). An assumption made with this method, however, is that the results obtained with the manikin can be generalized to humans.

Burkhard[2] has demonstrated recently that this assumption is basically invalid for the case of hearing protector evaluation. Specifically, he[2] found that attenuation data obtained from a manikin tended to overestimate the attenuation determined subjectively for the same hearing protector placed on human ears. In addition, the American standard restricts the application of the secondary method to muff-type protectors only.

At present, it appears that what is needed is a real-ear method that evaluates hearing protectors at both low and high noise levels. If it is not possible or practical to test at both low and high intensities, the goal should be to develop a real-ear test method that evaluates the effectiveness of hearing protectors at noise levels comparable to those in which the protector is to be worn. Such a test procedure requires no assumptions about the linearity of attenuation or the generalization of physical data to human subjects.

METHODS AND RESULTS

Three methods of hearing protector assessment are in the process of being evaluated at the Auditory Research Laboratories of the Division of Hearing and Speech Sciences at Vanderbilt University. At this time, the data to be reported for each method are only preliminary in nature. At present, each of the methods to be described is being evaluated on a large sample of subjects and for a variety of hearing protectors through a project supported, in part, by the National Institute of Occupational Safety and Health. Each of the methods to be described is a real-ear procedure that permits the assessment of hearing protector attenuation at both low and high sound levels. The methods to be discussed are: (1) cross-modality matching; (2) masked bone-conduction threshold; and (3) real-ear probe-microphone measurements.

<u>Cross-modality Matching</u> The theory underlying the psychophysical procedure of cross-modality matching will not be reviewed in detail here. Stevens[3] provides an excellent contemporary review and discussion of this material. Briefly, however, cross-modality matching enables the experi-

menter to scale subjective sensations that have magnitude or quantity, such as loudness. Cross-modality matching is similar in concept to procedures such as magnitude estimation or magnitude production. In fact, Stevens[3] argues that magnitude estimation and magnitude production are special cases of cross-modality matching. Rather than assigning numbers to sensations as in the latter two scaling techniques, however, cross-modality matching involves the direct matching of sensory magnitude "A" to sensory magnitude "B", where "A" and "B" are prothetic continua from two different sensory modalities.

In a pilot study conducted recently in our laboratories[4] a cross-modality matching technique was applied to the assessment of hearing protector attenuation in the following way. Each subject (N=10) was instructed to match line length to the loudness of the narrow-band noise presented in free-field, such that the louder the noise, the longer the line. Noise levels were selected to cover a range from 10 to 110 dB SPL. Narrow-band center frequencies of 500 and 1750 Hz were selected for use in this pilot study. A reference function relating line length to noise level was obtained in the unprotected condition. Next, either earplugs or earmuffs were placed on the subject and a similar function defined. Figure 1 shows the mean data obtained in this manner at 1750 Hz. One unprotected and two protected functions are displayed in this figure. Consistent with expectations of the theory underlying cross-modality matching, the functions are linear when plotted on log-log coordinates. Note the convergence of the unprotected and protected functions in Figure 1 at high noise levels. The implications of this convergence are discussed below.

Figure 2 displays some hypothetical functions similar to the converging functions in Figure 1. Figure 2 depicts the manner in which the cross-modality matching data are used to provide estimates of hearing protector attenuation at low and high noise levels. A line parallel to the abscissa is first drawn between the unprotected and protected cross-modality matching functions. By dropping vertical lines down to the abscissa from the points at which the parallel line intersects each of the functions one

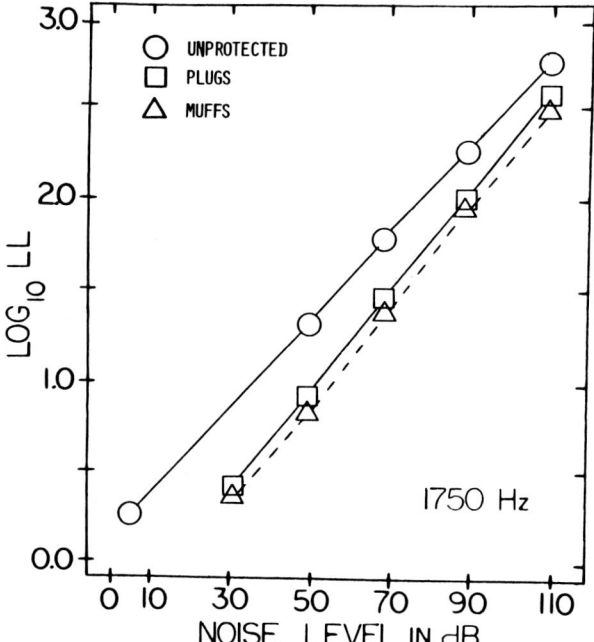

Figure 1. Graphic representation of the cross-modality matching data for a narrow-band noise having a center frequency of 1750 Hz. Line length (LL) and noise level are both plotted on log scales. Three matching functions are depicted; one unprotected and two protected. Data points represent mean values from ten normal-hearing young adults.

can determine the noise level required in the protected and unprotected conditions to evoke the same magnitude of loudness. The difference in intensity between these two points along the abscissa represents the attenuation provided by the protector. If the unprotected and protected functions run parallel to one another throughout the range of noise levels, then attenuation for the protector is constant regardless of noise level. If, on the other hand, the functions converge at high intensities, then attenuation decreases at high noise levels. The latter type of function was observed for both protectors in this preliminary study.

The decrease in attenuation at high noise levels determined from the cross-modality functions in the manner described above is made more apparent in Figure 3. In this figure hearing protector attenuation is plotted as a function of noise level. The attenuation values depicted as

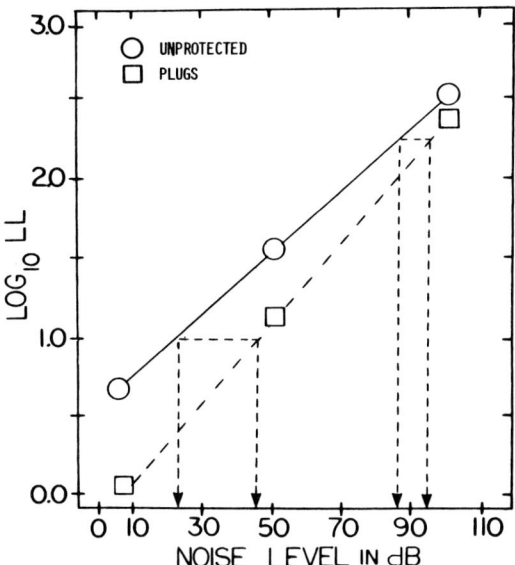

Figure 2. Hypothetical matching functions for an unprotected (circles) and protected (squares) condition. Consistent with the data shown in Figure 1, these functions were drawn so as to converge at high noise levels. The length of the horizontal dashed lines drawn between the two functions and parallel to the abscissa reflect the amount of attenuation provided by the plug-type protector at low and high noise levels.

solid circles were derived from the data for the plug-type protector for the 1750 Hz center frequency (Figure 1) using the method described graphically in Figure 2. The open circles show comparable data for the 500 Hz center frequency. In that the plug-type and muff-type protectors yielded very similar results (Figure 1), only the data for the plug-type protector are shown in Figure 3. The squares in this figure represent attenuation values determined for the same protector at the same frequencies using the primary real-ear method of ANSI S3.19-1974. The difference between the mean attenuation values determined with the two different methods at comparable noise levels (30 dB SPL) was not significant statistically, whereas the attenuation estimate at 110 dB SPL was significantly different from that obtained at 30 dB SPL using either the cross-modality estimate or the estimate obtained from the primary method of the American standard to obtain the latter attenuation value.*

*Editor's Comment: This data is, however, open to other interpretation.

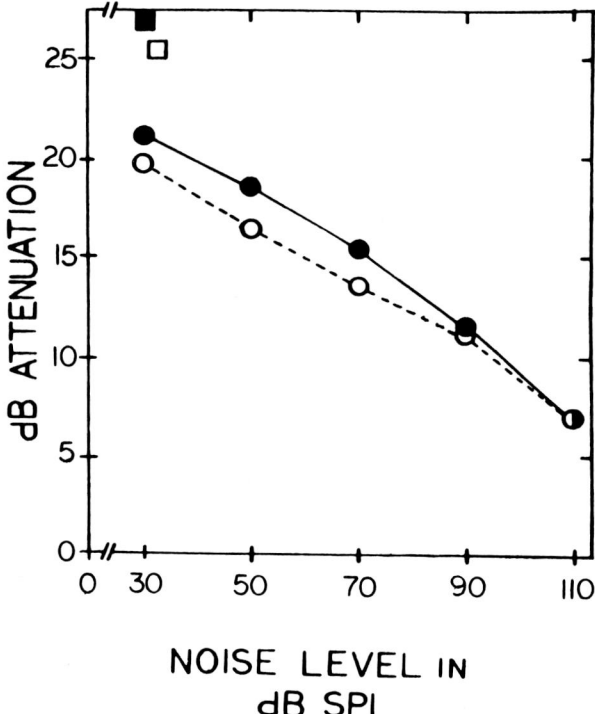

Figure 3. Attenuation values determined for the real-ear data in accord with the scheme described in Figure 2 for the earplug protector. Solid circles: 1750 Hz (Figure 1); Open circles: 500 Hz. The squares represent attenuation values determined with the real-ear threshold-level method of ANSI S3.19-1974. Solid square: 1750 Hz; Open square: 500 Hz.

The practical significance of a nonlinear attenuation characteristic associated with hearing protectors is obvious. These data, for example, suggest that a hearing protector rated according to the American standard as being capable of providing 25 dB of noise attenuation may, in fact, only provide 5-10 dB of protection in actual industrial settings where much higher noise levels are encountered.

The preliminary nature of this study, however, cannot be overemphasized. Only two protectors were evaluated. The frequencies selected for evaluation were low-to-mid frequency. Information at higher frequencies is of interest. Finally, the cross-modality matching procedure utilized exhibited considerable between-subject variability. We are

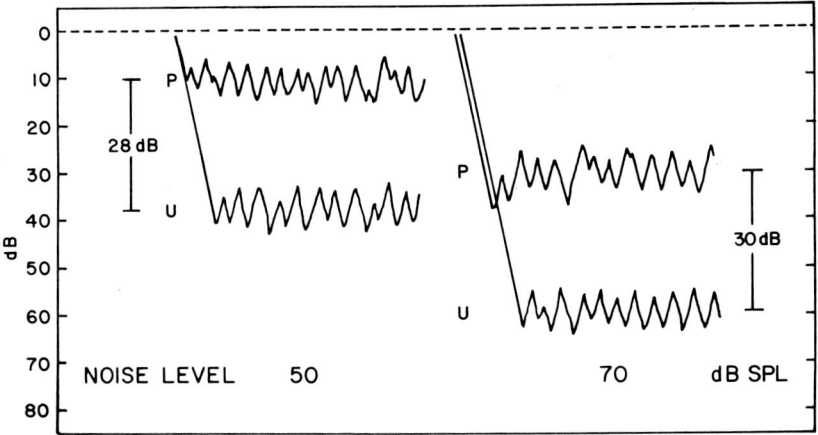

Figure 4. Example of a threshold tracing for one subject using the masked bone-conduction procedure. Tracings labeled "U" were obtained without protectors while those labeled "P" were obtained with protectors in place. A pair of tracings were obtained at each of two noise levels (50 and 70 dB SPL). The difference in the "U" and "P" at each noise level tracings reflects the amount of noise attenuation (28 and 30 dB).

presently revising the procedure in an effort to reduce variability and increase the efficiency of the technique for this particular application.

Masked Bone-Conduction Threshold A second technique that we have only recently begun to evaluate involves the measurement of bone-conduction threshold for pure-tone signals masked by broad-band noise. In this procedure, the subject is seated in a sound field with a bone-conduction vibrator placed on the forehead. The subject begins by tracing threshold for pure tones using a Bekesy tracking procedure. The protectors are then placed in both ears and the threshold tracing is repeated. At present, only frequencies above 1500 Hz are utilized so as to avoid the possible confounding influence of the occlusion effect. The first set of unprotected and protected threshold measurements is performed simply to confirm the absence of the occlusion effect at the frequencies studies. Next, the protectors are removed and various levels of broad-band masking noise are introduced. Bone-conduction threshold is then determined for the pure-tone signals in the presence of the broad-band noise. Once masked bone-conduction threshold is established, the protectors are placed on the subject and masked bone-conduction threshold is redetermined. Figure 4 shows an example of the results obtained with this technique for a signal frequency of 4000 Hz and overall noise levels of 50 and 70 dB SPL. The tracings labeled "U" reflect masked thresholds without protection and those labelled "P" reflect masked thresholds obtained under protected conditions. Because of the direct relationship between masker intensity and masked pure-tone threshold for noise maskers having supra-critical bandwidths[5], the difference in masked thresholds between the unprotected and protected conditions provides an indication of the reduction in masker intensity in the frequency region of the pure-tone test signal. Thus, we have a direct reflection of the attenuation provided by the hearing protector at varying noise levels.

There are restrictions, however, on the range of noise levels one can employ with this method. First of all, the linear relationship between masking and masker level for maskers of supra-critical bandwidth only holds for masker intensities above 0 dB effective masking. As a result, noise levels must be selected so that they are still effective maskers once they are attenuated in level by the hearing protector. In our preliminary study, masker levels below 40-50 dB SPL could not be used. A second restriction applies to the other end of the continuum and has to do with the maximum possible stimulus level deliverable through a typical bone vibrator. Masker levels in excess of 80 dB SPL produced masked bone-conduction thresholds beyond the output limits of our clinical bone-conduction apparatus. Thus, in this preliminary work masker intensities were restricted to a range from 40 to 80 dB SPL. The limited data available from a few subjects and for only one protector suggest that attenuation at 2000 and 4000 Hz is constant across this range of noise levels. These early findings stand in opposition to the conclusions reached from the cross-modality matching paradigm. Efforts are underway, however, to extend the range of test frequencies and noise levels that can be evaluated with this method. Only when this is accomplished can an adequate comparison be made between these two sets of data.

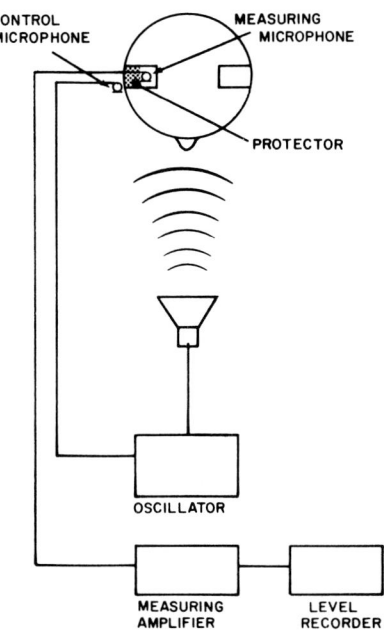

Figure 5. Schematic representation of the measurement situation employed with the real-ear probe-microphone method. The protected condition is depicted here.

Real-Ear Probe-Microphone Measurements The final method of hearing protector assessment that we have begun to investigate makes use of tiny probe microphones that can be placed in the ear canal of the subject. Figure 5 displays schematically a typical measurement situation. Two microphones are used in this procedure. As shown in Figure 5, one microphone, the measuring microphone, is placed in the ear canal and is used to monitor the sound levels at this location. A second microphone serves as a control microphone and feeds the compressor circuit of the signal generator. As shown, this microphone is positioned adjacent to the concha of the external ear and is used to assure a constant sound pressure level at a position just lateral to the protector. The subject is seated in an anechoic chamber and the frequency response of the unprotected ear is established using pure tones of various input levels. Next, the protector is placed in the ear canal over the microphone wires and the response is redetermined for the same input levels. This protected condition is shown in Figure 5. Subtraction of the protected and unprotected frequency responses obtained at the same input levels yields the attenuation provided by the hearing protector. Preliminary data from two subjects for input levels of 50 to 80 dB SPL indicate that attenuation does not depend upon input level over this restricted range of intensities. Much more data are needed from a larger number of subjects and a variety of protectors, however, before a definitive statement can be made. This work is presently in progress. We are also working on extending the upper end of the range of input levels to 100 dB SPL.

CONCLUSION

Three methods of hearing protector evaluation have been described. Each method is a real-ear method that can be used at both low and high sound levels thereby minimizing the key assumptions inherent in the real-ear auditory threshold procedure. Of the three methods described, the masked bone-conduction threshold procedure is probably the most promising. Unlike the cross-modality matching technique, it represents a simple supplement to the traditional real-ear threshold method in that the nature of the listening task is very similar. The limitations discussed above regarding our experience with this method, moreover, are not insurmountable.

The real-ear probe-microphone technique is also an attractive method. An assumption made with this technique, however, is that the appropriate sound level can be measured in the ear canal. This assumption minimizes the roles of compressional bone-conduction, and to some extent, inertial bone-conduction in the development of noise-induced hearing loss. In addition, calibration of the measuring microphone for use under a plug-type protector is difficult. A method that could be applied universally to all types of protectors is desirable.

ACKNOWLEDGEMENT

This work is supported, in part, by a research grant from the National

Institute of Occupational Safety and Health (1 R01 OH00895-01) and the University Research Council of Vanderbilt University. Thanks are expressed to Barb Coulson for typing the manuscript and to Don Riggs for assistance in preparing the illustrations.

REFERENCES
1. American National Standards Institute. Method for the measurement of real-ear protection of hearing protectors and physical attenuation of earmuffs. ANSI S3.19-1974. American National Standards Institute: New York (1974).

2. Burkhard, M.D. Non-hearing aid uses of the KEMAR manikin. In Burkhard, M.D. (Ed.), Manikin Measurements. Industrial Research Products: Elk Grove Village, Illinois, 63-65, 1978.

3. Stevens, S.S. Psychophysics. John Wiley and Sons, New York, 1975.

4. Jay, R.E. Determination of ear protector attenuation by cross-modality matching and numeric estimation. Unpublished Ph.D. thesis, Vanderbilt University, 1977.

5. Hawkins, J.E. and Stevens, S.S. The masking of pure tones and of speech by white noise. J. Acoust. Soc. Amer., 22, 6-13, 1950.

13
Hearing Protectors Attenuation Measurement by Means of Bone Conduction Testing

André Damongeot and Robert Lataye

INTRODUCTION

The measurement of the acoustic attenuation provided by individual hearing protectors can be performed by subjective or by objective methods. At present, the subjective methods are considered as the most accurate. The most common is the method of the threshold of audibility shift, but there are also superliminal methods such as the "binaural balance" method, used in South Africa[1] or the French method using a reference sound transmitted by means of bone conduction.

PRINCIPLE OF THE METHOD

The method worked out at the "Institut National de Recherche et de Securite (I.N.R.S.) and which is now the basis of the French standard AFNOR NF S 31 062 of September 1978[2] allows measurement of the attenuation due to individual protectors in backgrounds where the sound level is of 100 decibels in each octave band. This method uses a pure reference sound, transmitted by means of bone conduction, with a sufficiently high frequency so that it is not modified when wearing the protector. This reference is compared to the airborne sound heard through the protector, and then without the protector to be tested. The comparison is done, with a good reproducibility, by means of recording the emergence threshold of the bone sound in the airborne sound (the bone sound is intermittent in order to make its identification easy). The principle of the measurement is described in Table 1.

METHODOLOGY

Testing Site

Though fundamentally different as far as the testing method is concerned, the French standard is as close as possible to the ISO standard[3], with regard to the characteristics of the testing site. The same third octave bands are used for the airborne sound and the same criteria are used for homogeneity of the diffuse acoustic field.

Table 1: Principle of the measurement (for a given frequency band).

	First step : patient wearing the protector	Second step : patient without the protector
Airborne sound	$L_o = 100$ dB	$L_o \searrow L_o - L$ (reemergence of the bone reference)
Bone reference	$L \nearrow L_o$ (emergence)	L_o (unchanged)

Background Noise

The admitted limits of background noise in the test room are as the ISO standard, though the attenuation measurements themselves do not require levels of background noise as low as the ones done with the method of the threshold of audibility shift. However, the same room is used to check that the wearing of the protector does not modify the bone reference. This is done with a measurement of the threshold of audibility by bone conduction, with and without the protector. The requirements, relative to the background noise, are then similar to the ones of the method of the airborne threshold of audibility shift. The limit values of background noise in the test room are mentioned in Table 2.

Table 2: Limit values of the background noise in the test room

Median frequencies of the third octave bands (Hz)	125	250	500	1000	2000	3150*	4000	6300*	8000
Maximal background level (dB)	14	6	2	1	2	-1	-4	3	10

Note: An interpolation has to be undertaken from these values for bands of intermediate frequencies.

* optional frequencies

Airborne Sounds

The airborne sounds have the same nature as the ones required by the ISO standard. Only their dynamic range is different. The characteristics of these sounds are given in Table 3.

Table 3: Median frequencies of the airborne sounds and dynamic range

(Hz)	\multicolumn{8}{c}{Median frequencies of the third octave band}

(Hz)	125	250	500	1000	2000	3150*	4000	6300*	8000
Minimal range of the acoustic signals (dB)	60 - 100				40 -100			20 - 100	

* optional frequencies

Bone Sound

The reference signal is introduced through a vibrator, of the same type as the ones used for bone audiometry, placed on the forehead of the subject as for the Weber test and held by means of an elastic strap. The vibrator is activated by a sinusoidal audiofrequency generator with an attenuator, matched to the vibrator. The intensity of the signal is recorded in decibels from an origin which can be arbitrarily chosen. The signal is pulsed at a rate of 3 to 4 pulses per second, in order to make its identification easy. There should not be any overintensity or any standing waves because of the pulser. The application force of the vibrator should be of around 5.4 N. The frequency of the reference bone sound to use for each band of the airborne sound is given in table 4.

The frequencies indicated in the second column of the table usually fit most of the cases. As they are higher or equal to 1500 Hz, the bone reference is in fact not modified by the wearing of the protector.
- In some cases of protectors having a strong attenuation, at low frequencies, the bone sound can emerge at its threshold of audibility (when a security gap of at least 5 dB is necessary). In

Table 4: Choice of the frequencies of the bone reference sound according to the frequency band of the airborne sound

Median freq. 3rd octave bands airborne sound (Hz)	Freq. of bone reference - pure sound - (Hz)	"Replacement" freq. for reference - pure sound - (Hz)
125	1 500	500
250	1 500	1 000
500	1 500	1 500
1 000	3 000	3 000
2 000	4 000	3 000
3 150*	5 000	5 000
4 000	6 000	6 000
6 300*	7 500	7 500
8 000	6 000	10 000

* Optional frequencies -

other words, it is not possible to cover the bone reference with the airborne sound, before detecting its emergence. At this range it is therefore necessary to use lower "replacement" frequencies, such as the ones shown in the third column of the table. The results can be corrected without any difficulty when following the measurement process indicated below.

Measurement Chain

The synoptic figure of the measurement chain used at the I.N.R.S. is shown on Figure 1.

Figure 2 illustrates a subject in the process of measurement, wearing the vibrator and the earmuffs to be tested.

Testing Procedure

The measurement procedure is performed as shown in Figure 3, to take account of the eventual influence of the protector being tested on the bone reference.

RESULTS

At the time of writing, more than a hundred protectors have been tested

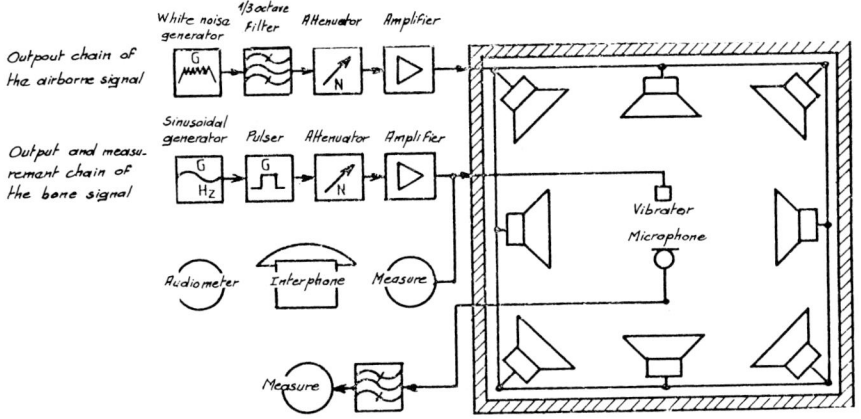

Figure 1.   Synoptic drawing of the measurement chains.

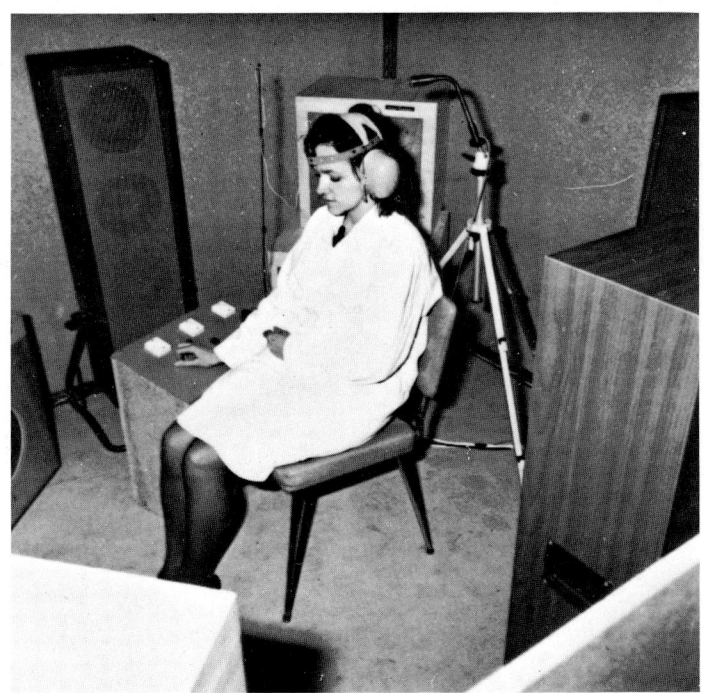

Figure 2.   Subject performing the attenuation measurement of earmuffs.

Test with the protector		Test without the protector	
Room : Silence	Room : $L_1 = 100$ dB	Room : Silence	Room : $L_1 \searrow L_2$
l_1	l_3	l_2	l_4
- Look for the threshold of audibility by bone conduction l_1	- Program $L_1 = 100$ dB in the room - Look for the emergence threshold l_3 of the vibrating reference	- Look for the threshold of audibility by bone conduction l_2	- Program the reference l_4 - Program $L_1 = 100$ dB then decrease until emergence of the reference, and L_2 is this value
— Note l_1	— Note l_3	— Note l_2 — Calculate : $\Delta l* = l_2 - l_1$ — Calculate : $l_4 = l_3 + \Delta l$	— Note L_2 — Calculate : $\Delta L = L_1 - L_2$

<u>Figure 3.</u>   Measurement procedure (for a given frequency band). The results for each subject, are easily filed, as shown in Figure 4.

in France by this method. The complete results of 40 of them are presented in the booklet "Efficacite et confort des protecteurs individuels contre le bruit" published in 1978 by the I.N.R.S.[4]. At the time of previous tests, in 1972, 60 devices had been tested with each of the methods: one using the threshold of audibility shift, and the other using the bone conduction reference in a high ambient noise.

Generally, it had been seen that:
-   In the case of ear-plugs, the attenuations recorded at 100 dB were lower than the ones recorded at the threshold of audibility, at low frequencies. The differences disappeared from 2000 Hz upwards.
-   In the case of earmuffs, the same tendencies were present, with however smaller gaps.
-   In the case of helmets, the values were not significantly different.

Device reference :
Subject reference :
Name of operator :
Date of measurements :

	VIBRATOR					LOUDSPEAKERS			
Frequency (Hz)	Threshold with protector l_1	Threshold without protector l_2	(Eventual) correction Δl	Emergence with protector l_3	Emergence without protector l_4	Frequency (Hz)	Level without protector L_2	Level with protector L_1	Attenuation ΔL
1 500						125		100	
1 500						250		100	
1 500						500		100	
3 000						1 000		100	
—	—	—	—	—	—	—			
6 000						8 000		100	

Figure 4. Example of measurement file

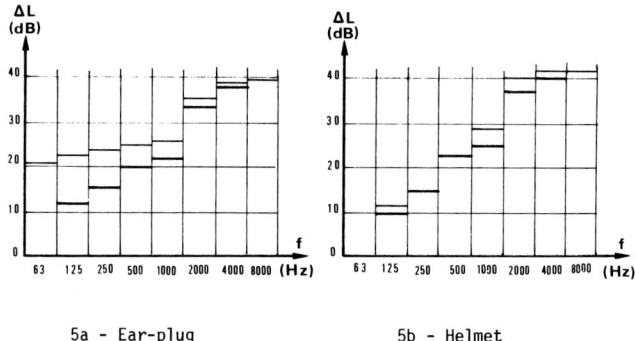

5a - Ear-plug   5b - Helmet

Figure 5. Example of attenuation recorded at threshold of audibility (thin line) and at high level (thick line)

Figures 5a and 5b show these differences in two examples.

DISCUSSION AND CONCLUSION

The method that is presented here gives largely reproducible results because of the accuracy with which the emergence point of the bone sound is detected in the airborne sound. However, the differences seen in the results, relative to the method of the threshold of audibility shift, lead to questions of the validity of one or the other method. It is our opinion that these differences may depend on the sound level at which the tests are performed. For example, at 100 dB, factors that are not relevant at the threshold of audibility, could come into play, such as the stapedial reflex or some other non-linear mechanisms. In such a case, the tests that are performed in an ambiance of 100 dB are more representative of the real conditions of the protectors' usage among an industrial population than the ones performed at the hearing threshold. It also seems difficult to us to admit that an ear-plug, whatever it is, could give an attenuation of 25 dB and more in the 125 Hz frequency band. Complementary tests have been attempted with an experimental set-up which allows simultaneously taking the ear-plugs out of the auditory canal and lowering the sound level in the room, until there is an impression of a similar loudness: the values then measured were closer to the 10 to 15 dB obtained through our supraliminary method than to the 25 dB obtained through the threshold of audibility shift method. The problem of these differences is worthy of study by research workers who can afford time and the necessary means. As each of the methods mentioned may lead to a controversy, it would be necessary to call for other methods, and eventually for more sophisticated ones, in order to decide between them. Supraliminary methods that have already been formerly tested, could then be resumed, such as the stapedial reflex shift measurement, the measurement of the noise which, without protector, gives the same temporary threshold shift, as the noise perceived with the protector. . . Measurement procedures using more recent techniques could also be set, especially with electrophysiological techniques.

REFERENCES
1.   Meij G.V., Hendrikse W.J., Breed J.A., Standardized Loudness Balance Method of Determining Attenuation of Ear Protectors, South African Bureau of Standards -Pretoria *

2.   AFNOR - norme enregistree NF S 31 062, Mesure de l'affaiblissement de perception sonore apporté par les protecteurs individuels contre le bruit (méthode subjective supraliminaire), AFNOR, Septembre 1978.

3.   ISO - projet de norme internationale ISO/DIS 4869 Acoustique - Mesurage de l'affaiblissement acoustique des protecteurs individuels contre le bruit - Methode subjective. ISO - 1977.

4.   Damongeot A., Lataye R., Krawsky G., Lievin D., Englert M., Efficacite et confort des protecteurs individuels contre le bruit. Travail et Securite, I.N.R.S., 361-381, mai/juin 1978.

*   Document with no date. It was handed to the members of the ISO/TC43/SC1/WG17 working group in 1975.

… *Personal Hearing Protection in Industry*, edited by P. W. Alberti, Raven Press, New York ©

14   SINGLE-NUMBER PERFORMANCE FACTORS FOR HEARING PROTECTORS

Paul L. Michael

INTRODUCTION

Prior to 1960 most hearing conservationists in the United States used octave band (O.B.) measurements of sound pressure level for describing potentially harmful noise exposures. Most of the damage risk criteria and personal hearing protector calculation procedures, were also based on O.B. data. An example of the so-called Long Method for calculating exposure levels under hearing protectors is shown in Table I, where protected and unprotected exposure levels are presented in octave bands.

The use of O.B. exposure levels is easily understood and for most steady-state noise exposures they afford adequate spectral detail, or resolution, with a reasonable number of measurements. However, octave band measurements are difficult or impractical to obtain with simple and inexpensive equipment when noise levels vary significantly in short time periods. The need for a single-number, overall measure of rapidly changing exposure levels became obvious in the mid to late 1960's during the development of workplace noise exposure regulations. In effect, a compromise was made at that time to exchange the detailed spectral information obtained with O.B. data for the practical advantage in measuring non-steady noise levels provided by the single-number procedure.

The use of single-number measurements of exposure led to the development of single-number performance descriptors for hearing protectors that are calculated with so-called Short Method calculations. The advantage of using single-number factors for both exposure measurement and protector performance is readily apparent from a comparison of the calculations in Tables I and II. The development and general use of the

221

single-number descriptors for hearing protector performance in the United States is the major focus of this paper.

Most hearing protector performance calculations, using Long or Short Methods, make use of adjustments for differences in attenuation values that can be expected between wearings on a given person or on different persons. Standard deviations around mean attenuation measurement data have been used for this purpose because of economic and various practical considerations. Standard procedures for developing these mean and standard deviation values were first specified by the American National Standards Institute (ANSI) in 1957 (ANSI Z24.22-1957)[1] and more recently in 1974 (ANSI S3.19-1974)[2].

Although most hearing protector attenuation measurements were made according to the ANSI Z24.22-1957 specifications in the period from 1957 to 1972, very little use was made of the standard deviation values. Suggestions to manufacturers and users of hearing protectors that standard deviations be used to afford a greater safety factor were generally ignored until the writer suggested this in a paper presented at a Mining Congress Meeting held in Cleveland in 1972.[3,4] In this paper it was suggested that two standard deviations could be subtracted from each mean attenuation value as shown in Table I to afford approximately 98 percent confidence limit instead of the 50 percent afforded by mean values (see Figure 1). Several mixed responses were received from this suggestion. A few protector manufacturers claimed the use of standard deviations would put them out of business while others welcomed the opportunity to show the superiority of their products. Most comments indicated that a one standard deviation adjustment would be more realistic than the two proposed.

A meeting with representatives of the American National Standards Institute (ANSI) Z-137 writing group, the U.S. Bureau of Mines (BOM), the U.S. National Institute for Occupational Safety and Health (NIOSH), and the U.S. Department of Labor (OSHA) was held following the Mining Congress meeting to develop a unified approach to this problem. The

Table 1: Sample calculations using the Long Method to determine the A-weighted sound exposure level under a given hearing protector that is used in a noise whose octave band levels have been measured.

COMPUTATION OF THE A-WEIGHTED NOISE EXPOSURE LEVELS

Octave Band Center frequency in Hz	125	250	500	1000	2000	4000 (1)	8000 (2)	
1. Measured octave band exposure levels in dB	98	100	101	101	98	94	88	
2. "A" weighting adjustments in dB	-16.1	-8.6	-3.2	0	+1.2	+1.0	-1.1	
3. Unprotected ear "A" weighted levels step #1 - step #2 in dB	81.9	91.4	97.8	101.0	99.2	95.0	86.9	$\Sigma = 105.1 dB^{(3)}$
4. Mean attenuation in dB at frequency	12	17	25	33	34	42	25	
5. Standard deviations in dB times 2	4	6	8	10	10	4	4	
6. Protected ear weighted levels in dB	73.9	80.4	80.8	78.0	75.2	57.0	65.9	$\Sigma = 85.5 dB^{(3)}$

[1] Average of 3000 and 4000 Hz values
[2] Average of 6000 and 8000 Hz values
[3] Use logarithms to determine dB sums

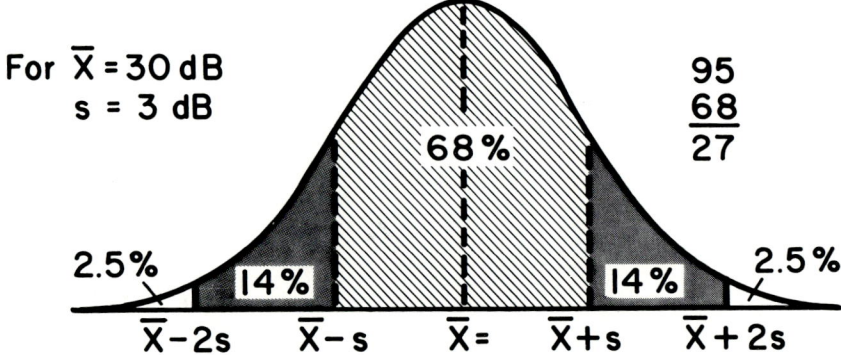

Figure I. Percentage of attenuation values for normally distributed set of data.

argument was made that an adjustment of one standard deviation would afford nearly the same confidence limits for protection as does the present OSHA noise exposure limits which are based on a dose equivalent to an A-weighted noise level of 90 decibels (dB) over an eight-hour period. The final consensus of the group, however, was that two standard deviations should be used to remove as much uncertainty as possible. A strong argument for the use of the more conservative two standard deviation adjustment was that the protection afforded in actual use is generally less than that measured in the laboratory. Since this time, most proposed Long and Short Methods for protector performance calculations have used two standard deviation adjustments.

Other than the standard deviation adjustments, Long Method calculations have changed very little in the past 11 years. There have been, however, several different Short Methods proposed that differ in both philosophy of use and in confidence limits for protection of the wearer. The Short Method for calculating single-performance descriptors for hearing protectors was first proposed by the Z-137 writing group in unpublished drafts of a proposed standard more than 10 years ago. This standard, which is intended to supplement the current ANSI S3.19-1974 Standard, has yet to be published although another "final" draft has been circulated recently.

The intended purpose of Short Method calculations in the beginning was to provide for the user a simple means for determining single-number (A-weighted) exposure levels while wearing specified protectors. In particular, the Short Method was intended for use when only A-weighted exposure levels are available, or more specifically when octave band data are not available (see Table II). The Long Method was generally recognized as the preferred method when octave band data were available because of its better accuracy. In the years following its introduction, however, the Short Method has become more complex and more importance has been placed on it as a primary descriptor of hearing protector performance.

Table II: An example of the use of hearing protector single-number performance factors.

Measured A-weighted Exposure Level to Unprotected Ear	102 dB
Minus the Single Number Protector Performance Factor	19 dB
A-weighted Exposure to Protected Ear	83 dB

THE DEVELOPMENT OF SINGLE-NUMBER DESCRIPTORS

The first step in the development of a single-number (Short Method) calculation procedure is to assume a noise exposure spectrum. In most cases a pink noise spectrum (equal sound pressure levels in octave bands) has been assumed because this spectrum correlates reasonably well with many industrial noises.[5] Other proposed spectra based on selected samples of industrial noises[6] have scientific merit but since the advantage is small considering the effects of other variables, pink noise spectra continue to be used for most calculations.

The absolute level assumed for each octave band is not critical because this number cancels out in the single-number calculations. In most cases, however, 100 dB is assigned for each octave band level as shown in Table III.

The next step in a Short Method calculation is to adjust each O.B. level of the assumed spectrum with the frequency weighting used for measuring or limiting noise exposures. In most cases the A-frequency weighting is used as shown in lines 2 and 3 of Table III. The logarithmic sum of the adjusted values shown in line 3 provides the assumed A-weighted exposure to unprotected ears. The exposure levels for each octave band under the hearing protector (line 6) is determined by subtracting the mean attenuation values (line 4) from the corresponding adjusted octave band levels (line 3) and adding two standard deviations (line 5). The logarithmic sum of the octave band levels in line 6 provides the assumed overll A-weighted sound pressure level under the protector.

A number of different procedures have been used to develop single-number descriptors following the calculations shown in Table III. The National Institute for Occupational Safety and Health (NIOSH)[7], the Mining Enforcement and Safety Administration (MESA)[8], the ANSI Z-137 writing group, and others have proposed specific calculation procedures similar to those in Table III but with modifications and adjustments that lead to single-number values having a range of several dB for any given protector. The confusion caused to both users and suppliers of hearing protectors has been made even worse by changes in proposed methods from within some groups. The Z-137 writing group and NIOSH have each proposed at least three different procedures during the past 12 years. Further confusion has been caused by the use of the same designation (R for example) for significantly different single-number descriptors.

Recently the U.S. Environmental Protection Agency (EPA) has promulgated general provisions of a regulatory program for labelling hearing protectors that includes a specific procedure for developing a single-number descriptor, the Noise Reduction Rating (NRR). This NRR factor should reduce the confusion surrounding the use of single-number descrip-

Table III: Sample calculation of a single-number performance factor (R) based on A-weighted exposure levels.

COMPUTATION OF THE NOISE REDUCTION RATING (R)

Octave Band Centre Frequency in Hz	125	250	500	1000	2000	4000 [1]	8000 [2]	
1. Assumed Pink noise levels in dB	100	100	100	100	100	100	100	
2. "A" weighting adjustments in dB	-16.1	-8.6	-3.2	0	+1.2	+1.0	-1.1	
3. Unprotected ear "A" weighted levels, #1-#2 in dB	83.9	91.4	96.8	100	101.2	101	98.9	Σ =107dB [3]
4. Mean attenuation in dB at frequency	12	17	25	33	34	42	25	
5. Standard deviations in dB times 2	4	6	8	10	10	4	4	
6. Protected ear weighted levels; line #3 - line #4+ line #5 in dB	75.9	80.4	79.8	77.0	77.2	63.0	77.9	Σ =86.1dB [3]
7. R = Σ line #3 values - Σ line #6 values - 2dB R = 107.0 - 86.1 - 2 = 18.9dB								

---

[1] Average of 3000 and 4000 Hz values
[2] Average of 6000 and 8000 Hz values
[3] Use logarithms to determine dB sums.

tors considerably and enable meaningful comparisons of hearing protectors because by this law all protectors or their containers produced after September 27, 1980 must be labelled with the NRR factor.

SPECIFIC SINGLE-NUMBER DESCRIPTORS NOW IN USE

NIOSH, MESA (now known as the Mine Safety and Health Administration (MSHA), and EPA are responsible for the major single-number performance factors for hearing protectors in use in the United States. The EPA NRR factor can be expected to be the primary single-number descriptor used in the United States in the near future. However, some of the other single-number descriptors will still be used during the next few years so their calculation procedures will be covered briefly.

NIOSH Method 1: Three single-number noise reduction (R) factors were introduced by NIOSH in 1975.[7] The most accurate of these is determined by their Method 1 shown in Table IV. This Method requires knowledge of the unprotected octave band noise exposure levels where the protector is to be used as well as the mean and standard deviation attenuation data measured in the laboratory for the hearing protectors being considered. The calculations are similar to those of the Long Method previously described except that the NIOSH Method 1 uses the difference between overall A-weighted exposure to unprotected and protected ears to specify the R factor (line 3 - line 6) while the Long Method is used to specify the A-weighted sound level under the protector (Σline 6).

NIOSH Method 2: Method 2 is the second-most precise of NIOSH's three methods. The development of the Method 2 formula

$$R = R_c - \delta$$
$$= 5.5 - 10 \log T - \delta$$

is complex but its use is relatively simple <u>if</u> the 10 log T value is provided for the particular protector being considered. Only the C-weighted (L_C) and A-weighted (L_A) unprotected noise exposure levels must be provided to calculate $\delta = L_A - L_C$ and, in turn, the R factor. If the 10 log T term

Table IV: Sample calculation of the NIOSH Method I single-number performance factor (R) based on A-weighted exposure levels.

COMPUTATION OF THE A-WEIGHTED NOISE EXPOSURE LEVELS

Octave Band Centre Frequency in Hz	125	250	500	1000	2000	4000 [1]	8000 [2]
1. Measured octave band exposure levels in dB	98	100	101	101	98	94	88
2. "A" weighting adjustments in dB	-16.1	-8.6	-3.2	0	+1.2	+1.0	-1.1
3. Unprotected ear "A" weighted levels, #1 - #2 in dB	81.9	91.4	97.8	101	99.2	95	86.9 Σ=105.1dB[3]
4. Mean attenuation in dB at frequency	12	17	25	33	34	42	25
5. Standard deviations in dB times 2	4	6	8	10	10	4	4
6. Protected ear weighted levels in dB	73.9	80.4	80.8	78.0	75.2	57.0	65.9 Σ=85.5dB[3]
7. R = Σ #3 values - Σ #6 values = 105.1 - 85.5 = 19.6dB							

[1,2] Average of 3000, 4000 Hz values and 6000 and 8000 Hz respectively
[3] Use logarithms to determine dB sums.

is not provided for this protector it must be calculated using the A-weightings for each octave band along with the mean and standard deviation attenuation values measured in a laboratory. A 3 dB safety factor is used in Method 2 for spectral uncertainty since a pink noise exposure spectrum is assumed. The complexity of Method 2 is shown by the three pages used by NIOSH to describe its development and use as compared to one and one-half pages used to describe Method 1 which is essentially the Long Method.

NIOSH Method 3: Method 3 is the least precise of the three NIOSH methods. It uses the formula

$$R = -1.5 - 10 \log T$$

to calculate this noise reduction factor (R). As with Method 2 it is simple to use if the term 10 log T is known for the protector under consideration. As with Method 2, if 10 log T is not provided it must be calculated from the A-weightings for each octave band along with laboratory derived mean annd standard deviation data for the particular hearing protector. This R factor is computed without measured noise level data as indicated by the above formula. In use it is subtracted directly from the unprotected A-weighted exposure level at the workplace to obtain the protected exposure level. An adjustment of 8.5 dB is used for spectral uncertainty in the development of the above formula since in effect an assumption of pink noise has been made.

MESA/MSHA Method: The MESA/MSHA single-number performance (R) factor was perhaps the first to be put into practical use and is, therefore, the oldest single-number factor in wide use today. The MESA/MSHA R factor is developed using pink noise exposure as a base unprotected level as shown in Table V, but this Method does not use the laboratory derived standard deviations nor the spectral uncertainty adjustments as does the NIOSH and EPA Methods.[8] Therefore, the MESA/MSHA R factors normally will be significantly higher than those of NIOSH and EPA for the same hearing protectors. MESA/MSHA noise measurement regulations do

Table V: Computation of the MESA/MSHA A-weighted attenuations value (R-factor)

Octave Band Center Frequency in Hz	125	250	500	1000	2000	4000 (1)	8000 (2)
1. Assumed Pink noise levels in dB	100	100	100	100	100	100	100
2. "A" weighting adjustments in dB	-16.1	-8.6	-3.2	0	+1.2	+1.0	-1.1
3. Unprotected ear "A" weighted levels step #1 - step #2 in dB	83.9	91.4	96.8	100	101.2	101	98.9 Σ =107.0dB[3]
4. Mean attenuation in dB at frequency	12	17	25	33	34	42	25
5. Protected ear weighted levels; step #3 - step #4 in dB	71.9	74.4	71.8	67	67.2	59	73.9 Σ =79.7dB[3]
6. R = Σ step #4 values - Σ step #5 values R = 107.0 - 79.7 = 27.3dB							

[1,2] Average of 3000 and 4000 Hz values, and 6000 and 8000 Hz values respectively
[3] Use logarithms to determine dB sums.

not require L_C measurements so the $L_C - L_A$ adjustment used by NIOSH Method 2 cannot be made unless changes are made in the MESA/MSHA noise measurement procedures.

EPA Method: The EPA Noise Reduction Rating (NRR) is the single-number performance factor used for labelling hearing protectors in EPA's Noise Labelling Rule.[9] According to the amended rule all hearing protectors or their containers produced in the United States shall be labelled with the NRR factor prior to September 27, 1980.

The NRR factor is calculated using many of the same assumptions and procedures used for calculating previously described single-number factors. Table VI shows a sample calculation of the NRR factor where unprotected pink noise exposure is assumed, A-weighting spectral adjustments are made, and laboratory derived mean attenuations with two standard deviation adjustments are made to determine the protected A-weighted exposure levels. The NRR factor is then determined by subtracting the protected overall A-weighted exposure level from the unprotected overall C-weighted exposure level and adjusting this difference by three decibels to account for spectral uncertainty.

The major difference between the NRR and other calculations of single-number factors is that the A-weighted exposure under the protector is subtracted from the C-weighted unprotected level. The unprotected C-weighted level (107.9 dB) and the unprotected A-weighted level (107.0 dB) used in other calculation procedures remain constant so the difference between these levels will remain at 0.9 dB. Therefore, the EPA NRR factor calculation is essentially the same as the earlier calculation shown in Table III where the A-weighted exposure under the protector is subtracted from the A-weighted unprotected level but with an adjustment of 2.1 dB instead of 2.0 dB for spectral uncertainty.

In use, the EPA NRR factor is to be subtracted from the A-weighted exposure level to unprotected ears at the user's location to obtain the exposure level to protected ears. A caution is given that "For noise

Table VI: Computation of the Noise Reduction Rating (NRR)

	Octave Band Center Frequency in Hz	125	250	500	1000	2000	4000 [1]	8000 [2]
1.	Assumed Pink noise levels in dB	100	100	100	100	100	100	100
2.	"C" weighting adjustments in dB	.2	0	0	0	-.2	-.8	-3.0
3.	Unprotected ear "C" weighted levels in dB	99.8	100	100	100	99.8	99.2	97.0 $\Sigma = 107.9$ dB
4.	"A" weighting adjustments in dB	-16.1	-8.6	-3.2	0	+1.2	+1.0	-1.1
5.	Unprotected ear "A" weighted levels, #1 - #4 in dB	83.9	91.4	96.8	100	101.2	101	98.9 $\Sigma = 107$ dB [3]
6.	Mean attenuation in dB at freqency	12	17	25	33	34	42	25
7.	Standard deviations in dB times 2	4	6	8	10	10	4	4
8.	Protected ear weighted levels; #5 - #7 in dB	75.9	80.4	79.8	77.0	77.2	63.0	77.9 $\Sigma = 86.1$ dB [3]

9. NRR = Σ step #3 values - Σ step #8 values - 3dB
   NRR = 107.9 - Σ step #8 values - 3dB
   = 107.9 - 86.1 - 3 = 18.8 dB

[1,2] Average of 3000 and 4000 Hz values and 6000 and 8000 Hz values respectively
[3] Use logarithms to determine dB sums.

environments dominated by frequencies below 500 Hz the C-weighted environmental noise level should be used".

SUMMARY AND CONCLUSIONS

A consistent single-number hearing protector performance factor would be a useful tool for the many hearing conservation programs using single-number exposure criteria. Several single-number performance factors have been introduced but considerable confusion has resulted because a given protector may have different dB ratings from the different calculation procedures. For example, the hearing protector attenuation data used in the Tables of this paper would have a NIOSH Method 3 R factor of 12.4 dB, an EPA NRR factor of 18.8 dB, and a MSHA R factor of 27.3 dB. To add to the confusion single-number factors calculated with different procedures have in some cases been assigned the same descriptor (i.e., the R factor) and the same group may have proposed more than one single-number calculation procedure.

The EPA NRR factor should provide more consistency in reported single-number factors in the future since by law all protectors must be labelled with this number after September 27, 1981. It can be expected, however, that there will be some groups who will add additional safety factors to the NRR factor to make up for poor performance due to poor hearing conservation programs. The philosophy of whether or not the performance factors for protective equipment should include an accounting, or acceptance, of improper fitting and wearing in general use will no doubt be argued for years to come.[10] Hopefully, any further changes in single-number performance reporting will be done in a way to minimize further confusion by the users of hearing protectors.

REFERENCES

1. American Standard Method for the Measurement of the Real Ear Attenuation of Ear Protectors at Threshold, Z24.22-1957, American National Standards Institute, New York, NY, 1957.

2. American National Standard Method for the Measurement of Real Ear Protection of Hearing Protectors and Physical Attenuation of Ear Muffs, S3.19-1974, American National Standards Institute, New York, NY, 1974.

3.	Michael, P.L., Hearing Conservation. Mining Congress 15, 74-82, 1972.

4.	Lotito, F. Methods of Measuring and Rating Hearing Protector Performance. Amer. Ind. Hyg. Assoc. J., 37, 590-595, 1976.

5.	Karplus, H.B., Bonvallet, G.L., A Noise Survey of Manufacturing Industries. Amer. Ind. Hyg. Assoc. 14, 235-263, 1953.

6.	Johnson, D.L., Nixon, C.L., Simplified Methods for Estimating Hearing Protector Performance. Sound and Vibration, 8, 20-27, June 1974.

7.	List of Personal Hearing Protectors and Attenuation Data. NIOSH Technical Information. HEW-NIOSH Publication No. 76-120, Sept. 1975.

8.	Personal Communications with the Pittsburgh Technical Support Center, MESA, April 1975.

9.	Noise Labelling Requirements for Hearing Protectors. Federal Register, 40CFR Part 211, Subpart B, 56139-56147, V. 4, No. 190, Sept. 28, 1979.

10.	Michael, P.L., Bienvenue, G.R., Hearing Protector Performance -- An Update. Amer. Ind. Hyg. Assoc. J., 41, 542-646, 1980.

15 SINGLE-NUMBER NOISE-REDUCTION FACTOR OF CIRCUMAURAL HEARING PROTECTORS BY DOSIMETRY

David Y. Chung, Jorge Menyhart, and R. Patrick Gannon

INTRODUCTION

In the evolution of hearing protectors various methods have been employed to evaluate the performance characteristics of ear muffs and plugs. There are basically two approaches. One is to use an artificial head or cadaver with insert or implanted microphone, and the other one is to use live subjects. In the latter approach it is done either by measuring the real ear threshold shifts for various acoustic stimuli, or by inserting miniature probe microphone within the ear canal. Alternatively the probe microphone may be placed through the shell of an ear muff. Unfortunately, the attenuation data obtained by these two approaches often do not correlate well with each other.

There are several reasons why different methods of measurement yield uncorrelated data. One important reason is that in measuring attenuation characteristics with live subjects the protection provided by hearing protectors is dependent upon a combination of many factors: shape and size of the external ear canal, head contours around the ear, and characteristics of skin which affect the seal of the hearing protector. Since these factors vary with individuals even the same model of ear protector can yield different amounts of protection for different wearers. The live-subject approach, therefore, represents a more realistic situation.

This is one of the reasons why the ASA Z24.22-1957 and the ANSI S.19-1974 are the two preferred methods for measuring the attenuation characteristics of hearing protectors. The former standard requires free-field pure-tone threshold measurements, of ten normal-hearing listeners, three times each with and without the hearing protector in an anechoic chamber. The latter standard prescribes the use of one-third octave bands of noise presented in a semireverberant room. It seems that if the tests are conducted by careful investigators in accordance with these standards, reliable results may be obtained.

The attenuation data obtained with the Z24.22-1957 or the S.19-1974 are usually arranged in table form with dB attenuation versus frequency. This kind of data cannot be interpreted readily by untrained viewers. Also, they offer little help in the comparison of one hearing protector to the other.

This led to the development of a single-number noise-reduction factor (SNNRF) for a hearing protector. There are basically two ways to obtain a SNNRF. The first requires an octave band analysis of the actual noise spectrum, together with the attenuation and standard deviation data of the hearing protector. This method has not gained popularity because it is complex and requires flat response octave-band levels from 125 Hz through 8 kHz with an octave band analyzer. Furthermore, this method assumes that a typical industrial worker stands practically still all day, every work day at the same place.

The other way to obtain a SNNRF is to assume one or more noise spectra that would represent frequently encountered industrial noise spectra. In this way each make of hearing protector can be assigned a precalculated SNNRF. This eliminates sophisticated instrumentation and laborious calculations and facilitates the process of hearing protector selection.

Since the risk for noise damage depends not only upon the intensity level but also upon the time period of exposure, it seems that a more realistic measure for the risk of noise damage, is noise exposure and not noise level alone. This is particularly important when the noise is intermittent and changes in level. A noise dosimeter can be used to obtain a single number for a prolonged exposure to variable noise. The single-number display on the dosimeter allows the computation of an equivalent intensity level (L_{eq}) for the exposure.

It was suggested by Rood and Baines[1] that noise exposure under circumaural hearing protectors can be measured with a dosimeter. In their prototype a Knowles electret type microphone with a dimension of 8 mm x 6 mm x 1.5 mm was connected to a dosimeter with a strip conductor which was only 0.25 mm thick. The strip conductor may be passed under the ear-muff seal without causing significant leakage. Therefore, if one attaches the small microphone of a dosimeter to the inside of an ear-muff and another to the outside of the same ear-muff, one should be able to calculate the attenuation provided by the ear-muff.

In this study, this method of evaluating ear-muffs was used both in the laboratory and in the field. Three different makes of ear-muffs were used and the results are compared with the attenuation characteristics provided by the manufacturer.

METHOD

Instrumentation: The basic equipment used is a pair of dosimeters (Quest M-8), modified to suit the need of this study. They were supplied by the manufacturer, each with a ¼-inch ceramic microphone. Two modifications were made in our laboratory. One is the connection of the ¼-inch microphone to a 15 cm long, 0.5 mm thick, three-wire cable, which in turn was connected to the regular 2.5 mm thick cable. This 15 cm part of the cable was the part that passed underneath the ear-muff cushion seal. The other modification was to convert the 40 dB response range from the normal range of 80 dBA - 120 dBA to 70 dBA -110 dBA. This was easily achieved by changing a resistor. The crest factor of the dosimeters is 10 dB. These two dosimeters had an exchange ratio of 3 dB, i.e. 3 dB increase for each doubling of the exposure time. A full description of the dosimeter is given in the instruction book provided by the manufacturer. Calibration was done in a Bruel and Kjaer hearing aid test box. The two dosimeters were calibrated to be as close to each other as possible in response to tonal stimuli. The Calibration data are shown in Table I. The response curves of the two dosimeters were very similar to each other and flat to 6 kHz.

Table 1: Calibration of the two dosimeters

Frequency	$L_{eq}A$	$L_{eq}B$	Actual dB A delivered to dosimeter
125	85.2	85.2	83.9
250	91.7	91.6	91.4
500	97.0	97.1	96.8
1000	100.0	100.2	100.0
2000	101.2	101.1	101.2
4000	99.7	99.2	101.0

Hearing Protectors: Three pairs of ear-muffs of different makes were used in this study. They were all rated as A class according to C.S.A. standard Z94.2-1974. Their attenuation characteristics, provided by the manufacturers, are depicted in Figure 1.

Experiment I: Laboratory Test

Subjects: Twenty male subjects participated in this part of the experiment. These volunteers were either staff members of the Workers' Compensation Board of British Columbia (W.C.B.) or claimants petitioning the W.C.B. for noise-induced hearing loss. Their ages ranged from 28 to 64.

Stimuli: The noise source was white noise generated by a Grason-Stadler 1701 audiometer via two loudspeakers. Octave band analysis of the noise at 107 dBA at ear level in the sitting position is shown in Figure 2.

Procedure: Each subject was seated inside a double-walled I.A.C. sound insulated room three feet from each of the two speakers which were located at 45° to either side of the 12 o'clock position. The microphones

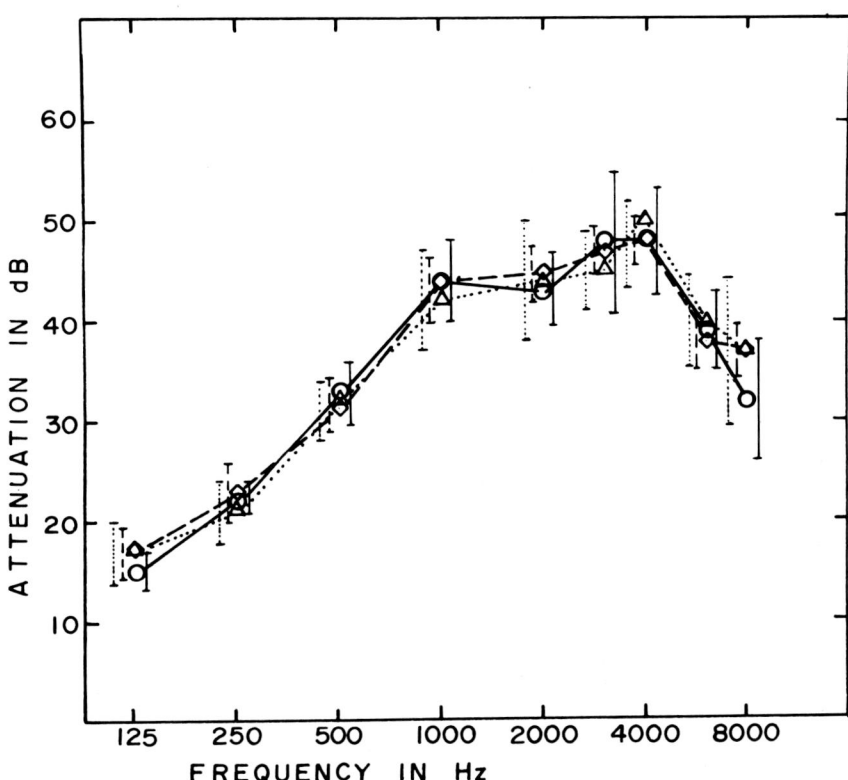

Figure 1. Attenuation characteristics of the three hearing protectors as provided by manufacturers. Hearing protector A: ◇--◇; B: ○——○; C: △···△. Vertical bars denote one standard deviation from the means.

of the dosimeters were attached to the ear-muff on the right, one inside the ear-muff, on the foam facing upwards and the other outside, on the top of the ear-muff facing forwards. The ear-muffs were then fitted carefully for maximum comfort and effectiveness. The 107 dBA noise was then turned on for a duration of five minutes and timed by a stopwatch. After the five-minute exposure, readings of the dosimeters were taken. The microphones were then reversed in position and the procedure was repeated. The readings for the four conditions, two positions x two dosimeters, were converted into L_{eq}. The average of the two difference L_{eq}'s between the outside and the inside of the muff, was considered as the attenuation provided by the muff. There were ten different subjects for each pair of ear-muffs but some of the subjects were tested with more

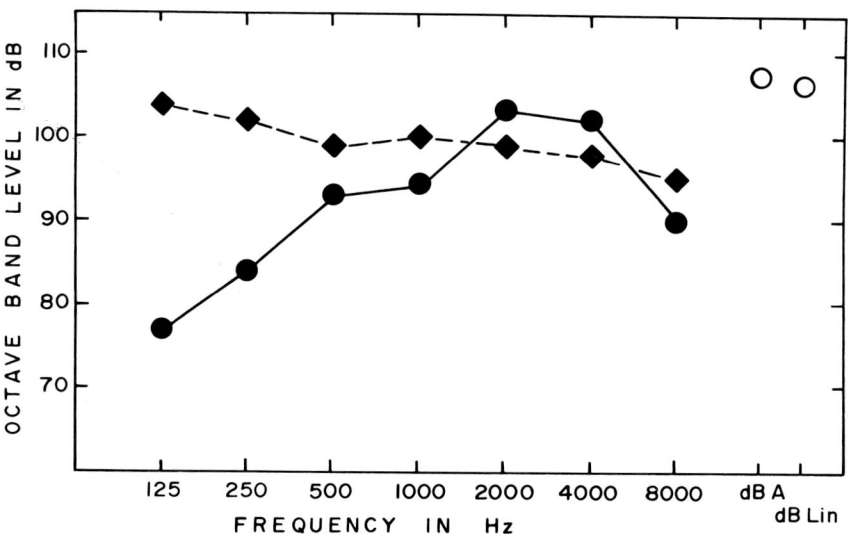

Figure 2. Octave band analyses of the laboratory noise used in this study: ●—● , and the typical noise of Tobias: ◆--◆. ○ denotes the dBA and dBLin of the laboratory noise.

than one pair of ear-muffs.

Experiment II: Field Test

Subjects: Thirty male volunteers were used in this experiment. They were workers from various plants, mainly in the lumber industry. Their ages ranged from 20 to 55. Their jobs varied from stationary ones (e.g. shingle sawyer) to very mobile ones (e.g. plant foreman).

Stimuli: The noise source in this experiment varied with the subjects position at a particular time. This represents a practical situation where a worker moves in the manner that he would normally do. The type of noise that these workers were exposed to was basically steady-state noise. The L_{eq} of the subject's exposure should be at least 90 dBA. Since the lower limit of the dosimeter was 70 dBA, any attenuation provided by the hearing protector to give a value of less than 70 dBA inside the muff, would not be registered on the dosimeter. Therefore, if the level inside the muff was consistently below 70 dBA in the field testing situation, the measurement inside the muff would tend to yield a lower L_{eq}, and hence, a slightly exaggerated attenuation number. On the other hand, peak noise levels exceeding 120 dBA will be internally clipped and act as if they were 120 dBA. In this experiment the L_{eq} in the workers studied, varied from 94 to 107 dBA.

Procedure: Typically, a subject would be called to the foreman's office during his shift and be told about the experiment by the investigator. The ear-muff-dosimeter assembly was then fitted on the subject. Any loose wire was later secured. The period of recording was dependent on the level of noise exposure. For a level of 107 dBA the dosimeter was saturated in about 10 minutes. The recording period, therefore, varied from 8 minutes for a chipper operator (107 dBA) to 30 minutes for a plant foreman (94 dBA). At the end of the recording period they were called into the foreman's office for a second time, and the positions of the two microphones were reversed, after the readings were recorded. They were then sent back to work for the same period of time at the end of which, the dosimeter readings were recorded. Three subjects were tested in each plant, one with each of the same three ear-muffs as in experiment I. The three subjects in the same plant usually had similar jobs in the same general area.

RESULTS AND DISCUSSION

The results of both experiments are shown in Table II. For comparison the table also shows the SNNRF calculated by the octave band method, assuming the laboratory noise and the "typical noise" suggested by Tobias and Johnson[2]. This typical noise is shown to be an appropriate representation of industrial noise. Attenuation characteristics used in the calculation were provided by manufacturers. It can be seen, that for all three hearing protectors, the least amount of attenuation obtained was by the field method. One has to be careful in making comparisons since the noise spectra used were different under different conditions.

When the attenuations from the laboratory data are compared with attenuations calculated with data provided by the manufacturers, assuming the laboratory noise spectrum (Figure 2) it can be seen that the former is a much smaller number than the latter. A plausible reason for this discrepancy is that no attempt was made to select subjects without glasses, and/or with short hair. Actually half of the subjects, in each of the three groups with different hearing protectors in the laboratory test, had glasses on. No significant differences, however, were found when the results of the two groups, with and without glasses, were tested by the t-test. The discrepancy also may be ascribed to the different methods used in the two cases. There is, however, no reason to believe that one method should yield results so different from the other.

Comparing the laboratory data with the field data is not a valid procedure since the noise spectra in both cases were very different. The typical noise of Tobias and Johnson was used to obtain a SNNRF for each hearing protector, with the attenuation characteristics provided by the manufacturers. Again the field data were much lower than the calculations using the typical noise. The fact that SNNRF calculated with the typical noise is much lower than that calculated with the laboratory noise, suggests that the reason the field data is lower than the laboratory data is at least partly due to the difference in noise spectra.

The important finding of this paper is not the discrepancy between the data from this study and those from manufacturers but that the hearing protectors, on the average, actually give more than 20 dB of protection in the field. Assuming that noise level below 85 dBA is "safe", the hearing protectors on the average, should be adequate for noise level below 105 dBA, if workers wear them properly. However, the standard deviations shown in Table II, suggest that there are people who actually get less than 20 dB of protection. For one subject in the field test wearing hearing protector C, the attenuation provided by the muff was only 13.5 dB. In this case, the hearing protector C did not offer adequate protection.

The question arises, how can one be satisfied that a person is obtaining adequate protection from a particular hearing protector. Different individuals have different head contours, hair style and also many of the

Table II: Means and standard deviations of attenuations provided by three hearing protectors as measured in this study. SNNRF denotes single-number noise-reduction factor and TTN, the typical noise.

Muff	Attn. in dB Lab. data	Std. dev.	Attn. in dB Field data	Std. dev.	SNNRF (Lab Noise)	SNNRF (TTN)
A	30.95	4.73	24.78	4.18	43.5	33.3
B	28.50	4.5	23.93	4.71	42.3	32.0
C	25.60	3.8	22.08	6.33	43.2	32.6

workers wear safety glasses. From our experience, it is difficult to predict which hearing protector is best for a particular individual. We feel that hearing protectors are like hearing aids; they need to be fitted. A dosimeter with the ¼-inch microphone attachment seems to be suitable for accomplishing such a task. Therefore, it is proposed that first, a large sample of circumaural hearing protectors should be tested by this method in the laboratory using a noise similar to the typical noise. Those with the highest attenuation and the lowest standard deviation would be recommended. Secondly, all workers exposed to noise levels above a certain intensity, e.g. 100 dBA, should be fitted with hearing protectors. Only those hearing protectors that reduce the level inside the muff to below 85 dBA should be given to the worker. This method also can determine whether a used pair of ear-muffs have lost some of their protective function due to hardening of the cushion seal, loosening of headband, etc.

The task of fitting is simple and can be carried out by a technician or first aid attendant. It only takes 10 to 30 minutes for testing, during which the worker would be able to work. One dosimeter with similar modifications made for this study would be adequate, since in that case all one needs to know is the noise exposure inside the muff.

The dosimeters used in this experiment are not suitable for impulsive noise since any peak noise levels exceeding 120 dBA will be internally clipped. In this respect the ear-borne sound level dosimeter described by Erlandsson et al[3] seems to have a tremendous potential for this type of measurement. The only drawback is that the read-out is not as direct as the pocket-borne dosimeter used in this study. This makes it inconvenient for practical use such as fitting of hearing protectors by technicians. The Bruel and Kjaer 4428 dosimeter seems to have the characteristics that are superior to the Quest M-8. It has a dynamic range of 60 dB and a crest factor of 30 dB. The only disadvantage of this dosimeter is its use of a ½-inch condenser microphone. This is too cumbersome to be placed inside the ear-muff.

For plants where insert-type hearing protectors are used real ear attenuation of hearing protection can be determined by specially designed circumaural headphone as used by Michael et al.[4]. Although this method of fitting involves perhaps more time loss from work than the method proposed here for circumaural hearing protectors, it also provides a reasonable estimate of the protection provided by ear plugs.

SUMMARY AND CONCLUSIONS

In this study a method of evaluating circumaural hearing protectors with the use of dosimetry is discussed. Three models of hearing protectors were used and it was found that on the average, a hearing protector would give more than 20 dB of attenuation. Since there are individual variations in head contours, head size, skin characteristics, etc., some wearers may not obtain adequate protection from a particular hearing protector. It is suggested that two measures should be taken:

(1) A laboratory test of all available models of circumaural hearing protectors should be done with a typical industrial noise. Those with the highest attenuations and the lowest standard deviations would be recommended to the industry.

(2) Workers exposed to noise levels above a certain intensity, e.g. 100 dBA, should be fitted with hearing protectors. Only those hearing protectors that reduce the level inside the muff to below 85 dBA should be given to the worker.

REFERENCES

1. Rood, C.M., Baines, D.C., A meter for the Measurement of Noise done under circumaural hearing protectors. Technical Memorandum FS

96, Royal Aircraft Establishment, 1976.

2. Tobias, J.V., Johnson, D.L., The typical noise: first step in the development of a short procedure for estimating performance of hearing protectors. J. Acoust. Soc. Amer., 63, 207-210, 1978.

3. Erlandsson, B., Hakansson, H., Ivarsson, A., Nilsson, P., Salem, B. Ear-borne sound level dosimeter. Rev. Sci. Instrum. 47, 1380-1382, 1976.

4. Michael, P.L., Kerlin, R.L., Bienvenue, G.R., Prant, J.H., Shampan, J.I. A real-ear field method for the measurement of the noise attenuation of insert-type hearing protectors. DHEW Publication No. (NIOSH) 76-181, June, 1976.

5. Edwards, R.G., Hanser, W.P., Moisecv, N.A., Brodersen, A.B., Green, W.W., Lempert, B.L. A Field investigation of noise reduction afforded by insert-type hearing protectors. DHEW Publication No. (NIOSH) 79-115, November, 1978.

16
The Advantages of Supplementing Conventional Static Noise Analysis Measurements with Personalized Sound Exposure Analysis

G. E. Menzies and R. F. Winn

INTRODUCTION

In industrial noise surveys, the aim of the sound measurement is to determine high noise areas and when possible, identify those occupations which potentially have excessive exposure. However, the accurate measurement of an employee's sound exposure has not previously been performed due to the absence of acceptable measuring devices.

In conventional sound surveys undertaken in the past two decades, a wide variety of instrumentation has been used, many different measuring techniques employed and several methods of reporting utilized, but all have proven to have deficiencies for establishing realistic occupational exposure. With the introduction of the <u>miniature</u> programmable sound dosimeter, one type of which has been used at Stelco for the past 18 months, it is now possible to measure noise accurately at the employee's ears, throughout his working area and over the entire shift. By correlating these results, over a broad base of industrial situations, it is possible to produce far more accurate sound exposure records than presently exist.

This paper discusses the advantage of using personalized hearing analyses over conventional static measurements in the accurate determination of an employee's potential noise exposure.

HISTORY

Since excessive noise was first recognized as a problem in the steel industry, our company's goal has been to protect the employees against the hazards of noise-induced hearing damage. To achieve this objective, a

Hearing Conservation Program was initiated in 1958 at the various Stelco plants, including the Hilton Works in Hamilton, Ontario, which is an integrated steel making and finishing facility with over 12,500 bargaining-unit employees.

At this plant, there is a wide variety of noise, most of it non-continuous in nature. There is a varied product mix and continual technological changes; many employees move around considerably in the performance of their duties. There has thus always been a problem in obtaining accurate representative noise exposure records for employees from year to year.

Initially, in 1958, noise was measured as a single overall dB level. Octave band surveys appeared in the early 60's, which were useful in the active engineering control aspect of our program, but did little to improve the measuring and understanding of occupational noise exposures. In the mid 60's, with a change in the Ontario Regulations for protection against excessive noise, the technique of using Average Speech Frequency (ASF) readings, that is, the average noise level in the three speech frequency octaves of 500, 1,000 and 2,000 Hertz, was used to identify the maximum levels permissible for eight hours exposure. Beginning with the 70's, our measuring concept changed again and dB(A) levels were obtained. This particular change, although intended to simplify things, confused those employees who had been exposed to extensive educational programs involving the ASF concept.

In the early 70's, most measurements consisted of short-term observations by a noise technician at specific stationary locations. Experience generally proved that in the presence of variable noise, the technician recorded, in most cases, a noise level which overstated the employee's exposure.

It became apparent that better methods and new instrumentation needed to be developed in order to establish the noise level more accurately over extended periods of time.

In the mid 70's, noise level analyzers (L_{eq} meters) were introduced into our program, and this made it possible to measure, on a geographical basis, noise over many hours and without operator interpretation.

At about the same time (mid 70's) another concept of measuring noise over time was introduced -- personal dosimeters. These early single reading outlet units appeared to be the ideal method needed to fulfill our requirements for measuring an employee's noise exposure in the variable setting characteristic of a steel industry. The microphone could be located adjacent to the employee's ears, it could accompany him throughout his normal working environment and could be worn for long periods of time. However, this concept had a rather limiting factor -- unless the employee was observed by a noise technician throughout his shift, there was no assurance that the level obtained was representative of his "typical" noise exposure. To the employee being tested, the whole procedure seemed to indicate that a "time study" was in progress. The instrument manufacturers were aware of the poor customer acceptance, hence, it became natural for a significantly improved dosimeter to be introduced, that is, microcomputerized noise dosimetry with hard-copy documentation.

This particular dosimeter system has been used at Stelco for the past 18 months and supplements the Hearing Conservation Program in several ways, which include the following:

1. It reduces significantly the need for personal observation by noise technicians.
2. Several units can be installed simultaneously, reducing staff work further.
3. The dosimeter is light-weight, small and can be worn comfortably by the employee for long periods of time.
4. Hard-copy documentation of various parameters, such as L_{eq}, L_{OSHA}, L_{OSHA} with specific cut-offs and exceedance levels, is provided for each occupation when the dosimeter is integrated with the printer.
5. System error or employee interference is documented on the

print-out.
6. Future changeability in the parameters being measured -simply by changing the "chip" in the dosimeter.
7. Versatility of the dosimeter function - it can also be used as a stationary noise level analyzer.

As with any instrumentation, there are limitations which must be recognized. These units are Type II measuring devices and do not respond with the same accuracy as Type I sound level meters. However, through our own comparative studies, we are satisfied that the readings are within acceptable standards for our program (Table 6). In fact, they provide useful information over a much broader base of noise situations than has ever been achieved in the past. The following examples will illustrate the advantages of personal hearing analysis over conventional static measurements.

COMPARISON BETWEEN STATIC AND DOSIMETER RESULTS
Static Measurements
In conventional geographical surveys, stationary noise level tests are taken at specific locations throughout a mill, power house, etc., and the levels obtained are used in the preparation of a noise map which delineates those areas where hearing protection is a posted requirement. Engineering noise controls and administrative controls are also recommended at this time.

This is a simplistic description of the geographical survey and it should be appreciated that factors such as varying product mix, nature of the noise (continuous, non-continuous, impulsive) and operating conditions are all taken into account prior to the final preparation of this noise map.

Described below are three cases which illustrate several factors which must be appreciated in any geographical noise measurement program. Two of the examples will include a historical look into the type of measuring devices and the parameters measured in the past.

Case 1 - Steady Noise: Coating Line - Operator's Station

Prior to 1980, very few changes had been made in this facility. The noise at the coating area has consistently exceeded 90 dB. The noise levels measured at the Operator's Station, for the same product, during the last eleven years are shown in Table 1.

Table 1: Steady Noise Levels Measured at The Operator's Station, Coating Line

Year	Type of noise measuring equipment used	Technician Recording instantaneous noise levels				Instrument compiling time weighted noise levels
		dB (ASF)	dB (L)	dB (C)	dB (A)	L_{eq} dB(A)
1967	Sound level meter (II), octave band Filter	96.5				
1968	Sound level meter (II)		99	98	97	
1973	Sound level meter (II)				96.5	
1977	Noise level analyzer (I)					95.3 (20 min. test)
1978	Sound level meter (II)				95	
1978	Noise level analyzer (I)					96.9 (20 min. test)

In the past eleven years, regardless of the measuring instrument or technique employed, the noise level has remained essentially the same. This is a result of the continuous nature of the noise in this area.

Case 2 - Varying Noise: Primary Rolling Mill

Continuous noise is the exception rather than the rule at Stelco. Judgment is required to estimate an employee's exposure by using the results obtained from stationary noise level tests conducted in a non-continuous noise environment. The data presented in Table 2 shows the wide variation of noise levels measured, as well as the noise parameters

Table 2: Varying Noise Levels Measured at One Test Location in a Primary Rolling Mill

Year	Type of noise measuring equipment used	dB (ASF)	dB (L)	dB (C)	dB (A)	L_{eq} dB(A)
1963	Sound level meter (II)	105				
1965	Sound level meter (II)			100		
1966	Sound level meter (II) octave band filter	103	108	108		
1966	Sound level meter (II)			104		
1969	Sound level meter (II) octave band filter	86	100	97	91	
1976	Sound level meter (II)				94 to 99	
1976	Noise level analyzer (I)					94.4 (20 min. test)
1978	Sound level meter (II)				92 to 102	
1980	Dosimeter (II)					92.9 (7 hrs.46 min. test)

measured, during the last 17 years at essentially one specific test location.

With the advances in instrument technology, specifically, the noise level analyzer, noise over time in a non-continuous noise environment is much improved. However, in this phase of our measurement program, noise levels at specific work stations are still being measured.

Case 3 - Varying Product Mix: Coating Line - Operator's Station

Another parameter which must be understood, in addition to the actual measurement of noise in continuous or non-continuous environments, is the variable product mix of a process. Table 3 illustrates this situation.

Table 3: Noise Levels Measured for three different Products at Various Locations along the Coating Line

Location Casting Area	Product A	Product B	Product C
15 feet NE	91.5 dB(A)	92.5 dB(A)	95.0 dB(A)
15 feet E	88.5 dB(A)	91.0 dB(A)	93.0 dB(A)
20 feet NW	88.5 dB(A)	92.0 dB(A)	95.5 dB(A)
25 feet NE	91.5 dB(A)	91.0 dB(A)	95.0 dB(A)
40 feet E	87.5 dB(A)	89.5 dB(A)	91.5 dB(A)

Even though steady noise exists, the variation in the product being coated causes up to a 7 dB(A) change over the course of just a few weeks.

Geographical surveys will continue to be useful in gathering noise data for use in posting of "excessive noise areas" and for the evaluation of engineering and administrative controls. However, they will be of limited use in determining potential employee noise exposure over a typical eight hour shift.

Dosimeter Measurements

The programmable dosimeter system has only been in use at Stelco for the past 18 months. Employees performing specific occupations are provided with a personal dosimeter which they wear throughout their shift. The objective of this part of our program is to identify those occupations for which potential exposure to noise exceeds our maximum exposure guideline. These studies identify "high risk" occupations and these are reported to the departments affected.

With this important new measurement tool, accurate information, useful for establishing a cause and effect relationship, will now be available to those involved in hearing conservation.

The overestimation and underestimation of employee noise exposure, as a result of static measurements, has already been indicated by dosimeter studies. The following are two examples.

Case I - Furnace Operation: Static vs. Dosimeter Values (Overestimating)

The most common occurrence is to overestimate employee exposure through a geographical survey. For many employees, their assigned work station is located in a posted noise area, yet the work practice may result in the employee being in this posted area for relatively short periods of time; the majority of the time is spent in quieter areas such as control rooms, lunchrooms, washrooms, offices, etc.

The noise levels on the operating floor of one of our large furnaces exceed 90 dB(A). Hearing protection is mandatory for employees working in this area. However, under the noise dose guideline, $L_{OSHA\ (90)}$, no employee is subjected to an eight hour average exposure of greater than 90 dB(A), as is shown in Table 4.

Table 4: Static and Dosimeter Measurements on the Operating Floor of a Large Furnace

Occupation	Dosimeter Values $L_{OSHA\ (90)}$ dB(A)	Static Values dB(A)
1	84	91 to 95
2	73	91 to 95
3	84	91 to 95
4	86	91 to 95
5	71	91 to 95

Considering the short duration dB(A) measurement program typical of industry today and assuming that $L_{OSHA\ (90)}$ provides a realistic measurement of an employee's noise exposure, then the company is potentially overestimating this exposure as well as overprotecting their employees in relation to existing regulations.

Case 2 - Mobile Equipment: Static vs. Dosimeter Values (Underestimating)

In our testing of large mobile equipment, such as, tractor trailers and ingot carriers, one dosimeter is placed in the cab (acts as a stationary noise level meter) and the second dosimeter is attached to the driver. Several tests, on different shifts, are taken for each occupation involved in order to approach normal working conditions as closely as possible. The duration of most of these tests is some 7 to 8 hours.

Our noise technician accompanies the operator of the vehicle for a period of about 30 minutes at the beginning of the shift, at which time, noise levels representing various operating conditions are measured (for example, idling, high RPM, normal driving, loading, unloading, etc.). Generally, the noise levels recorded inside the cab vary from 75 to 95 dB(A). The results of the concurrent occupational and equipment noise measurements are shown in Table 5.

Table 5: Static and Dosimeter Measurements in the Cab and on the Driver of Four Different Types of Mobile Equipment

Unit	Test Location	$L_{OSHA(90)}$ dB(A) Dosimeter Values	Static Values
Stake	Driver	80.7	
	Cab		74.4
Disposal Truck	Driver	78.0	
	Cab		75.2
Large Float	Driver	73.9	
	Cab		66.5
Tractor Trailer	Driver	72.5	
	Cab		60.2

The noise levels encountered by the drivers are consistently higher than those recorded from the stationary dosimeter studies performed inside the cab. This is because the operator of the unit must occasionally leave the truck, whereas, the stationary dosimeter records only the level in the cab.

Two other components in our measurement program are important to note at this time, namely, dosimeter accuracy and employee co-operation.

Dosimeter Accuracy

The noise levels obtained from the dosimeters are reasonably accurate. To verify this fact, several twenty minute studies were performed in different types of noise to check the dosimeter readings with those of a Type I noise level analyzer. Table 6 lists these results.

Table 6: Comparative Study between the Noise Levels Obtained from a Dosimeter and those Recorded on a Noise Level Analyzer in Different Types of Noise

	Type of Noise	Parameter Measured	Noise Analyzer (type I)	Dosimeter (type II)
a)	Steady	L_{eq}	79.4 dB(A)	79 dB(A)
		L_I	83.0 dB(A)	84 dB(A)
b)	Continuous, but varies widely	L_{eq}	87.2 dB(A)	86 dB(A)
		L_I	92.8 dB(A)	93 dB(A)
c)	High energy impacts, high background noise	L_{eq}	90.6 dB(A)	89 dB(A)
		L_{MAX}	106.0 dB(A)	108 dB(A)
d)	High energy impacts, low background noise	L_{eq}	91.0 dB(A)	89 dB(A)
		L_{MAX}	110.0 dB(A)	110 dB(A)

EMPLOYEE CO-OPERATION

Employee co-operation has been excellent. More than 500 individual tests have been completed and documented. The success rate is approximately 90% as is indicated in Figure 1. Of the 10% of the tests which have not been considered to be acceptable, 7% can be attributed to mechanical failure and 3% to employee problems.

These figures clearly indicate that the co-operation from our bargaining

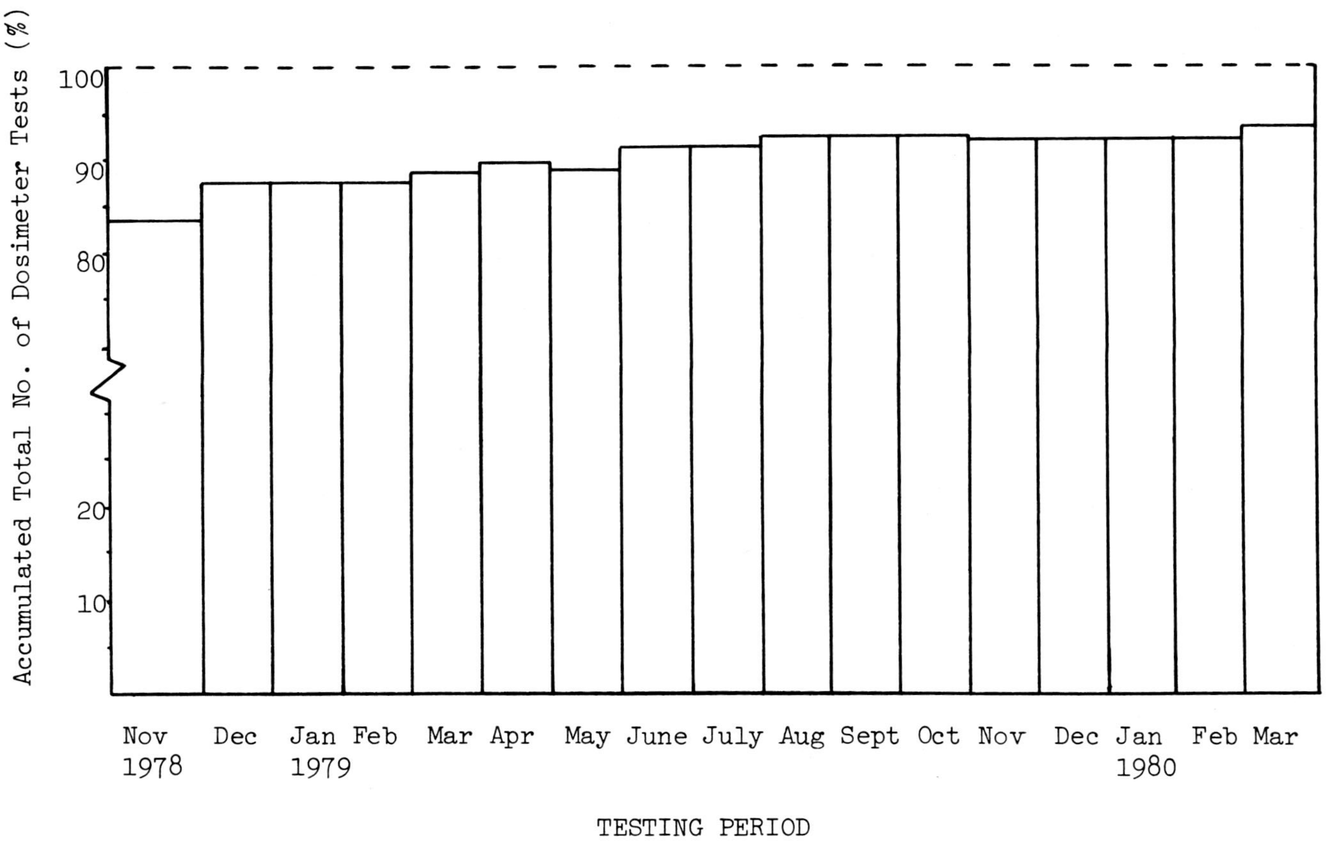

Figure 1. Success Rate of Stelco's Occupational Noise Survey Program

unit employees has been outstanding. For more than 10 years, our employees have been very aware of the various phases in our Hearing Conservation Program and realize that the testing which they are participating in will benefit them.

The key to this success is that nothing is hidden or appears to be hidden from the employee. Before each test, the purpose and the operation of the dosimeter is explained fully to them. The results of the test, if they so desire, are shown to the employee along with an explanation. Finally, all tests are voluntary and if, for any reason, the employee feels uncomfortable wearing the dosimeter, this fact is accepted and the noise technician finds another employee performing the same occupation.

The following points are significant, relative to our occupational noise survey program.

1. With the introduction of the programmable dosimeter system, it is now possible to measure accurately an employee's potential noise exposure on his job throughout a typical shift (assuming ear protection was not being worn in posted areas).
2. There are approximately 1,800 different occupations at our particular plant. A knowledge of the duties for each occupation is time consuming but necessary when it comes to interpreting the hard-copy results.
3. A knowledge of the process and the product mix is needed prior to studying each occupation. With so many different operations in the steel complex, it takes time to understand the particular jargon involved in each phase of the process.
4. The noise readings from the personal dosimeters are sufficiently accurate, for our program.
5. Employee co-operation has resulted in greater than 90% of the dosimeter tests being considered successful.

Conclusions

The programmable dosimeter system is now an integral part of our Hearing Conservation Program. With this sytem it is now possible to measure accurately noise at the employee's ears, throughout his working area and over his entire shift. By correlating the results from these occupational studies, with the data obtained from the geographical surveys, it is helping to ensure that STELCO employees have the maximum hearing protection, that the Hearing Conservation Program will meet and exceed government noise regulations, and that employees' hearing is preserved.

Personal Hearing Protection in Industry, edited by P. W. Alberti, Raven Press, New York ©

17 THE EFFECTIVE ATTENUATION OF HEARING PROTECTORS AS A FUNCTION OF WEARING TIME

Roland Tengling and Rune Lundin

There are many factors which influence the choice of a hearing protector, including attenuation, price, weight, comfort and disposability. Attenuation is frequently considered the most important: for the Safety Officer high attenuation may mean a good protector and for the buyer high attenuation may mean low cost per decibel of noise reduction but this is only true if the protector is worn.

Clearly a hyper-effective protector that is too uncomfortable to use, defeats its purpose.

RISK

As shown by Robinson (1968)[1] the risk for occupational deafness can be predicted from the total A-weighted noise dose received by the exposed person during the working day (Leq), and the effectiveness of a hearing protector is governed more by its ability to reduce the total A-weighted noise dose rather than the instantaneous sound level. When calculating equivalent continuous sound levels we know that even very short periods of high noise levels will have a dramatic effect on the Leq.

Two examples illustrate this point.

In the first example a man is subjected to the soundpattern shown in fig. 1, namely 95 dB(A) for 5 hours, 105 dB(A) for 45 minutes and 115 dB(A) for 10 minutes. For the remainder of the day the sound level is 70 dB(A) and can be safely ignored. The Leq is 100 dB(A).

In the second example a man wears hearing protectors practically the

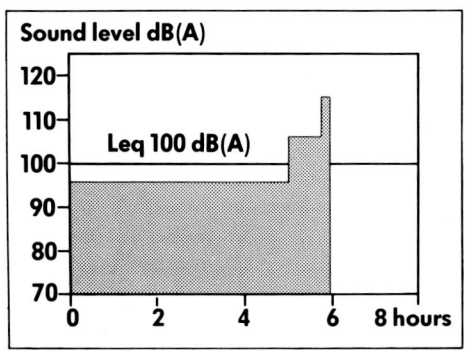

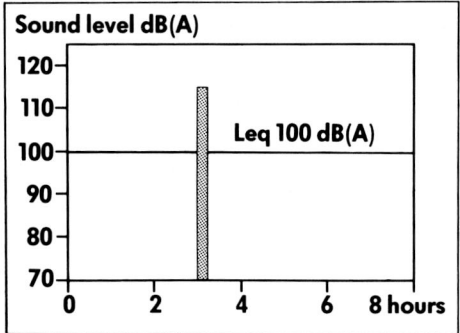

Figures 1 and 2. Examples of noise exposure in dB(A) as a function of time.

whole day in a steady noise level of 115 dB(A). The protectors are capable of attenuating the sound to the maximum permitted level, but the man removes them for a few minutes at a time - in all 16 minutes per day. He would then be exposed to the same hearing damage risk as if he went with unprotected ears in a continuous sound level of 100 dB(A) during an 8-hour day. In other words, only 16 minutes a day without protectors in a 115 dB(A) noise level is equivalent to the same noise dosage as the first example, Leq 100 dB(A)!

The danger of wearing hearing protectors for only part of the noise exposure time is not readily appreciated. The fact that the unit of sound level, the decibel, is based on a logarithmic scale is perhaps the main reason for this. Unless one knows exactly when intermittent periods of extremely intense noise may occur, protectors must be worn at all times.

EFFECT OF REMOVING PROTECTORS

The foregoing examples show that relatively short exposures to high noise levels involve a serious risk of hearing damage. It has also been shown that the effective protection of hearing protectors can be expressed in terms of the reduction in Leq achieved by the wearing of them.

Else (1973)[2] has previously demonstrated that the removal of hearing protectors for short periods during noise exposure seriously reduces the protection afforded by the protectors. This effect is illustrated in fig. 3.

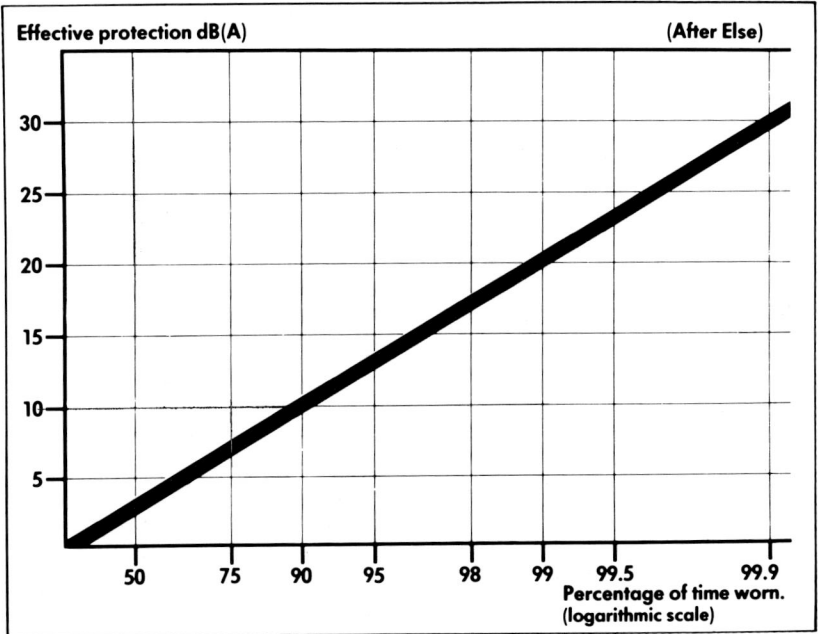

Figure 3. The protection in dB(A) as a function of the percentage of the expsoure duration for which the hearing protectors are worn.

The hearing protector is assumed to provide infinite attenuation - no sound energy at all reaches the ears while they are worn.

For example, take an exposure with an equivalent continuous noise level (Leq) of 107 dB(A). From the graph fig. 3 it can be seen that to reduce the Leq to 90 dB(A) - or by 17 dB(A) - infinite attenuation protectors would have to be worn for as much as 98% of the total exposure time. Consider another situation where the Leq is 105 dB(A) and the theoretical protectors are used for 90% of the exposure time. The graph shows that despite the infinite attenuation of the protectors the actual protection achieved is insufficient - no more than 10 dB(A).

The practical result of these findings is further illustrated in comparing two contrasting types of hearing protectors. One is a "super" muff with high attenuation, particularly in the low frequency range. The other is of the insert type. For convenience, we have used the attenuation data for a mineral down earplug which is generally accepted as a comfortable protector but with relatively low attenuation. The effective protection curves for the respective protectors are shown in figures 4 and 5. It can be seen that if the "super" muffs were to be removed for 10% of the noise exposure, the effective protection would be no more than 10 dB at all frequencies. And there is every reason to assume that they would be removed - frequently and for long periods. To begin with, high attenuation muffs - practically by definition - are uncomfortable to wear for any length of time. Moreover, because of their high attenuation at speech frequencies, and the way they affect normal hearing, i.e. impair sound localisation, there would be a tendency to take them off during conversations. As the mineral down plugs (figure 5) have none of the inherent disadvantages of "super" muffs, they are more likely to be used for the entire exposure time. Their nominal attenuation values would then be the same as their effective protection, with high attenuation of the high-frequency components of the noise, but with limited low frequencies performance.

THE PRACTICAL NOISE SITUATION
Frequency spectra vary greatly in industry. Consequently the protection provided by a given protector will also vary.

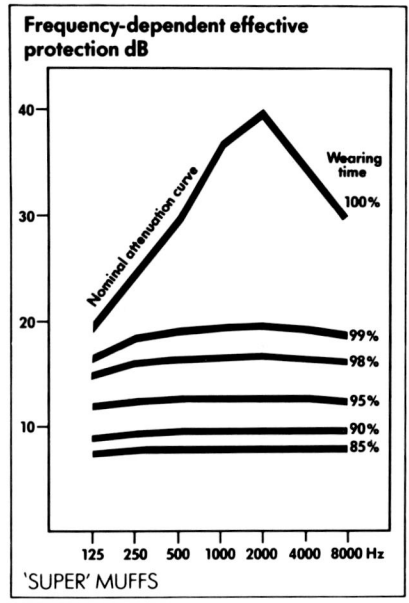 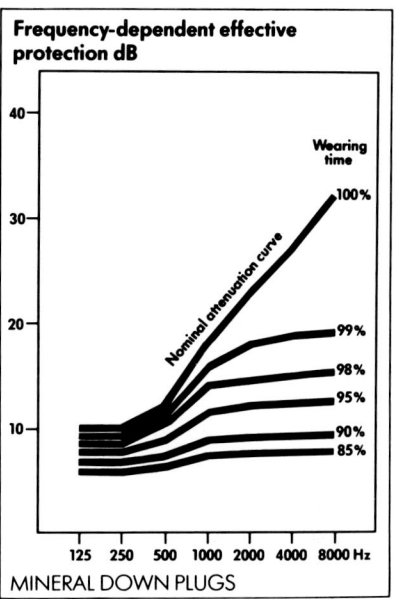

Figures 4 and 5. Effective protection curves for 'Super' muffs and mineral down plugs. The attenuation values for both protectors are as tested by Karolinska Institutet in Stockholm, the upper limit of the lower quartile being taken as the nominal attenuation. The formula used to obtain the frequency dependent effective protection in relation to the time worn is as follows;

$$\Delta L_{eff} = -10 \log \left[\frac{t2}{T} \cdot 10^{\frac{-\Delta L}{10}} + \frac{t1}{T} \right]$$

where:
ΔL_{eff} = the effective protector
ΔL = the nominal attenuation of the hearing protector
t1 = exposure duration without hearing protector
t2 = exposure duration with hearing protector
T = t1 + t2 = total duration of noise exposure

In figure 6 the A-weighted sound levels of 100 noise spectra have been plotted against the difference between their C-weighted and A-weighted sound levels ($L_C - L_A$). The greater the difference, the more powerful the low-frequency components and vice versa. The spectra are those selected

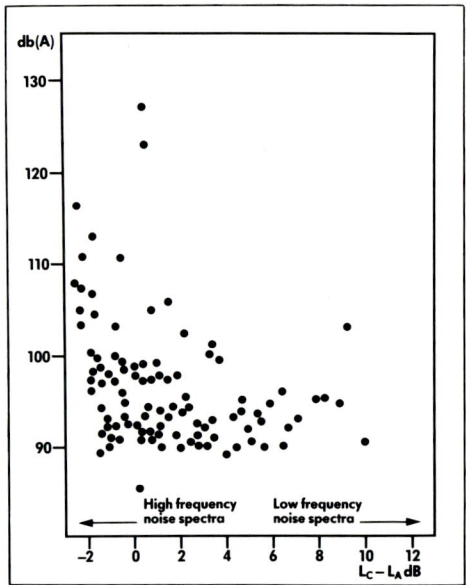

Figure 6. A-weighted sound levels of 100 NIOSH noise spectra as a function of the difference between their C-weighted and A-weighted sound levels (L_C-L_A).

by the National Institute for Occupational Safety and Health (NIOSH) as being typical for industry in the USA. They are chosen from the 579 noise spectra published by Karplus and Bonvallet (1953)[3] for which the octave levels were presented by Johnson and Nixon (1974)[4]. Waugh (1973)[5] has also published 619 spectra typical for the Australian industry divided into 5 classes according to the difference between C-weighted and A-weighted mean sound level. A comparison of the NIOSH-spectra mean levels, classified and weighted in the same way, shows a good measure of accordance. It is therefore relatively safe to assume that the NIOSH-spectra also are typical for other industrialized countries.

The first thing to be noted is that the vast majority of these spectra represent sound levels below 100 dB(A). It is also clear that the high sound levels apply predominantly where the L_C-L_A value indicates powerful high frequency components. The next stage is to evaluate the performance of the two types of protector (figures 4 and 5) in the context of the 100 typical spectra.

Table 1: Comparison of Waugh and NIOSH spectra.

Class	L_C-L_A dB	Mean level in dB(A) for the class	
		Waugh	NIOSH
1	< 0	98.0	99.8
2	0.1 – 2.0	96.5	97.9
3	2.1 – 4.0	94.8	94.1
4	4.1 – 9.0	94.5	93.7
5	> 9.0	92.1	"92.6"

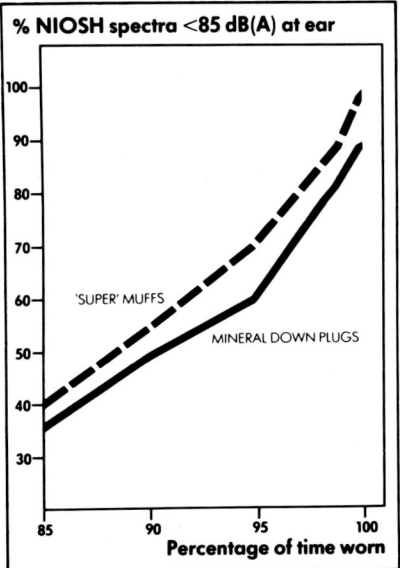
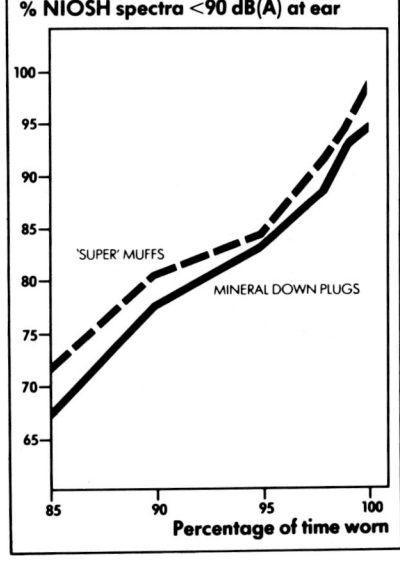

Figures 7 and 8. The percentage of NIOSH-spectra reduced to an equivalent sound level at ear of < 85 and 90 dB(A) respectively by the wearing of the subject hearing protectors as a function of time worn.

THE POTENTIAL DANGERS OF OVERPROTECTION

Figures 7 and 8 show the influence of wearing time on the performance of hearing protectors in practical noise situation.

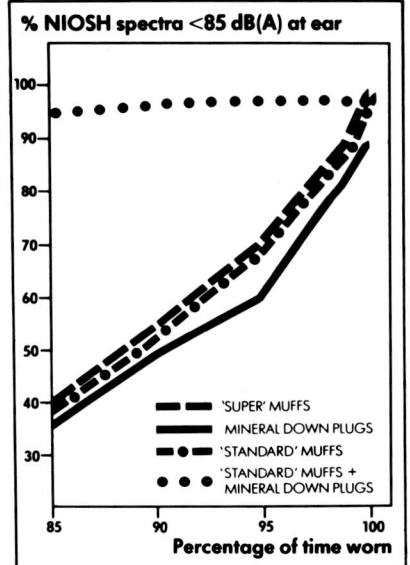 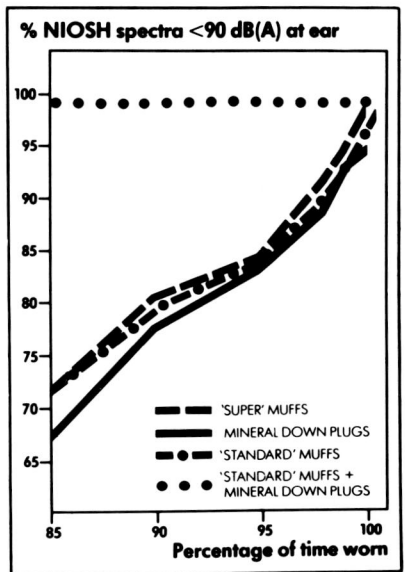

Figures 9 and 10. The percentage of NIOSH-spectra reduced to an equivalent sound level at ear of < 85 and 90 dB(A) respectively by the wearing of the subject hearing protectors as a function of time worn.

The curves were arrived at by calculating the percentage of the 100 NIOSH-spectra reduced to an Leq below the risk criteria of 85 and 90 dB(A) respectively by the wearing of hearing protectors for different fractions of the exposure time. The dotted curve represent the "super" muffs and the other curve the mineral down earplugs. It can be seen that in practice the benefit of the high nominal attenuation of the "super" muffs will be nullified if the mineral down plugs are worn as little as 1-3% more of the total exposure time. As very high attenuation and comfort appear to be incompatible characteristics in hearing protectors, it is suggested that the mineral down plugs would be worn considerably longer than the "super" muffs and thereby give better overall protection.

However, in certain noise situations there is a need for high attenuation hearing protectors. And there is a way of optimising attenuation and comfort, namely by combining two comfortable hearing protectors - earplugs and earmuffs. When using this combination, it must be assumed that the earplugs are so comfortable that they can be used for 100 percent of the exposure time. As seen from the figures the combination allows removal of the earmuffs for quite a long time and still give adequate protection, thus increasing the probability of achieving proper protection.

CONCLUSIONS

If a high-attenuation hearing protector is not worn for the full duration of an exposure, then the same degree of protection, or greater, can be achieved with a hearing protection, which provides less instantaneous reduction in sound level, provided that it is worn for a sufficient percentage of the exposure duration.

A recent comparative investigation of the difference in protection efficiency between earplugs and earmuffs carried out by the University of Lund [6] in a large Swedish shipyard provides statistical support for this hypothesis. The results indicate that the workers who wear protectors with relatively high attenuation (earmuffs fitted to helmets) generally have more severe hearing impairment than those who use more comfortable earplugs with 10-15 dB less nominal attenuation. The study concludes that this paradoxical situation arises from the fact that the high attenuation protectors are often removed during noise exposure.

The conclusion which can be drawn is that the attenuation needs to be adequate - but no more than adequate. An attempt to over-protect may in fact defeat its own purpose, if the higher attenuation is achieved at the expense of comfort.

REFERENCES
1.   Robinson, D.W., Relations Between Hearing Loss and Noise Exposures, Teddington, England, National Physical Laboratory, Aero Report, AC32, 1968.

2.   Else, D., 1973, A Note on the Protection Afforded by Hearing Protectors - Implications of the Energy Principal. Ann. Occup. Hyg. 16, 81-83, 1973.

3.   Karplus, H.B., Bonvallet, G.L., A Noise Survey of Manufacturing

Industries. Indust. Hyg. Quart., Dec. 14, 235-263, 1953.

4.   Johnson, D.L., Nixon, C.W., Simplified Methods for Estimating Hearing Protector Performance. Sound and Vibration, 8, 20-27, June 1974.

5.   Waugh, R., dB(A) Attenuation of Ear Protectors. J. Acoust. Soc. Amer., 53, No. 2, 1973.

6.   Erlandson, B., Hakansson, H., Ivarsson, A. and Nilsson, P. The Difference in Protection Efficiency Between Earplugs and Earmuffs. An Investigation Performed at a Workplace. Scand. Audiol., 9, 215-221, 1980.

18 HOW REALISTIC ARE STANDARD SUBJECTIVE TEST METHODS FOR EVALUATING HEARING PROTECTOR ATTENUATION?

Alan Martin

INTRODUCTION

The progressive growth of excessive occupational noise over the past 100 years has resulted in an increase in the provision of personal hearing protection as a method of noise reduction. The proper and efficient application in industry of personal protectors requires that an accurate and consistent measure of their acoustic attenuation is known and readily available. Such knowledge is essential for the accurate comparison of the efficiency of different protectors, and the types most suitable for a particular noise environment to be chosen in the light of the noise spectra and the noise limits currently in force. The method by which the attenuation characteristics of protectors are evaluated must not only be amenable to standardisation and produce consistent and reliable data, but also provide a realistic measure of the noise reduction to be expected in the real industrial situation.

The more practical problems involved in setting up and running a hearing protection programme in industry, such as selection, getting the protection worn and the effects of the percentage time worn on the overall protection supplied are obviously important. However before these can be considered, it is essential to ensure that the basic attenuation data upon which the programme is founded are directly and realistically applicable to that situation. This paper is concerned with examining the extent to which standard subjective test procedures reproduce and simulate the various acoustical factors involved in wearing hearing protectors in the real-life industrial situation.

The types of sound field and stimuli and the protector fitting procedures employed, the effect of physiological noise on the resulting attenuation data, and the variation of attenuation with incident sound level are considered. Such an assessment must bear in mind the necessary requirement that standard tests must be accurately specified and reproducible by different laboratories.

TEST PROCEDURES

Subjective national standard methods for evaluating the attenuation of hearing protectors, for example the British[1] and the American standard[2], rely in the main on determining the differences between the average binaural free-field thresholds of hearing of a number of subjects with the protector under test being worn and with ears unoccluded. They are generally known as real ear at threshold (REAT) methods.

Although tending to differ somewhat in experimental detail, the majority of national standard measurement methods relying on the REAT approach have broadly similar test procedures. Subjects are situated in a closely specified laboratory sound field and their responses to a series of free-field acoustic stimulus presentations result in the determination of their thresholds of hearing over a specified range of discrete frequencies. Of particular relevance to the realism of this procedure and the degree to which it simulates the practical industrial environment is the way in which the subjects fit the protectors on or in their ears and the types of stimulus and sound field employed.

PROTECTOR FITTING

It has been shown that widely differing mean and standard deviation values of attenuation are obtained for different types of fitting procedure especially in the case of earplugs. Table I compares these data for a prefabricated plastic earplug fitted following two distinct procedures. The first may be described as an "experimenter best fit" approach. Here the person carrying out the attenuation measurements actually selects and fits the earplug in the ear canal of the subject, and ensures a best fit and acoustic seal with little regard to the discomfort that may be experienced after a few hours of wear. The second approach is a "subject fit" procedure where the subject selects and fits the protector himself

Table 1: Comparison of mean and standard deviation values of attenuation, in dB, of a prefabricated earplug for two fitting procedures, obtained by the real-ear at threshold measurement method[3].

Fitting		Test Frequency Hz							
		1/4	1/2	1	2	3.1	4	6.3	8
Experimenter Fit	Mean	25.1	25.8	29.1	34.1	38.6	34.7	32.3	30.9
	S.D.	4.3	4.9	3.7	4.3	5.6	5.7	6.0	5.8
Subject Fit	Mean	16.9	16.4	18.8	24.0	30.0	28.4	28.1	29.7
	S.D.	9.3	12.1	8.4	7.8	9.9	8.1	11.3	10.5

following the manufacturer's instructions consistent with reasonable comfort. The experimenter only checks visually that no gross misfit or error has occurred.

It is immediately apparent from Table 1 that the "experimenter best fit" procedure produces markedly higher mean attenuation values, particularly at the lower test frequencies, and the standard deviations are about half those of the "subject fit" values. The reduced mean attenuations at the lower test frequencies in the latter case are due to the lack of adequate seal and resulting enhanced acoustic leaks around the earplug because of the relatively poor fit.

This is of course a comparison of extremes, but it does illustrate the need for rigorously defined fitting procedures in standard methods and, more importantly, the need for general agreement as to which type of fitting procedure should be specified.

In the practical industrial context it may perhaps be assumed that an enlightened and reasonable worker, who has had the benefit of education about hearing protection and its use would don his protection before entering the noisy environment and then adjust the fit to give optimum noise reduction consistent with reasonable comfort. This is the approach taken in the British standard[1] for example, which specifies that subjects shall select and fit the protectors following the manufacturer's instructions (if any) and then adjust them for the best attenuation consistent with reasonable comfort whilst listening to pink noise at 70 dB(A). The American standard[2] specifies a very similar procedure, although it also provides the alternative choice of an "experimenter best fit" procedure as well.

For the results of any standard test to be directly relevant to the real practical situation, the procedures involved must simulate as closely as possible those that occur in practice. The "subject fit" procedure is a good example of this requirement and represents a good compromise between practical realism and experimental accuracy. Attenuation data obtained with this procedure tend to be somewhere between the extremes illustrated in Table I, and provide a realistic measure of the protection likely to be afforded to a worker who follows a reasonable fitting procedure at the workplace.

Test Stimuli and Sound Field

In the past, early standard methods of evaluating hearing protectors, such as the superceded (1957) American standard[4], specified pure tones as the test stimuli for determining free-field thresholds of hearing. These were presented by a single loudspeaker directly facing the experimental subject under anechoic conditions, thus producing a plane-wave stimulus.

However the use of pure tones in progressive-wave free-field threshold determinations had certain drawbacks. Owing to diffraction at the subject's head, the sound level at the ears may vary considerably, thus introducing errors; particularly at the higher test frequencies and when the subject is wearing earmuffs. Also in the case of earmuffs pure tone signals may well produce resonances within the muff shell. So that at, or near to any of these resonant frequencies, small changes in absolute frequency may produce disproportionately large changes in apparent attenuation. More importantly in the present context, the majority of industrial-type noises are not pure tones but are generally broad-band in nature, although some may contain tonal components. Thus pure-tone stimuli cannot be regarded as either conducive to experimental accuracy or providing a realistic simulation of the common practical industrial noise environment.

Similarly plane-wave radiation under anechoic conditions, although simply specified, does not represent the diffuse reverberant or semi-reverberant type of sound field that usually occurs in most industrial environments.

Both these aspects have been improved considerably in later national standards by the specification of 1/3-octave bands of random noise as the test signal, presented to the subject as a diffuse homogeneous sound field. For example, the British standard[1] recommends that the diffuse sound field is produced by four matched single-source loudspeakers arranged in a symmetrical tetrahedral array around the subject in an anechoic room, with the subject's head at the centroid of the array. This arrangement is illustrated in Figure 1, which also shows the type of equipment used to generate the 1/3-octave band noise stimuli and record the subjects' responses. The American standard procedure[2] recommends a different method for generating the diffuse sound field, which involves three sets of three loudspeakers orientated orthogonally in a reverberation chamber.

The 1/3-octave bands are centred on the frequencies 63, 125, 250, 500, 1000, 2000, 3150, 4000, 6300 and 8000 Hz, and represent a reasonable compromise between the need for frequency-specific attenuation data and the practical noise environment. The diffuse sound field although derived differently in different national standards, ensures that sound is incident upon the protectors under test from all directions, as is usually the case in industry.

Thus these aspects of standard subjective tests, can be considered to simulate the industrial noise environment in a realistic manner consistent with the need for experimental accuracy.

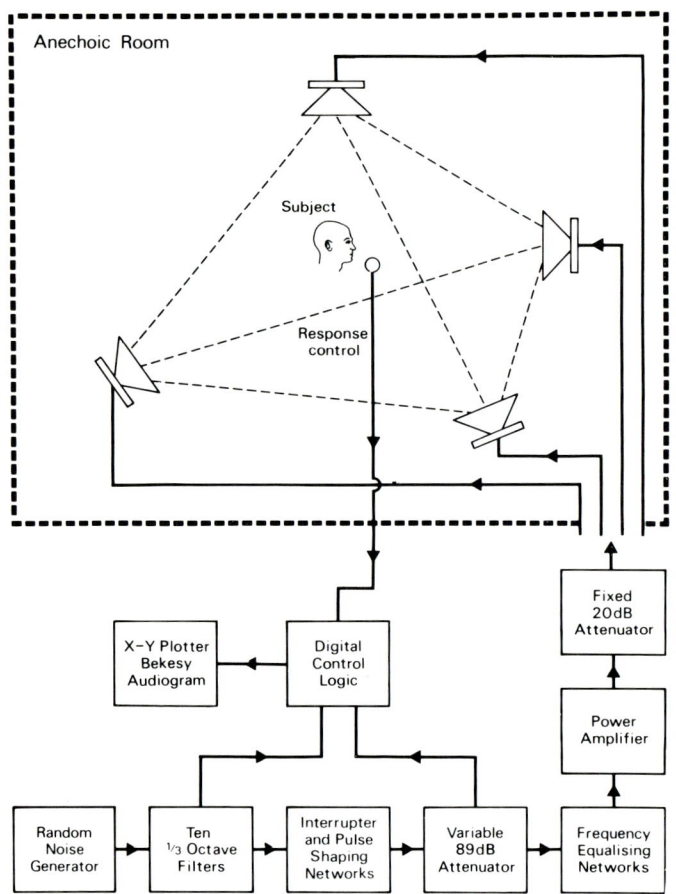

Figure 1. Block diagram of experimental set-up for the measurement of protector attenuation following the British Standard procedure(1). The tetrahedral array of loudspeakers is shown together with one channel of a four-channel self-recording audiometer(5) designed specifically for the standard test.

ATTENUATION LINEARITY AND PHYSIOLOGICAL NOISE

Real ear at threshold methods necessarily measure attenuation at low incident sound levels, with the concommitant problem of physiological noise. As such data are applied to the occupational situation where hazardous high-level noise is present, often with impulsive components, the questions raised are: how do protector attenuation characteristics vary with incident sound level, and how important is the effect of physiological noise on the resulting data?

An experiment was undertaken to examine the relationships between protector attenuation-frequency characteristics and incident sound level over a range of hazardous levels typical of those commonly experienced in industry, including both steady state and impulse noise. If it can be shown that protector attenuation characteristics are essentially constant over this range, then attenuation data obtained in the laboratory may be applied realistically and with confidence to the industrial situation.

Standard subjective measurement procedures do not permit examination of the variation of attenuation with increasing sound levels, neither do they allow the attenuation of impulse noises nor the characteristics of non-linear amplitude-sensitive protective devices to be evaluated.

The use of an artificial ear or head to examine these particular protector characteristics is an appropriate measurement technique. However, the problems of simulating accurately the many complex dynamic, physical and acoustical properties of the human head and external ear canal have not been completely solved so far.

In order to overcome these problems, while still retaining the versatility and flexibility of an 'artificial head' approach, freshly prepared and instrumented cadaver ears have been used. A small measurement microphone was introduced through the postero-superior wall of the deeper bony part of the cadaver external meatus, so that its diaphragm was flush with the meatus wall external to the intact eardrum. This enabled the sound level in the region of the eardrum to be measured under various experimental conditions.

Measurements were carried out, using this technique, of the attenuation-frequency characteristics of seven hearing protectors for pure tone, 1/3-octave bands of random noise, and impulses, with sound levels in the range 75-175 dB. The linearity of attenuation characteristics of the protectors, of which two are amplitude-sensitive devices, were examined over this range, and average attenuation data are compared with the results of standard subjective tests.

Methods

Nine cadavers were tested following the course of a normal post-mortem examination, which involved the removal of the skull roof and brain thus giving access to the internal aspects of the skull. The preparation technique has been described previously by Forrest and Coles[6].

A metal sleeve was inserted from within the cranial cavity through a hole drilled downward and slightly anteriorly through the squamopetrous suture so that the lower end of the sleeve was flush with the skin of the meatus just lateral to the eardrum. The sleeve fixture was made strong and airtight with dental cement further surrounded with plasticine. A tightly fitting Bruel and Kjaer "quarter-inch" condenser microphone was then inserted into the sleeve so that its diaphragm was flush with the external meatus wall. The general arrangement is shown in Figure 2.

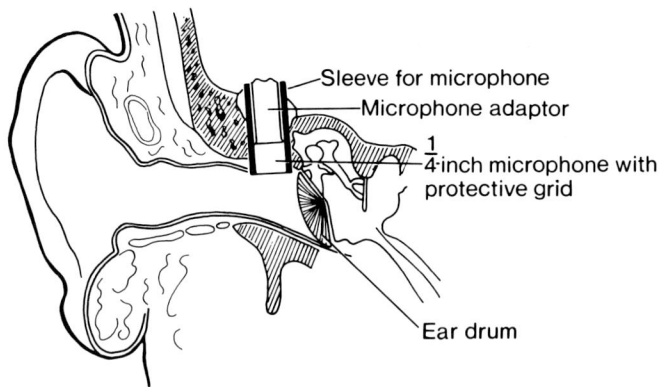

Figure 2. Cadaver ear instrumented with "¼-inch" condenser microphone. After Forrest and Coles(6).

Measurements of acoustic impedances of the cadaver ears made before and after instrumentation gave results which were not statistically significantly different, and which also came within the clinically accepted normal limits for live ears.

Preliminary tests to ensure that acoustic and vibration pathways to the measurement microphone, other than those of interest, were minimised by the preparation technique showed that attenuation for individual protectors were not influenced significantly by such pathways.

The equipment used for the generation, recording and the analysis of the acoustic stimuli employed during the experiment is shown in Figure 3. Impulse noises were generated with a starting pistol using either 0.22 or 0.32 inch cartridges and the pressure-time waveforms were recorded on a two-channel storage oscilloscope. After preparation and instrumentation of the cadaver ear with the internal 1/4-inch condenser microphone (microphone A in Figure 3), the external 1/4-inch condenser microphone (microphone B) was set up at a standardised distance of 150 mm from, and directly in line with, the cadaver ear canal.

The sound levels were measured at positions A and B for pure tones and 1/3-octave bands of random noise with centre frequencies of 125, 250, 500, 1000, 2000, 3150, 4000, 6300 and 8000 Hz for incident sound levels varying in steps of 10 dB in the range 75-125 dB. Similar measurements were also made at these positions using impulses with peak sound levels in the range 135-175 dB(P). This range was obtained by using 0.22 and 0.32 inch cartridges and by varying the distance between the starting pistol and the cadavers for the seven different types of hearing protector described in Table 2. The sound levels at the two microphone positions were also measured on the nine cadaver ears in the unoccluded condition (without fitted protector).

In general, measurements of the sound levels at microphone positions A and B, with and without a protector occluding the ear, allow three separate but independent quantities to be deduced. These are the transmission loss of the protector, the insertion loss of the protector, and the transfer function of the open ear.

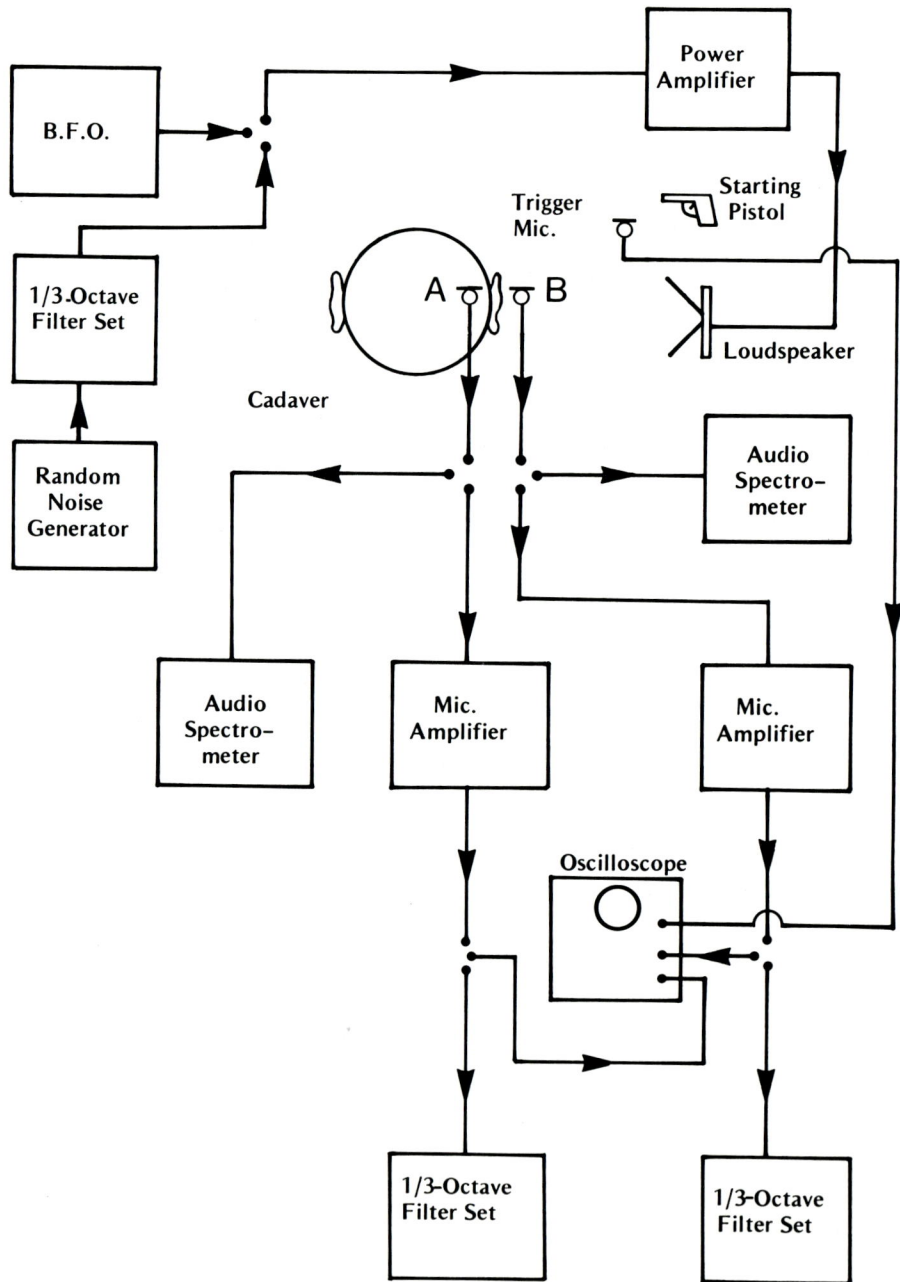

Figure 3. Block diagram of equipment for the generation, recording and analysis of steady-state and impulse stimuli used during experiment.

Table 2: Hearing protectors included in study

Code	Type	Characteristics
A	Mine Safety Appliances V51-R type earplug	Prefabricated solid plastic.
B	E.A.R. earplug	Semi-disposable plastic foam.
C	Racal Gunfender earplug	Prefabricated plastic, non-linear device.
D	Norton Sonic Ear Valve earplug	Non-linear valve in rubber capsule.
E	Mine Safety Appliances Comfo 500 earmuffs	Symmetric plastic shells, foam-filled cushion seals.
F	Welsh 4530 earmuffs	Symmetric plastic shells, foam-filled cushion seals.
G	Racal Sonogard earmuffs	Asymmetric plastic shells, liquid-filled cushion seals.

Both transmission loss and insertion loss are measures of attenuation but, from a practical viewpoint, the insertion loss is the more important parameter. This is the measure evaluated by standard subjective procedures and is the value most relevant to the wearer in industry in the context of hearing conservation. It provides a measure of the reduction in sound level at the eardrum which occurs when a protector is fitted to the ear.

Time limitations and attempts to reduce errors caused by repeated refitting of the protector, precluded direct measurement of the insertion loss of each protector. However, this was deduced from the transfer function of the open ear from the transmission loss of the protector, Martin[7].

Hearing Protectors Tested

The general characteristics of the hearing protectors tested are summarised briefly in Table 2. Of the four earplugs tested, two (C and D), were intentionally non-linear amplitude-sensitive devices intended for protection against gunfire noise, while allowing steady-state sounds to be partially transmitted.

As far as possible, test hearing protectors were fitted to cadaver ears in a similar manner to that for normal live subjects. Earmuff shells were placed over both ears with the tensioning headband over the top of the head, while the correct size of earplug was individually fitted to the ear canal where this was appropriate.

Results
Open-ear Measurements.
The results of measurements made on cadavers with the ear unoccluded by any protectors provide a measure of the acoustic transfer characteristics of the human ear between a point adjacent to the eardrum and the external sound field, as well as factors to correct transmission-loss measurements to insertion-loss attenuation values.

In the case of the steady-state stimuli the attenuation (the experimental measure of the acoustical transfer characteristics) of the unoccluded ear was found to be constant with external sound level over the range studied, as shown by linear regression analyses undertaken at each test frequency. Consequently, the data were combined to give estimates of the mean value at each test frequency. Figure 4 shows the means and standard deviations of the attenuation for pure tones and for 1/3-octave bands of random noise, each point being the mean of 37 measurements. Figure 4 shows that there is a gain in the system above 500 Hz, which is maximally about 10 dB in the case of pure tones between 2 and 6 kHz and maximally about 13 dB for the 1/3-octave band of random noise centred on 2 kHz.

The observed gain is assumed to be caused by resonances in the external ear and ear canal and may be regarded as quite substantial. Certainly, a hearing protector must overcome this gain before actually providing attenuation of the sound reaching the eardrum. This presumably is

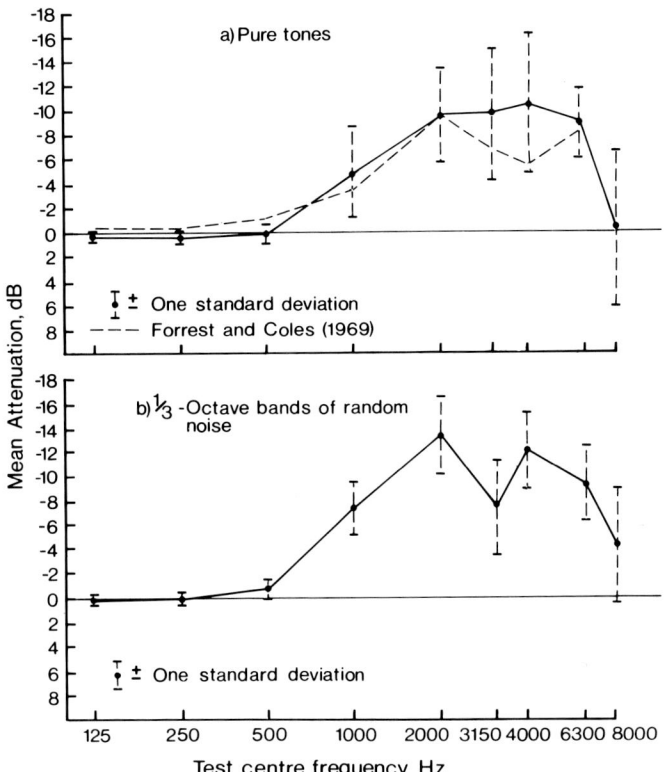

Figure 4. Means and standard deviations of attenuation of unoccluded ear for (a) pure tones, and (b) 1/3-octave bands of random noise.

achieved, partly by its actual presence on or in the ear, thereby reducing and possibly changing these resonances, and partly by acting as a simple acoustic barrier.

In the case of impulse-noise stimuli, a linear regression analysis of 17 measurements of attenuation produced a correlation coefficient which was not significant. Consequently, as in the case of steady-state stimuli, the transfer characteristics of the unoccluded ear may be regarded as constant with incident peak sound level over the range 135-175 dB(P). The mean attenuation (reduction in peak level) was found to be -11.1 dB with a standard deviation of 3.03 dB. Thus a gain of 11.1 dB in the initial peaks of impulses was observed and this is entirely consistent with the results for steady-state stimuli. This is to be expected, as the frequency spectrum of the impulse noise is generally broad-band over the frequency range of interest, with considerable energy at the higher frequencies.

Steady-state Noise Measurements.

The attenuation characteristics of the seven hearing protectors were determined for pure-tones and 1/3-octave bands of random noise with incident sound levels between 75 and 125 dB. Attenuation linearity was examined for the results at 250, 500, 1000, 4000 and 8000 Hz. At each test frequency, linear regressions of the attenuation data with incident sound level were deduced for individual cadaver ears. Of interest here is the gradient of the regression line, which should be zero if the attenuation does not change with incident sound level, or have a value significantly different from zero if it does. Mean values of the gradient were determined for each protector and test frequency for pure-tone stimuli and 1/3-octave bands of random noise. It was found that all values of the gradient were small varying between -0.14 and 0.15 with a mean of 0.036.

Students' 't' tests showed that all the hearing protectors considered generally provide attenuation which is constant with incident sound level for the range of steady-state sounds examined here.

Having established the linearity of acoustic attenuation with incident sound level over the range so far considered, it is now permissible to reduce the available attenuation data for each protector to a single mean value at each test frequency. Thus, each estimate of the mean attenuation for a particular test frequency is based on approximately 20 measurements of the attenuation made over the range 75-125 dB.

Figures 5 - 11 show the mean attenuation frequency characteristics of the seven protectors for pure-tones and 1/3-octave bands of random noise, in terms of the insertion loss.

As a comparison, attenuation data measured by national standard subjective procedures are also shown in the Figures where appropriate and available (Martin, 8). Pure-tone attenuation data are compared with those obtained from measurements following the American subjective standard[4] which itself uses pure-tone stimuli, while the attenuation values determined with 1/3-octave bands of random noises are compared with results of the British standard[1] which also uses these noise stimuli.

Impulse Noise Measurements.
The basic measure of attenuation was taken as the difference in decibels between the peak sound pressure levels of the high initial peaks of the impulse sound pressure wave forms recorded by microphones B and A. Between 13 and 21 measurements were made of attenuation for each of the seven hearing protectors over the range 135-175 dB(P). These values were then corrected to the insertion loss with the open-ear transfer function data.

The linearity of attenuation with incident peak sound level was examined, as before, in terms of linear regression between these two quantities for each protector. The number of measurements, the gradient of the regression equation and the regression correlation coefficient are given in Table 3 for each protector. Students' 't' tests of the significance of the correlation coefficients were also carried out. As indicated in Table 3, with the exception of results for earplugs C and D, the correlation coefficients are not significant. This shows that the five protectors that are intended to have linear attenuation characteristics do, in fact, have such characteristics for impulse sounds in the range 135-175 dB(P). The two intentionally non-linear earplugs C and D provide linear regressions with significant correlation coefficients ($p < 0.001$), thus vindicating the manufacturers' claim for these devices.

The non-linear attenuation characteristics of earplugs C and D are shown in Figures 12 and 13 respectively, in which the individual points are ploted in terms of the measured transmission loss. The regression equation is plotted for the data in each case. These figures also show the insertion losses of the protectors. As before, these data are derived from the results of the unoccluded condition for impulse noises. Earplug C provides attenuation which appears to vary monotonically

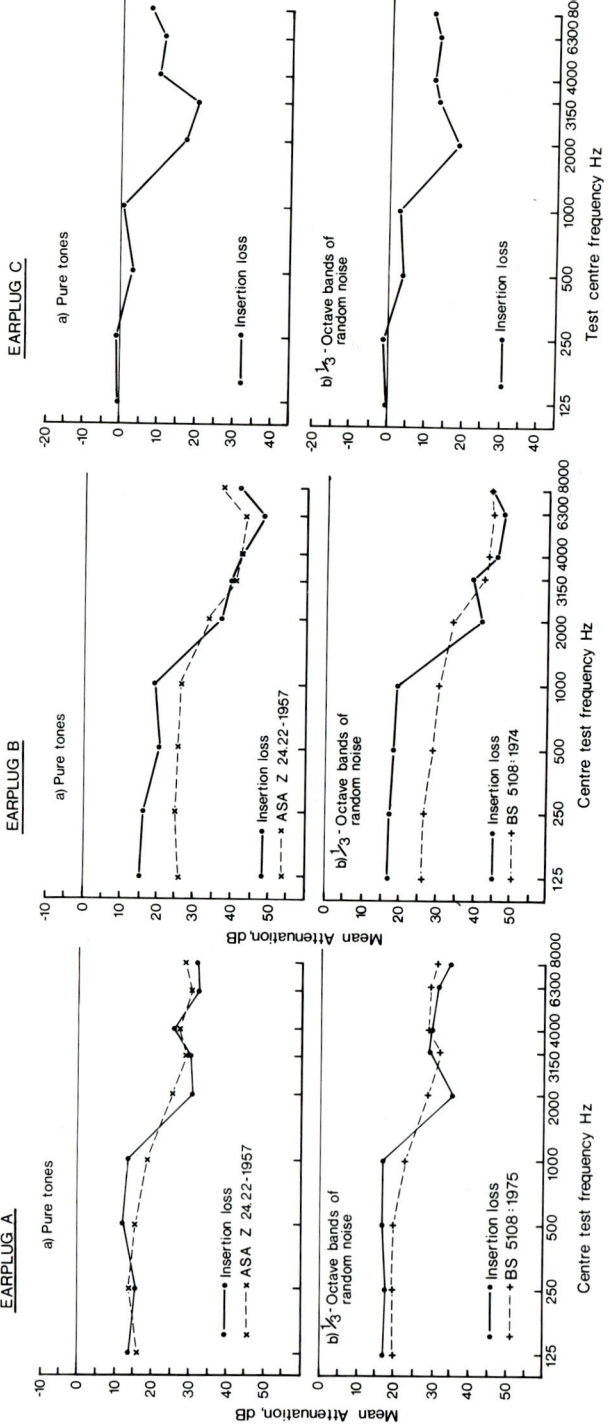

Figures 5-7. Mean attenuation-frequency characteristics of hearing protectors A, B and C for steady-state stimuli.

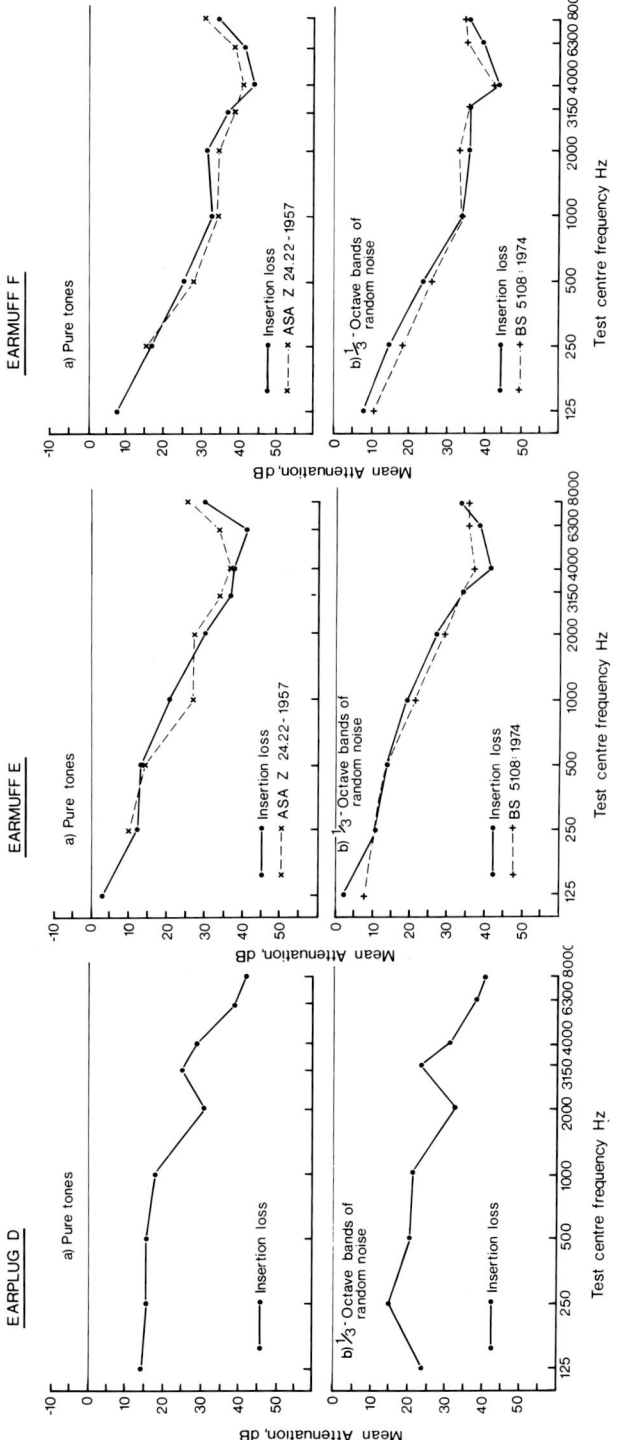

Figures 8-10. Mean attenuation-frequency characteristics of hearing protectors D, E and F for steady-state stimuli.

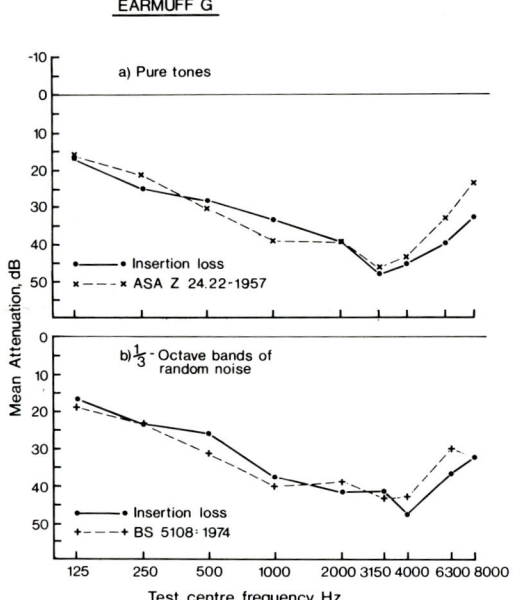

Figure 11. Mean attenuation frequency characteristics of hearing protector G for steady state stimuli.

Table 3: Relevant results of linear regression analyses of attenuation with incident peak sound level for impulses in the range 135-175 dB(P)

Hearing Protector	Number of measurements	Gradient(m)	Correlation Coefficient(r)	Mean insertion loss dB
A	16	0.109	0.229	25.1
B	14	-0.014	-0.024	38.4
C	13	0.430	0.950*	-
D	21	0.314	0.510*	-
E	19	0.110	0.217	32.1
F	20	0.025	0.044	39.0
G	18	0.024	-	39.8

$p < 0.001$

from about 18 dB for an incident peak sound level of 135 dB(P) to 35 dB for incident sound at 175 dB(P). Similarly, attenuation of the earplug D varies from about 20-34 dB over this range of incident peak sound level. The results reported by Forrest[9] obtained by similar experiments are also given in Figures 12 and 13 for earplugs C and D. There is good agreement between the transmission loss values reported by Forrest and those observed in the present study, with less than 5 dB difference between the two lines for both earplugs within the range of impulses considered.

With regard to the five hearing protectors shown to have linear attenuation characteristics for the range of impulses studied, the data points may now be combined to give an estimate of the mean value for each of these protectors. The mean attenuations of these protectors are given in Table 3.

DISCUSSION

In the case of steady-state stimuli all seven protectors in general provide substantially constant acoustic attenuation characteristics over the range of incident sound levels between 75 and 125 dB. This is in fact the most important range for practical industrial hearing conservation purposes.

However, protectors are usually evaluated by one of the national standard subjective test procedures, which involve low incident sound levels in the region of 0-40 dB SPL; therefore the question remains of attenuation linearity between these ranges (between about 40 and 75 dB) and whether attenuation data from standard tests are directly applicable to hazardous noise levels. Examination of the differences between attenuation data obtained by standard REAT procedures and those from the present study may provide further information on attenuation linearity over this range.

Figures 5, 6, 9, 10 and 11 compare the attenuation data obtained in the present study with those from the two national standard procedures, and there is generally good agreement between them. Figure 14 shows the differences in attenuation between results of the two approaches, expres-

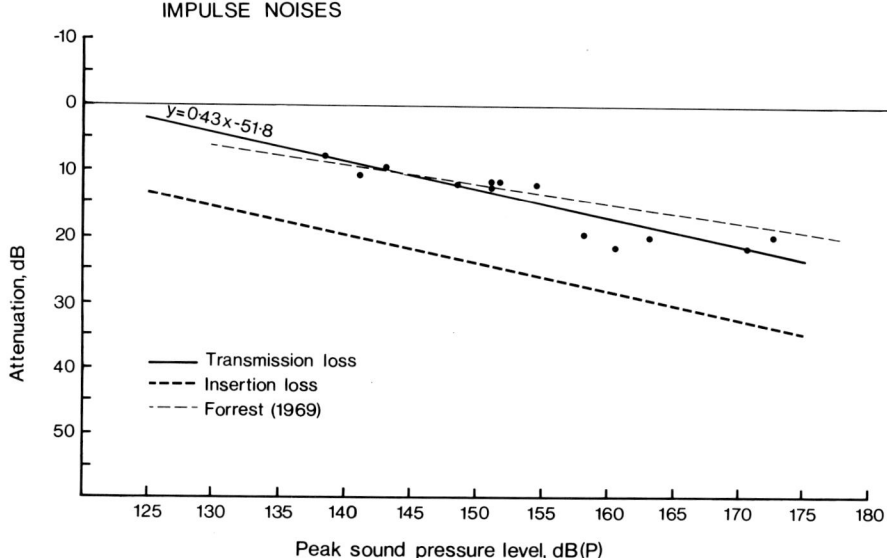

Figure 12. Variation of attenuation with incident peak sound level of earplug C for impulse noise stimuli.

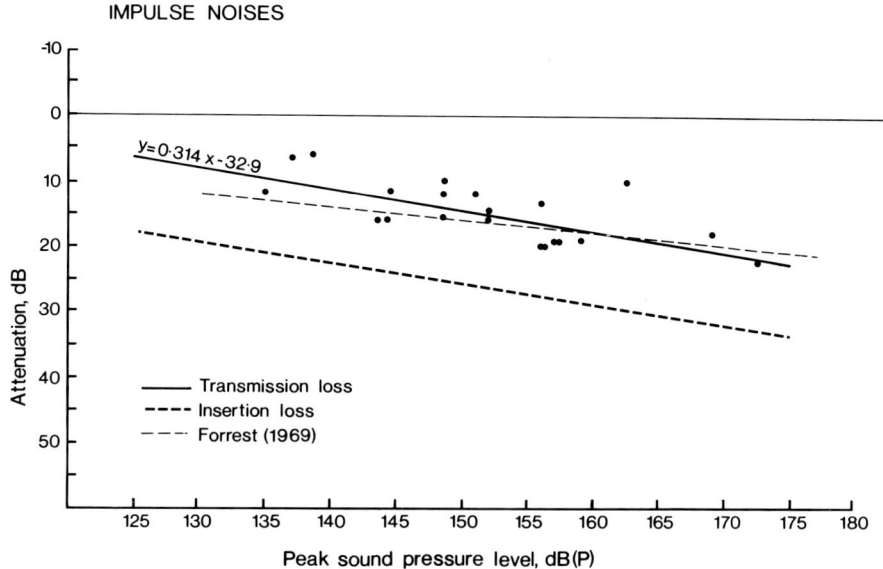

Figure 13. Variation of attenuation with incident peak sound level of earplug D for impulse noise stimuli.

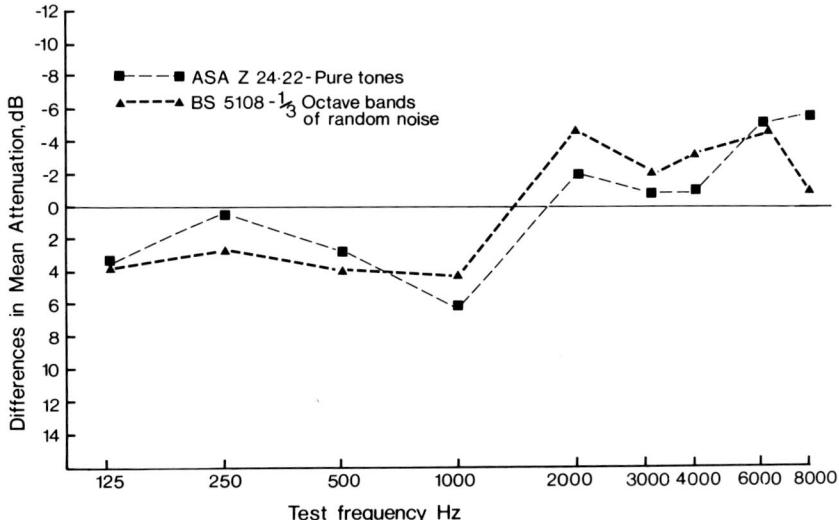

Figure 14. Differences between mean attenuation values obtained by standard REAT procedures and those measured on Cadaver ears, averaged over results for hearing protectors A, B, E, F and G. Results of ASA Z24.22-1957(4) are compared with pure-tone data, and results of BS5108: 1974(1) are compared with 1/3-octave band random-noise values. Positive difference indicates that result of standard test is greater.

sed as the average differences for the five hearing protectors. These are plotted separately for the pure tone and 1/3-octave band random noise comparisons. Positive differences indicate that the results of the standard subjective procedures are greater than those obtained from cadaver ear measurements. There is little difference between these comparisons, both curves following a similar pattern. In general, the subjective standard procedures give attenuation values which are greater, on average by 3.4 dB, than those observed in the present study for the lower test frequencies between 125 and 1000 Hz. On the other hand, for test frequencies of 2000 Hz and above, the reverse tends to occur, wehre the present data from cadaver ears are on average 2.8 dB greater than those measured with the standard subjective procedures. These are small differences, considering the diverse nature of the experimental procedures involved in these comparisons. Nevertheless they are, in the main, explicable in terms of known auditory physiological phenomena.

The former observations for frequencies below 1000 Hz may be explained in terms of the artefact introduced into the standard subjective REAT methods because of the enhancement of physiological noise by the presence of the protector. In this regard, the data measured in the present experiment may be considered to be nearer the true attenuation provided by hearing protectors. Similar differences of the order of 3-5 dB have been reported by Webster[10] and Weinreb and Touger[11] in the case of comparisons between the American standard method and loudness-balance and insert microphone techniques. Anderson and Whittle[12] investigated in considerable detail the differences between hearing thresholds determined using free-field and earphone-generated signals. They reported that the difference varied monotonically between about 15 dB and zero over the frequency range 100 - 1000 Hz, and concluded that it was caused by physiological noise of vascular origin generated in the external ear canal. They also showed that the level of physiological noise was inversely proportional to the effective volume of the occluding device. Furthermore, the presence of an earplug in the ear canal will enhance the noise by providing additional sound-radiating surfaces. Thus, it is likely that the differences between subjective free-field threshold measurements of protector attenuation and those employing objective techniques are greater for earplugs than for earmuffs. This is exemplified in particular by the relatively large differences between data from standard subjective and cadaver ear procedures observed at the lower test frequencies for earplug B shown in Figure 6. Indeed this device appears to enhance physiological noise to a greater extent than the other protectors assessed in this study and if its results are excluded from this analysis, the overall mean difference reduces from 3.4 to about 2.4 dB.

The fact that the results of the present study are, on average, slightly greater than those obtained from the standard subjective procedures for test frequencies above 1500 Hz may be explained by the ultimate limitation of attenuation provided by bone conduction in the latter more realistic situation. Incident sound will reach the inner ear via the bones and tissue of the head as well as by air conduction. According to Tonndorf[13] there are three main routes by which bone-conducted sound may reach the cochlea: (i) by vibration of the ear canal walls; (ii) by inertial vibrations of the ossicles and (iii) by mechanical distortion of the cochlea walls. Thus, in the present study the internal microphone would pick up the first of these signal routes, and possibly some portion of the second via vibration of the eardrum, but not the third. Consequently, these secondary paths are not completely accounted for in the present measurement technique, whereas they will obviously be included in subjective standard test procedures.

Perhaps the most important conclusion to be drawn from this part of the study is that, notwithstanding explicable average differences of the order of ± 3 dB, the attenuation data measured by national standard procedures are in very good agreement with those obtained in the present study. Consequently, protector attenuation would also appear to be constant for incident steady-state sound levels between 40 and 75 dB.

With regard to the results of measurements with impulse noises, the five protectors with intentionally linear characters have been shown to provide constant attenuation for impulses with peak sound levels between 135 and 175 dB(P). This result, coupled with the results for steady-state sounds, extends the range of measured attenuation linearity to include incident sound levels between 75 and 175 dB. Consequently, as discussed above, the general inference is that these protectors provide attenuation which appears to be approximately constant over the range of incident sound levels between about 40-175 dB.

Overall, therefore, this experiment has shown that the attenuation characteristics of hearing protectors are essentially constant for the range and types of noise commonly experienced in industry. Furthermore, although the effect of physiological noise does appear to enhance attenuation values derived by standard subjective test procedures for frequencies at 1000 Hz and below the resulting artefact is relatively small, being on average of the order of 3 dB. When considered in the light of the potential reductions in protection to the wearer due to the many practical problems often experienced in industry at the present time, such as percentage time worn and the use of damaged and ill-fitted protectors, and the fact that the higher frequencies are most hazardous to hearing, such artefacts may be considered to be relatively negligible.

CONCLUSIONS

To consider the question: how realistic are standard subjective test methods for evaluating hearing protector attenuation, those aspects of the test procedures have been examined which are considered to influence the realism of the resulting attenuation data.

Current standard REAT test procedures specify the use of sound fields and stimuli which simulate as realistically as possible those which typically occur in the real industrial environment, consistent with the requirements for experimental accuracy and reproducibility. Likewise the protector fitting procedures employed also simulate how an enlightened and reasonable worker should fit his protectors at the workplace. They attempt to take some account of the need for comfort, although it may be argued that the relatively short duration of the wear time during a standard test compared to, say, an 8-hour work shift, is not an ideal representation of the real practical situation. However, without radically increasing the duration of the standard test and the variability of the results, or altering the basis of the test procedures, the current approach may be viewed as a reasonable compromise between realism and the requirements of laboratory experimentation. Nevertheless there remains a need to develop a separate laboratory-based measure of a comfort index of protectors, which may subsequently be related to the REAT test procedure and to the protection afforded the wearer in the practical industrial environment.

It has been demonstrated that, for the protectors considered here at least, the effect of physiological noise on the attenuation measured by REAT methods occurs at the lower test frequencies and is relatively small, being of the order of 3 dB. When examined in the light of the many practical problems which tend to influence the noise hazard to the wearer in industry, such an artefact does not materially affect the realism of such test procedures for the majority of industrial noises. In extreme cases, where protection may be required against high-level low-frequency noise and where detailed knowledge of low-frequency attenuation figures may assist protector selection, some correction to the standard data might be appropriate along the lines discussed above.

Finally it has been shown that the attenuation-frequency characteristics of conventional protectors measured on instrumented cadaver ears are essentially constant for a wide range of incident sound levels and, notwithstanding explicable differences, are in very good agreement with the results of low-level REAT measurement methods. Consequently the results of standard test procedures may be applied with confidence to occupations where hazardous high-level noises are present.

Thus in general standard REAT test methods may be considered to provide a realistic assessment of hearing protector attenuation. The estimation of the actual noise reduction supplied to the wearer in practice, however, is often a different matter and depends upon many factors governing protector usage which are beyond the control and scope of the standard test. It is perhaps these factors which now need to be considered and improved if the full benefits of hearing protectors are to be realised in the future.

REFERENCES

1. British Standards Institution, BS5108: 1974. Method of Measurement of the Attenuation of Hearing Protectors at Threshold. British Standards Institution, London, 1974.

2. American National Standards Institute, ANSI S3.19-1974. Method for the Measurement of Real-Ear Protection of Hearing Protectors and Physical Attenuation of Earmuffs. American National Standards Institute, New York, 1974.

3. Martin, A.M., Methodology of the measurement of the attenuation of hearing protectors. Proc. Brit. Acous. Soc. $\underline{1}$(3), 71-85, 1971.

4. American Standards Association, ASA Z24.22:1957. Measurement of Real-Ear Attenuation of Ear Protectors at Threshold. American Standards Association, New York, 1957.

5. Whitham, W.M., Martin, A.M., The ISVR facility for the British

Standard method for the evaluation of hearing protectors. Tech. Memo. 558, Institute of Sound and Vibration Research, University of Southampton, 1976.

6. Forrest, M.R., Coles, R.R.A., Use of Cadaver ears in the acoustic evaluation of ear plugs. Royal Navy Personnel Research Committee, Report HeS/34. Medical Research Council, London, 1969.

7. Martin, A.M., Dependence of Acoustic Attenuation of Hearing Protectors on Incident Sound Level. Brit. J. Industr. Med. 36 1-14, 1979.

8. Martin, A.M., The acoustic attenuation characteristics of 26 hearing protectors evaluated following the British Standard procedure. Ann. Occup. Hyg. 20, 229-246, 1977.

9. Forrest, M.R., Summary report on the development of an improved amplitude-sensitive earplug. Royal Navy Personnel Research Committee, Report HeS/135. Medical Research Council, London, 1969.

10. Webster, J.C., Ear defenders: Measurement methods and comparative results. Noise Control 1, 34-42, 1955.

11. Weinreb, L., Touger, M.L., Variation in ear protector attenuation as measured by different methods. J. Acoust. Soc. Amer. 32, 245-259, 1960.

12. Anderson, C.M., Whittle, L.S., Physiological noise and the missing 6 dB. Acustica 25, 261-272, 1971.

13. Tonndorf, J., Bone Conduction. In Foundations of Modern Auditory Theory, volume 2, 197-237. Edited by Tobias, J.V., Academic Press, New York, 1972.

Personal Hearing Protection in Industry, edited by P. W. Alberti, Raven Press, New York ©

19 LABORATORY ESTIMATES OF THE REAL WORLD PERFORMANCE OF HEARING PROTECTORS

E. H. Berger

INTRODUCTION

The accurate quantification of hearing protective device (HPD) performance is key to appropriate selection for specific applications. A dilemma exists as most existing manufacturers' literature, and much research data developed from standard laboratory test procedures, consistently overestimate the real world (RW) performance of HPDs.

Our hypothesis is that the discrepancy is due to subject selection, training and motivation procedures practiced by many test facilities rather than with experimental methodology. In order to examine this hypothesis, we are currently conducting HPD attenuation experiments in our laboratory and reviewing existing studies in the literature.

APPROXIMATING REAL WORLD HPD PERFORMANCE
IN A LABORATORY SETTING

In the laboratory[1] the attenuation of HPDs is usually measured by performing absolute threshold shift attenuation tests on trained and motivated subjects using optimally fitted HPDs. The crucial questions are: 1) How does this relate to the real world? and 2) Should it? The answer to question number one, as has become increasingly apparent in recent years, is poorly[2-8]. Employees are seldom adequately motivated or sufficiently instructed in how to wear HPDs properly, and if the devices require special fitting techniques or are uncomfortable to wear, the problem is compounded.

The answer to question number two involves a discussion of testing concepts and philosopy. It may be argued that exacting subject selection, training, and motivation procedures are necessary to see how well HPDs can perform, and that the only performance benchmark which may be accurately quantified is the best attainable HPD performance. Furthermore, it has been suggested that if varying degrees of misuse occur, or particularly hard to fit subjects are included, there is no limit to how poorly a device can be shown to perform. However, these arguments ignore some critical factors.

Significantly greater discomfort can be tolerated by highly motivated test subjects who wear HPDs for only 5-10 minutes per test than will be endured for long term use by employees. Thus laboratory subjects may wear a device "perfectly" for a test in a way that they might not consider for longer use. Furthermore, even with the best possible industrial fitting, training, and motivational programs, the performance will not approach the high values attained with exacting laboratory fittings[9]. Therefore, we feel that exacting laboratory procedures should be modified or augmented to generate representative real world data. The purpose of this study was to examine that possibility by measuring the attenuation for a single HPD on a large group of untrained, unselected subjects, given minimal instruction and supervision.

Experimental Procedure

All HPD attenuation measurements were conducted in a previously described[10,11] 113 m^3 acoustically treated reverberation room specifically constructed for that purpose. The room and the associated equipment comply with the requirements of ASA STD1-1975 (ANSI S3.19-1974)[12], the new American hearing protector attenuation measurement standard.

All testing was by self-recording audiometry, 30 seconds at each test band, with an attenuator rate of 5 dB/sec. Retesting occurred for at least one frequency on each test. TDH-50 drivers mounted in MX41-AR cushions were used.

The 65 subjects were chosen at random from new and existing E-A-R Corporation employees, visitors to our laboratory, and friends of E-A-R

Corporation employees. The only restriction was an otoscopic examination showing an outer ear free from impacted cerumen and/or infection. All subjects were questioned concerning their familiarity with HPDs. Of the 65 subjects, 45% had never used a HPD, 28% had some experience but no supervised instruction and the remaining 28% used HPDs regularly, most often the E-A-R™ Plug. Most (95%) of the subjects were white and 62% were male. About 5% of the ear canals were extra small and about 9% were extra large as determined using the American Optical Eargage.

All subjects were administered a battery of four tests in the sequence shown in Table I. The complete set of tests, including the instruction, took 55-70 minutes per subject. Test A characterized the subjects' left and right ear hearing levels and familiarized them with self-recording audiometry. Tests B, C, and D constitute the HPD attenuation measurement series as outlined in ANSI S3.19, except that only 1 instead of 3 measurements of each fit were performed due to time limitations. The data are nevertheless valid due to the large number of subjects and due to evidence indicating that intersubject variability is significantly greater than intra-subject variability[13].

Table I: Test Sequence and Description

Test	Sound Field	Test Signal	Treatment
A	TDH-50/MX41-AR	Pure Tones	Unoccluded
B	Diffuse	1/3 OB Noise	Unoccluded
C	Diffuse	1/3 OB Noise	Occluded - Subject fit
D	Diffuse	1/3 OB Noise	Occluded - Experimenter fit

The order of Tests B, C, and D was fixed due to the nature of the experiment. Since the experimenter fit in Test D would necessarily influence the subject fit of Test C, D was forced to follow C. Test B, the unoccluded ear test, was presented first due to the lack of experience of the subjects and the observation that an occluded ear diffuse field threshold test is typically more difficult than an unoccluded pure tone audiogram test. Furthermore, learning effects[14] would tend to cause the test sequence to err in the direction of minimizing measured attenuation, since learning effects would improve thresholds on subsequent tests, and therefore minimize the unoccluded/occluded ear differences.

The hearing protector chosen for use in the experiment was the E-A-R Plug, a user formable, expandable foam insert. Since the device is available in only one size, .54" diameter, sizing was eliminated as a variable in the experiment. Also, due to the plugs delayed expansion, which enables the plug to adapt to the shape of the ear canal, it was necessary to wait after the plug has been inserted, before beginning testing. This precaution is sometimes neglected in laboratory tests of foam plugs and can spuriously reduce attenuation values by as much as 10 dB. The expansion time allowed in these tests was 4 minutes.

For the subject fit treatment, the subjects were handed a set of detailed instructions, including line drawings demonstrating plug roll down and insertion[15]. They were told to read the instructions carefully and insert the plugs however they thought correct. The experimenter offered no assistance and no comments about the fit prior to the test. For Test D, the experimenter fit, the experimenter rolled down and inserted the plug as he deemed correct. In most cases this meant that about 1/2 the axial length of the plug was compressed in the ear canal with the remainder of the plug protruding into the concha.

Experimental Results

In Figure 1 the mean attenuation and standard deviation data for tests C and D are plotted. It is clear that the subject fit provided significantly poorer attenuation below 2 kHz than did the experimenter fit. Notice that the experimenter fit on the 65 subjects gave mean attenuation results closely approximating a test in the same laboratory using 10 standard trained subjects, with an experimenter supervised fit. However, the data for the 10 trained subjects demonstrate lower variability at all

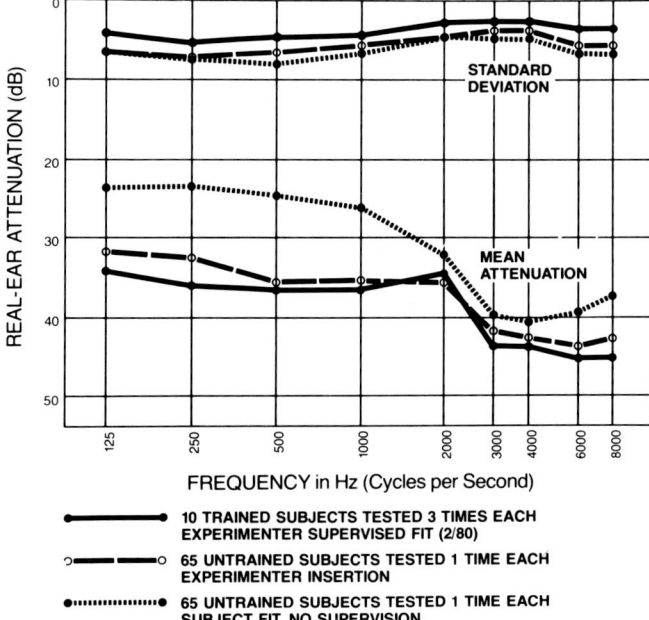

Figure 1. E-A-R plug attenuation data for 65 untrained listeners with two insertion methods, compared to data for 10 trained listeners.

frequencies.

As mentioned earlier, 28% of the subjects had regularly worn HPDs, mostly E-A-R Plugs. To determine whether these subjects unduly influenced the values determined for the subject fit, the data for these 18 subjects were compared to the remaining 37. At all frequencies the results agreed within 1.5 dB. Therefore further analyses combined these two groups.

In Figure 2 the mean attenuation for the experimenter fit is again plotted, but this time the 5th and 95th percentiles are also included. The 5th percentile is also plotted for the subject fit and demonstrates worst case attenuation that is $\geq$ 12 dB at any frequency.

OTHER MEASURES OF REAL WORLD PERFORMANCE
The experiments described can be compared to the work of other

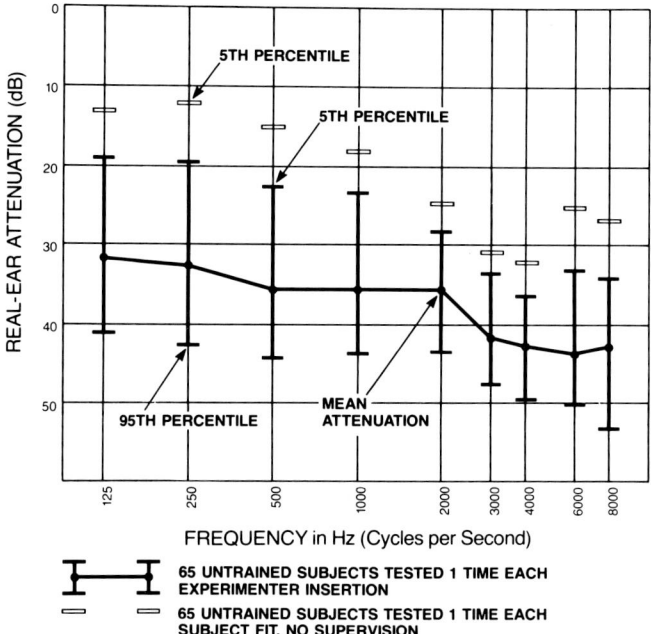

Figure 2.   E-A-R plug attentuation data for 65 untrained listeners with percentile data included.

researchers. Waugh, of the National Acoustic Laboratories (NAL) in Australia, has attempted to model his laboratory tests after actual usage conditions[16]. In a recent publication[17], the NAL reports attenuation data for 75 earmuffs and 19 inserts which were all tested at the facility.

The NAL has a subject pool consisting of 35-40 of its employees. Each HPD is tested once on 15 people. Devices also undergo a series of physical tests (vibration, impact, temperature cycling, etc.). Subjects are given the manufacturers' instructions and little experimenter supervision. The test procedure is an absolute threshold shift method similar in detail to the ANSI Z24.22[18] standard, with the data corrected[19] to 1/3 octave-band values. The NAL tests yield lower mean attenuations and higher standard deviations than data gathered for manufacturers in U.S. testing laboratories.

At least three experimenters have performed HPD attenuation tests[2-6] by

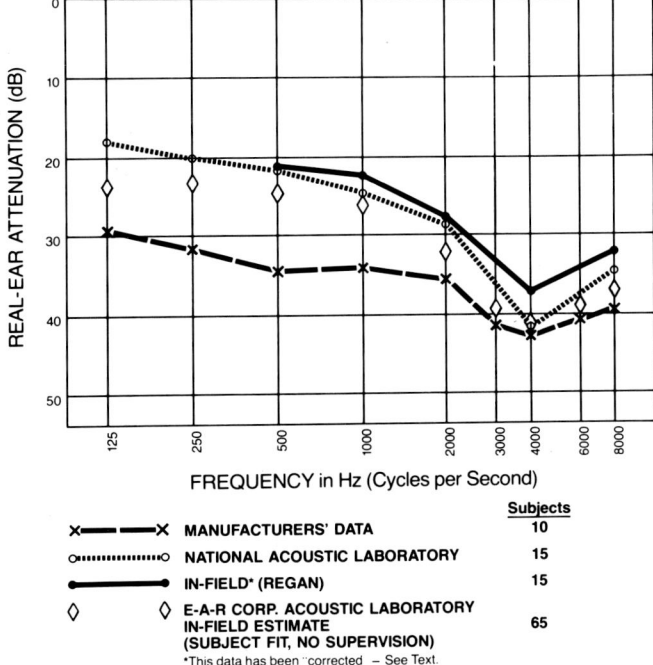

Figure 3. Attenuation data for foam insert protector by four methods.

setting up their measurement facilities at industrial plant sites and using noise exposed employees as their subjects. Although the employees were aware that they would be subjects, they were not aware of the exact times of their tests and were carefully monitored to assure that they did not readjust their protectors once they had been notified to proceed to the test booth. These three experiments included 613 subjects at 7 different plant sites using 5 inserts and 1 earmuff. Although the 3 studies varied in their exact measurement techniques, appropriate controls were incorporated to insure the validity of the results.

Data Comparisons

In Figure 3, the results of this study (subject fit) are compared to three other sets of data. The manufacturer's data is E-A-R Corporation's reported data as measured by an independent test laboratory. The NAL data were described previously. The field data, from Regan, are for E-A-R Plugs that were early prototypes, sold in limited quantities, and considerably more difficult to use than the present model, available since 1974. His data were conservatively corrected by adding 1 to 5 dB, figures derived from laboratory data comparing the prototype and current model foam plugs. There is good agreement between the three RW estimates - this study's subject fit, the NAL data, and the Regan in-field measurements.

Another recent RW estimate of HPD attenuation exists in the literature. This study, conducted by Alberti, et al[8] in conjunction with the Workman's Compensation Board of Ontario, utilized workmen in a laboratory setting. Each workman brought his HPD to the test site and "fitted the device himself as he would wear it at work". E-A-R Plugs were among the HPDs tested and the results, as expected, show less attenuation than manufacturer's data, but in this case even lower (by an average of 8 dB) than the three RW estimates in Figure 3. In fact, these results approximate the lower 5 percentile subject fit in Figure 2. These very low results demonstrate how a protector may be severely misused by untrained workers.

The important point to be gleaned from Figure 3 is that with appropriate protocol, laboratory data can yield a reasonable estimate of RW performance.* It appears that the very comprehensive NAL report may provide such data. Figures 4 to 8 investigate this possibility further.

In Figure 4 there is good agreement between the NIOSH[2,3] and Padilla[6] field studies at 500 Hz (Padilla only measured at 500 Hz). The field attenuation data are only about 40-60% of the decibel values of the

---

* Editor's comment: Figure 3 omits the Alberti et al[8] data which are discussed in the text; the adjustments to Reagan's Data do not sit comfortably with the editor, although repeated unpublished experimental data demonstrate that the current .54" diameter E-A-R^{TM} plugs perform 4-11 db better at all frequencies than the earlier prototype .61" diameter E-A-R plugs (Berger - personal communication).

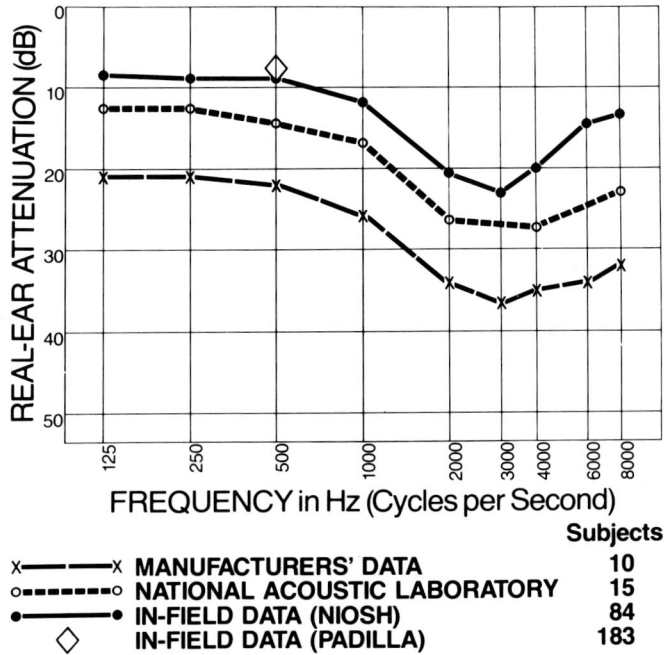

Figure 4. Attenuation data for V-51R insert protector by four methods.

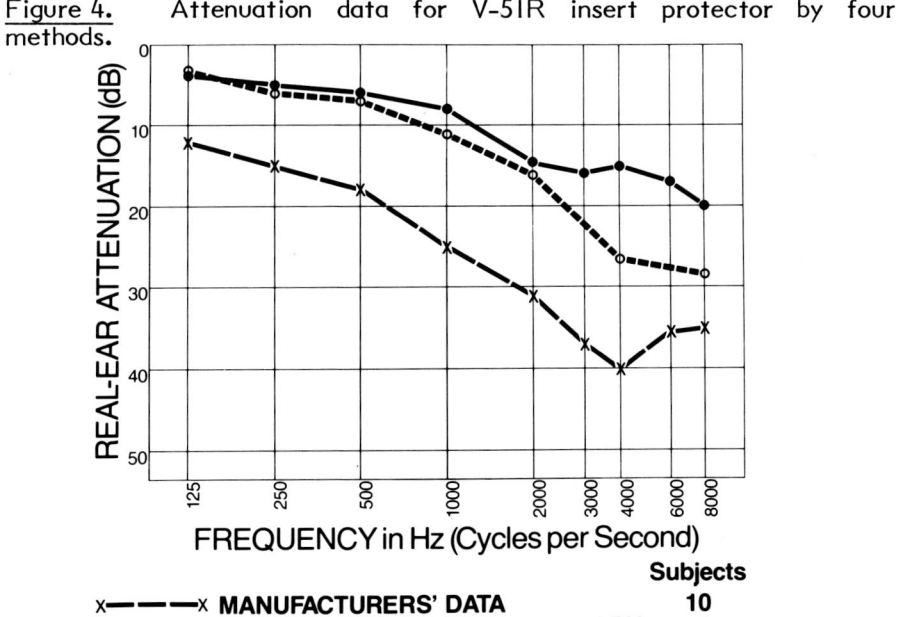

Figure 5. Attenuation data for Swedish wool insert protector by three methods.

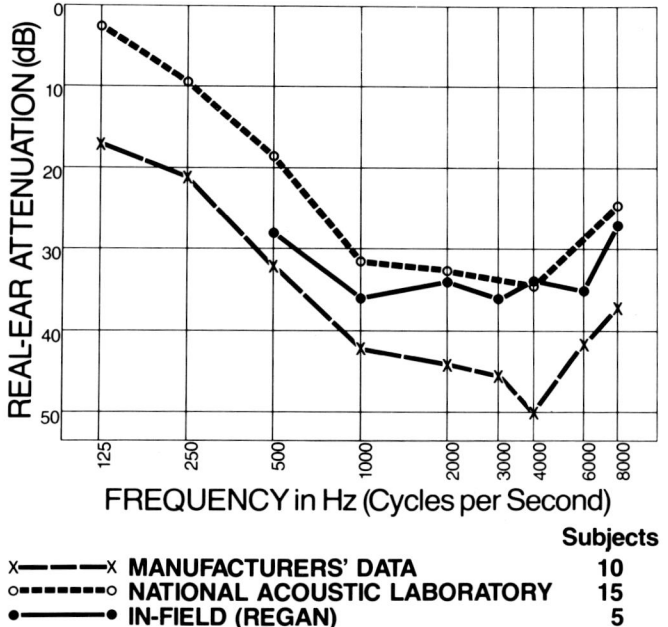

Figure 6. Attenuation data for earmuff protector by three methods.

manufacturer's reported attenuation data. NAL's data fall between these two data sets, only about 5 dB above the field data, except at the two highest frequencies. This may be due to better sizing techniques used at NAL than in industry. Figure 5 shows similar results for Swedish wool, with good agreement between NAL and field data, except at 4 kHz and 8 kHz. Figure 6 compares Regan's[4,5] field data for an earmuff to NAL data. Agreement is within 4 dB except at 500 Hz where NAL data are low. Thus manufacturers' laboratory data also over-estimate the RW performance of earmuffs, as confirmed by Alberti, et al[8], and a soon to be released MSHA[7] study that used miniature microphones to measure earmuff performance in the field.

The results of the latter study indicated performance of only 20-75% of the decibel values of the laboratory data with larger discrepancies at lower frequencies.

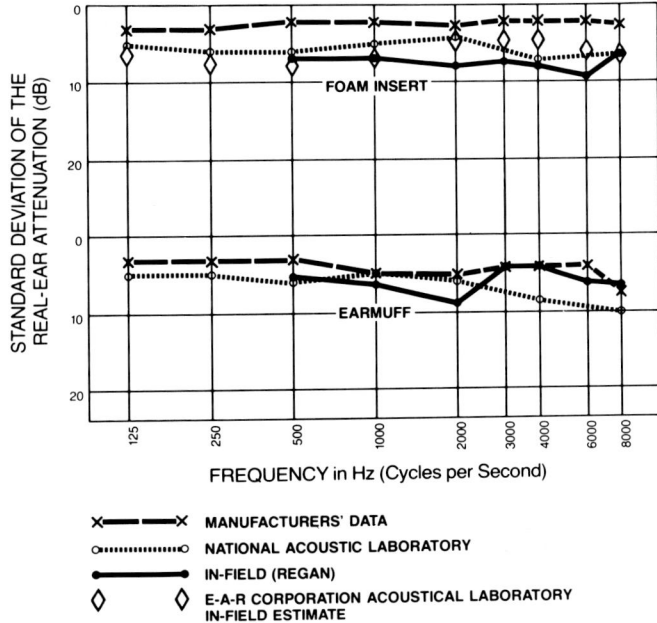

Figure 7. Standard deviation data for an earmuff and an insert by four methods.

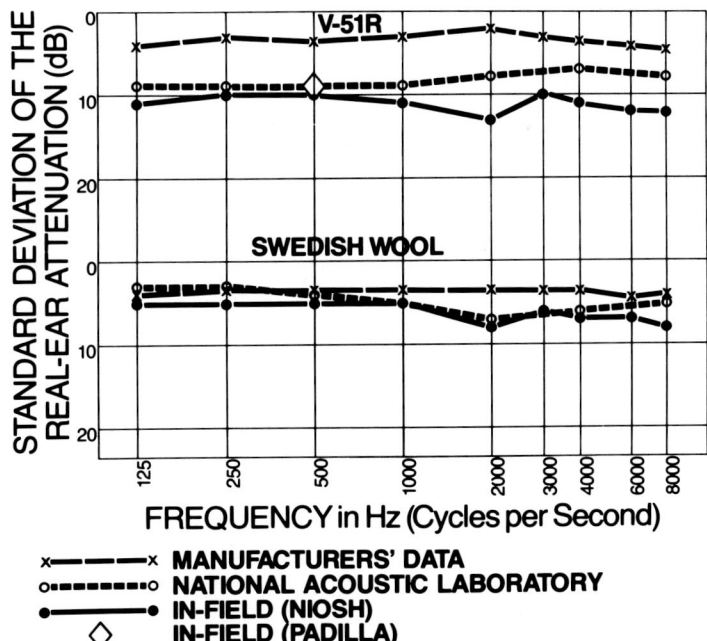

Figure 8. Standard deviation data for two insert protectors by four methods.

Figures 7 and 8 depict standard deviation data for the various devices measured via the four test methods. The general trend is for the field and NAL data to be in reasonable agreement and both somewhat higher than manufacturers' laboratory data. That this is not always the case, is partially explained by the fact that the standard deviation tends to vary in proportion to the mean attenuation, so that devices with lower mean attenuations have a reduced expected range of attenuation values as well.

SINGLE NUMBER RATINGS APPLIED TO REAL WORLD DATA

It is useful to be able to collapse hearing protector data to a single number rating suitable for use with dBC or dBA sound level measurements. Eleven of these methods are discussed by Berger[20], with the conclusion that the United States Environmental Protection Agency descriptor, the NRR[21], is a useful accurate method. The NRR, which assumes a pink noise spectrum, incorporates a 2 standard deviation (2σ) correction and a 3 dB spectral safety factor. These corrections are intended to insure protection for 98% of the population who "correctly" wear the HPD in 98% of the environments where the devices will be used. By "correctly" we mean, wear the HPD in the same manner as did the subjects who were used to generate the test results.

In Table 2, the NRRs for the four HPDs that have been discussed are presented. These NRRs were calculated using the manufacturers' laboratory data as well as the NAL data. Note that for two devices the NRR based on the NAL data is ≤ 1, i.e., 2% of the population will receive 1 db or less attenuation.

It may be that with RW or estimated RW data, a 2σ correction is too severe and that we should examine a 1σ correction (84% protection, i.e., 16% will get less than this number). These values are also shown in Table 2. (In fact, the single number rating listed in the NAL report is the SLC_{80}, which is very similar in concept[20,22] to the NRR, except that it uses a 1σ correction and lacks a spectral safety factor.) Even these more "optimistic" values demonstrate that certain protectors are only appropriate for lower levels of hazardous noise, a supposition substantiated by a

Table 2: NRR Values Based on Manufacturers' Laboratory Data and NAL Data

Hearing Protector	NRR* mfg	NRR** NAL	NRR*** NAL, 1σ
V-51R	18	0	9
Swedish Wool	16	1	6
Earmuff	25	6	13
Foam Insert (E-A-R Plug)	29	14	19

* based on manufacturers' laboratory data with 2σ correction.
** NRR based on NAL data with 2σ correction.
*** NRR based on NAL data with 1σ correction.

number of studies investigating the hearing levels of industrial noise exposed populations[9,23,24].

REFERENCES

1. Berger, E. H. (1979). EARLog #1 - The Threshold Shift Method of Measuring Hearing Protector Attenuation. Available upon request from E-A-R Corporation.

2. Edwards, R. G., Hauser, W. P., Moiseev, N. A., Broderson, A. B., Green, W. W., Effectiveness of Earplugs as Worn in the Workplace. Sound and Vibration, 12, No. 1, 12-22, 1978.

3. National Institute for Occupational Safety and Health. A Field Investigation of Noise Reduction Afforded by Insert-Type Hearing Protectors. U.S. Dept. of HEW, Report No. 79-115, Cincinnati, Ohio, 1978.

4. Regan, D. E., Real Ear Attenuation of Personal Ear Protective Devices Worn in Industry. Audiology and Hearing Education, 3, No. 1, 16-17, 1977.

5. Regan, D. E., Real Ear Attenuation of Personal Ear Protective Devices Worn in Industry. Doctoral Thesis, Kent State University, 1975.

6. Padilla, M., Ear Plug Performance in Industrial Field Conditions. Sound and Vibration, 10, No. 5, 33-36, 1976.

7. MSHA Denver Technical support Center - Field evaluation of earmuffs. To be published, 1980.

8. Alberti, P. W., Riko, K., Abel, S. M., Kristensen, R., The Effectiveness of Hearing Protectors in Practice. J. Otolaryn., 8, 354-359, 1979.

9. Royster, L. H., An Evaluation of the Effectiveness of Two Different Insert Types of Ear Protection in Preventing TTS in an Industrial Environment. Am. Ind. Hyg. Assoc. J., 41, 161-169, 1980.

10. Berger, E. H., The Measurement of Hearing Protector Attenuation via ASA STD1-1975 (ANSI S3.19-1974). J. Acoust. Soc. Amer., 67, Suppl. 1, p. S58, 1980.

11. Berger. E. H., Qualification of the E-A-R Corporation Hearing Protector Attenuation Testing Facility re ASA STD1-1975 (ANSI S3.19-1974). Report available upon request from E-A-R Corporation, 1979.

12. Acoustical Society of America. Method for the Measurement of Real-Ear Protection of Hearing Protectors and Physical Attenuation of Earmuffs. Standard ASA STD1-1975 (ANSI S3.19-1974), New York, N.Y., 1975.

13. Howell, K. Martin, A. M., Experimental Design for the Standard Measurement of the Acoustic Attenuation of Hearing Protectors. ISVR Memo. No. 472, Univ. of Southampton, England, 1973.

14. Robinson, D. W., Shipton, M. S., Whittle, L. S., Audiometry in Industrial Hearing Conservation - II. NPL Report AC 71, England, 1975.

15. Berger, E. H., The E-A-R Report. Report #EP3-9. Available upon request from E-A-R Corporation, 1980.

16. Waugh, R., Personal Communication, 1980.

17. National Acoustic Laboratories, Attenuation of Hearing Protectors (2nd Edition). Commonwealth Department of Health, Australia, 1979.

18. American National Standards Institute, Method for the Measurement of the Real-Ear Attenuation of Ear Protectors at Threshold. Standard Z24.22-1957 (R1971), New York, N.Y., 1957.

19. Waugh, R., Pure-Tone, Third-Octave, and Octave-Band Attenuation of Ear Protectors. J. Acoust. Soc. Am., 56, 1866-1869, 1974.

20. Berger, E.H., EARLog #2 - Single Number Measures of Hearing Protector Noise Reduction. Available upon request from E-A-R Corporation, 1979.

21. EPA. Noise Labeling Requirements for Hearing Protectors. Federal Register, Vol. 42, No. 190, 40 CFR Part 211, 56139-56147, 1979.

22. Waugh, R., Calculated In-Ear A-Weighted Sound Levels Resulting from Two Methods of Hearing Protector Selection. Ann. Occup. Hyg., 19, 193-202, 1976.

23. Royster, L.H., Effectiveness of Three Different Types of Ear Protectors in Preventing TTS. J. Acoust. Soc. Amer., 66, Supp. 1, DD 16,

1979.

24.   Royster, L.H., Lilley, D.T., Criteria and Procedures for Evaluating Industrial Audiometric Test Data. J. Acoust. Soc. Amer., 64, Supp. No. 1, p. S110, 1978.

20 User Fitting of Hearing Protectors: Attenuation Results

S. M. Abel, P. W. Alberti, and K. Riko

INTRODUCTION

It has been established that the attenuation provided by hearing protectors in the work place is significantly lower than the figures specified by the manufacturer[1-8]. In a preliminary report, Alberti and co-workers[9] suggested that the poor average performance and wide variation in score across individuals for three types of earplug were due to idiosyncrasies in fitting, especially with regard to sizing and technique for insertion. The present study is a continuation of this work. In particular, we wished to compare the attenuation provided by a wide variety of plugs and muffs when fitted by the worker. The number of individuals tested in each group was large enough to make valid estimates of attenuation scores at each frequency tested.

METHOD

The subjects for the experiment were 347 workmen referred for assessment of noise-induced hearing loss by the Workmen's Compensation Board of Ontario. They ranged in age from 35 to 65 years. Most were miners and steelmakers, who had worked in potentially hazardous levels of noise for 5 to 20 years. The type, location and duration of noise exposure varied widely.

Each subject brought his own hearing protectors from his place of work, which he fitted himself, without further instruction. In all, ten commonly used protectors were represented. As shown in Table I there were six types of plug and 4 different muffs. Across categories the smallest number of individuals tested was 15, and the largest number, 58.

Table 1: Types of Hearing Protectors

Plugs	N	Muffs	N
Comfit	18	MSA Mark IV	47
Custom	48	No Noise	58
Deci-Damp	24	Safety Supply	15
Ear	55	Straightaway	17
MSA	20		137
Willson	45		
	210		
Total:	347		

The apparatus and procedure used to measure the attenuation has been described previously[9]. The test was conducted in a double walled, soundproof booth. Free-field hearing thresholds were determined by the method of limits for each of eight digit test sounds with the open ear and with protectors fitted binaurally by the subject. The test sounds were narrowband noises centered at 125, 250, 500, 1000, 2000, 3000, 4000 and 6000 Hz.

RESULTS

Attenuation was calculated by taking the difference between the protected and open ear threshold at each frequency. The average open ear free-field hearing thresholds for the workmen in each of the 10 groups are presented in Figure 1. The data for the subjects using plugs are presented in the left panel, and for those using muffs, in the right panel.

The 10 groups are fairly similar. The change in threshold with frequency is typical of the more than 5000 claimants with noise-induced hearing loss seen in our department. At 125 Hz the threshold is about 30 dB SPL and at 6000 Hz, 55 dB SPL.

Figure 2 shows the average attenuation score obtained for each plug and muff type. The data for the muffs, indicate that the four models investigated give only 5 to 10 dB attenuation at 125 Hz. Attenuation increases sharply from 10 to 30 dB for frequencies between 125 and 1000

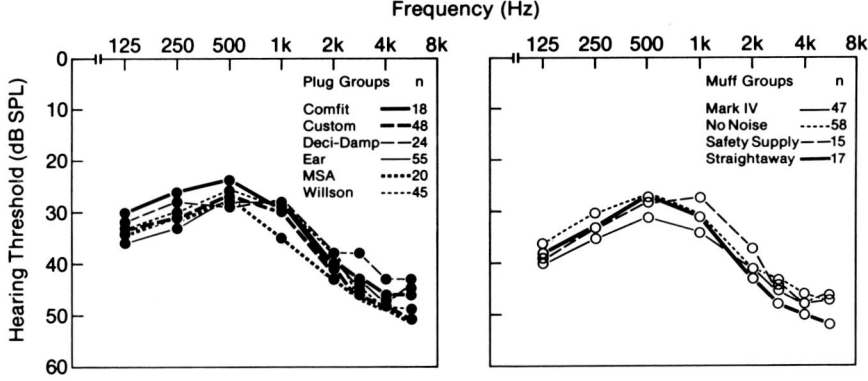

Figure 1. Free-field hearing threshold: Unprotected.

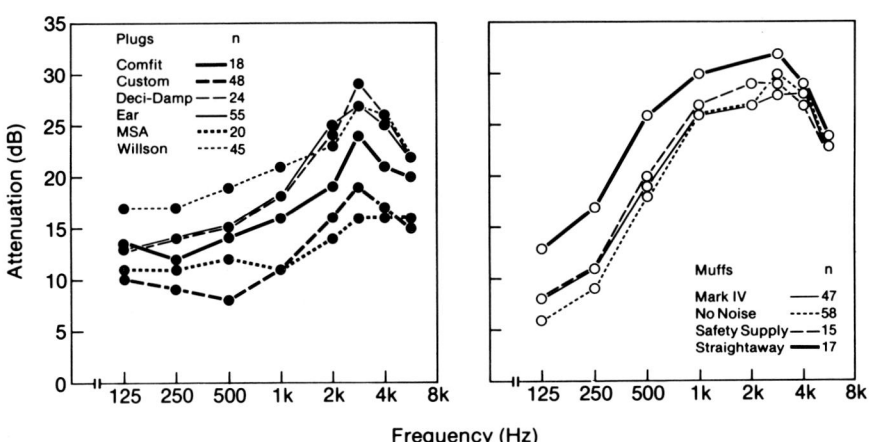

Figure 2. Attenuation for 10 hearing protectors.

Hz, remains fairly constant to about 3000 Hz, and then begins to decrease. The attenuation scores for the plugs show less change with frequency, but there is a wide variation across the 6 types studied. The greatest attenuation is provided by the Willson sound silencer, with the Ear and Deci-Damp running a close second. For these, average attenuation scores range from about 15 to 27 dB across frequency.

The average attenuation scores together with standard deviation values are listed in Tables 2 and 3 for ear plugs and muffs respectively. The standard deviations shown in these tables provide an index of the variation in attenuation scores measured for individuals in the group. This is shown more directly in figures 3 and 4 by means of histograms of attenuation in the muff and plug with the greatest sample size. The data are presented for each of four frequencies: 500, 1000, 2000, and 4000 Hz for Ear plugs and No Noise muffs on helmet. For both the plug and the muff, the distribution of attenuation scores is relatively broad, sometimes ranging from 0 to 45 dB. Wearing the muff, 80% of subjects obtain 15 dB of attenuation or better at 500 Hz, and 25 dB or better at 4000 Hz.

DISCUSSION

The data presented above attest to the wide variation in attenuation score which can be expected both within and between a broad class of hearing protector types. The difference in free-field hearing threshold, measured with and without the protector worn, may range from 0 to 45 dB in selected signals from 500 to 4000 Hz.

No doubt the relatively low average attenuation score, compared with the manufacturer's specification, and the wide variation across individuals for a given protector type are the result of the conditions of fitting, wearing and maintenance in everyday use[4,9]. Within our own clinic, we find that attenuation increases by about 7 or 8 dB across frequencies, when the audiologist fits the ear protector. These values are 3 to 4 dB less than the manufacturer's specification, again independent of frequency.

A comparison of plugs and muffs shows characteristic differences

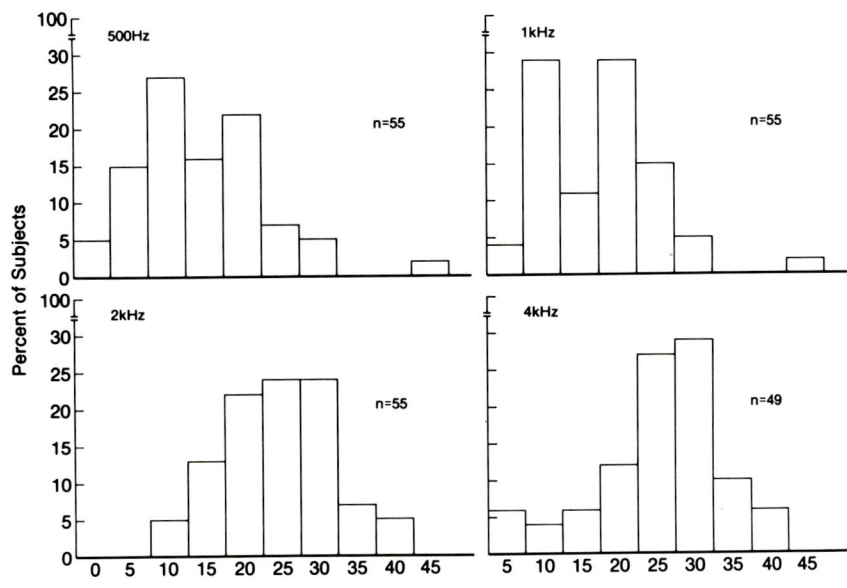

Figure 3. EAR plug frequency histograms.

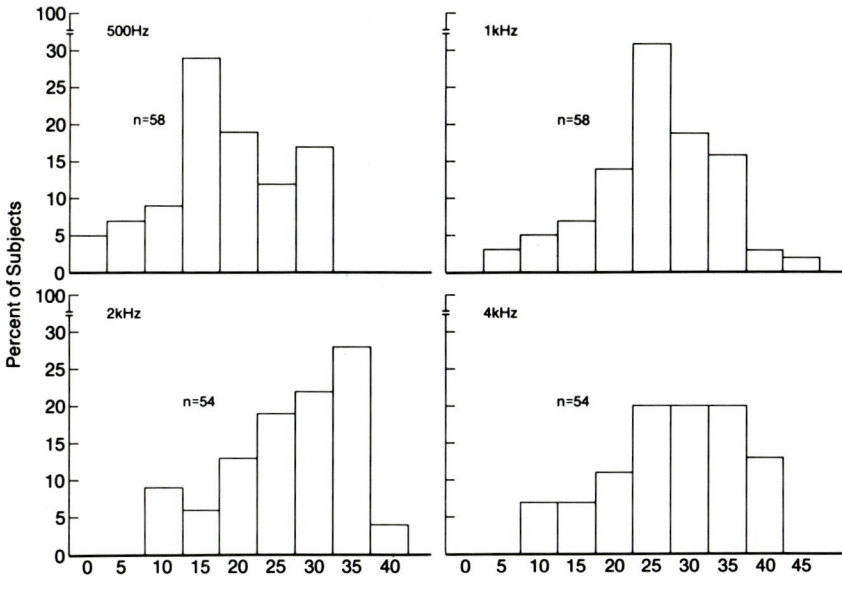

Figure 4. No Noise muff frequency histograms.

Table 2: Attenuation Scores for Six Types of Ear Plug

Frequency (Hz)

Plug Type	125	250	500	1K	2K	3K	4K	6K
Comfit	13.6 ± 7.4	12.2 ± 7.1	14.4 ± 7.6	16.4 ± 7.2	18.6 ± 7.0	23.6 ± 9.8	20.8 ± 9.1	19.7 ± 12.7
Custom	9.8 ± 9.0	9.1 ± 7.5	8.0 ± 6.2	10.6 ± 7.5	15.9 ± 8.7	18.5 ± 8.6	17.4 ± 8.8	15.2 ± 9.8
Deci-Damp	13.1 ± 7.8	14.0 ± 9.3	14.6 ± 8.7	17.5 ± 8.5	24.4 ± 9.8	29.3 ± 8.8	26.4 ± 10.0	22.3 ± 9.6
EAR	12.8 ± 8.3	14.2 ± 10.0	14.5 ± 8.7	18.0 ± 7.7	24.5 ± 7.5	27.1 ± 8.0	25.2 ± 8.5	21.8 ± 9.2
MSA	10.8 ± 10.2	13.3 ± 10.1	12.3 ± 9.5	10.5 ± 9.3	13.9 ± 8.6	16.4 ± 10.5	15.6 ± 9.4	15.9 ± 10.3
Willson	16.5 ± 10.8	17.4 ± 9.9	18.7 ± 9.3	20.9 ± 9.8	23.2 ± 9.3	26.9 ± 9.2	28.8 ± 9.6	22.0 ± 10.2

Table 3 Attenuation Scores for Four Types of Ear Muff

Frequency (Hz)

Muff Type	125	250	500	1K	2K	3K	4K	6K
MSA Mark IV	7.8 ± 9.6	11.2 ± 9.2	18.5 ± 9.6	25.7 ± 8.7	27.2 ± 7.1	27.7 ± 9.3	28.2 ± 10.1	23.1 ± 10.0
No Noise	6.3 ± 6.1	9.0 ± 7.1	17.9 ± 8.3	25.5 ± 8.5	26.9 ± 8.3	29.8 ± 9.7	27.6 ± 8.7	22.5 ± 8.9
Safety-Supply	6.7 ± 6.7	11.0 ± 8.7	19.3 ± 7.5	26.7 ± 8.1	29.3 ± 6.8	29.6 ± 9.3	26.5 ± 5.2	22.9 ± 7.3
Straight-away	12.9 ± 7.5	16.8 ± 9.3	25.9 ± 9.4	29.7 ± 9.4	28.5 ± 8.2	31.9 ± 7.5	31.9 ± 9.1	23.7 ± 10.3

between the two categories of protector. The four muffs studied give poor low frequency attenuation but provide in the order of 20 to 30 dB for frequencies between 500 and 6000 Hz. Plugs, on the other hand, are fairly constant in performance for a broad range of frequencies. For the six types studied, the attenuation values are on the average 12 to 20 dB. There is no significant difference in the variation of attenuation between plugs and muffs.

The reasons for the poorer attenuation of protectors in the work place are multiple; they include both protector and fitting factors. Plugs may be of an inappropriate size, be deformed either by use or deliberately, or the material altered by either dirt or by time. Muffs may have faulty seals, absent liners, inappropriate spring pressure, etc. The device may be faultily fitted, or other safety devices such as the temple bars of safety glass may prevent proper seal of muff to head, the shape of the head, ear or ear canal may preclude proper fitting. The factors are fully reported elsewhere in this symposium[10]. To be effective, the protector must be properly fitted and maintained. Attention to these factors is an important but frequently neglected feature of a hearing conservation programme.

The choice of an appropriate protector is affected by many factors, which include the intensity and spectrum of all noise. This is in part recognized by the Canadian Standards Association classification of hearing protectors[11]. However other factors such as comfort, which affects length of wearing time - an important factor[12], intermittency of noise, individual anatomical factors, working conditions and the need to wear other protective devices. There is no one protector which is THE correct one for all conditions and all subjects, and the attenuation figures described here are only one part of a complex equation.

ACKNOWLEDGEMENT

We wish to express our appreciation to the Workmen's Compensation Board of Ontario for their financial support and cooperation. Particular thanks are due to the staff of the Division of Audiology for undertaking the tests.

REFERENCES

1. Edwards, R.G., Hauser, W.P., Moiseev, N.A. et al. Effectiveness of earplugs as worn in the workplace. Sound vibration 12; 12-22, 1978.

2. Flaugrath, J.M., Wolfe, B.N. The effectiveness of selective earmuff-type hearing protectors. Sound and Vibration, 25-27, May 1971.

3. Martin, A.M. The acoustic attenuation characteristics of 26 hearing protectors evaluated following the British standard procedure. Ann. Occup. Hyg., 20; 229-246, 1977.

4. Russell, M.F., May, S.P. Towards the objective test for earmuffs. Lucas Engineering Rev., 7; 54-64, 1978.

5. Tobias, J.V. Earplug rankings based on protector-attenuation rating (P-AR), FAA-AM-75-11, October, 1975.

6. Waugh, R. Effect of ambient noise level on threshold-shift measures of ear-protector attenuation. J. Acous. Soc. Amer. 48; 597-599, 1970.

7. Webster, J.C., Thopmson, P.O., Beitscher, H.R. Noise bands versus pure tones as stimuli in measuring the acoustic attenuation of ear protective devices. J. Acous. Soc. Amer., 28; 631-638, 1956.

8. Whittle, L.S., Robinson, O.W. On the measurement of real-ear attenuation of hearing protectors by standardised test methods. NPL Acoustics Report AC 79, Feb. 1977.

9. Alberti, P.W. Riko, K., Abel, S.M., Kristensen, R. The effectiveness of hearing protectors in practice. J. Otolaryngol. 8; 354-359, 1979.

10. Riko, K., Alberti, P.W. How ear protectors fail: A practical guide. Personal hearing Protection in Industry. ed P.W. Alberti. New York, Raven Press, 1981.

11. Shaw, E.A.G., The Canadian Standards Association Classification of Hearing Protectors: History and Practical Problems in P.W. Alberti ed: loc cit.

12. Martin, A.M. Hearing conservation and noise reduction. In Hinchcliffe, R. and Harrison, D. (Ed.) Scientific Foundations of Otolaryngology. Heinemann Medical Books, London, 1976.

21
How Ear Protectors Fail: A Practical Guide

K. Riko and P. W. Alberti

INTRODUCTION

Personal hearing protectors are the most common means of preventing hearing loss in a workforce exposed to hazardous noise levels when engineering and administrative controls are inadequate for reducing noise to acceptable levels. Various standardized techniques have been developed to describe the attenuation characteristics of hearing protectors[1,2,3] and are used by manufacturers to describe the attenuation of any particular hearing defender. Manufacturers also specify very exactly how a particular protector is to be fitted and maintained in order to achieve these published attenuation figures. A 1975 NIOSH document on hearing protectors stressed that "it is necessary to maintain the same fit under actual working conditions to obtain the expected protection" and that factors other than calculated noise reduction must be considered if a device is to be accepted and used properly by the worker[4]. Is it realistic to expect the performance characteristics of hearing protectors as they are actually used by an individual, to equal the optimum results obtained by manufacturers using new and properly fitted devices on trained listeners?

A number of recent studies of protector performance have, in fact, demonstrated that the practical effectiveness of hearing protectors rarely matches ideal published attenuation figures and that employee misuse of protective devices is alarmingly high[5,6,7,8,9]. Alberti et al[10,11] recently evaluated the attenuation of hearing protectors brought by a large group of industrially noised exposed workmen when the device was fitted by the user himself. At least ten different types of protectors were tested and the mean attenuation figures obtained were lower than the figures generally accepted for both muffs and plugs. Furthermore the range of protection provided by individual protectors was found to be extremely wide. These results were disturbing but not unexpected.

Because it was suspected that both the condition of the hearing protectors and poor fitting habits were contributing to the low attenuation being obtained, a record was kept in the above study of how individual workers used their hearing protectors, what problems they had and what the condition of the protector was. Clear patterns of misuse and abuse emerged: poor placement technique, improper fit, maintenance problems, deliberate abuse, multiple protector requirements and poor hygiene were common hearing protector problems in practice.

Publications[12,13], and manufacturers instructions exist which clearly outline the various stages of proper choice, fitting, use and care of personal hearing protectors. However the tremendous variability in wearing patterns found, strongly supports the belief that the information is not reaching the user in an effective way.

We have even found that Hearing Conservation personnel are not always aware of the common pitfalls in the use of hearing protectors. Without such knowledge it is impossible to achieve optimum performance from hearing protectors or, ultimately, to conserve hearing.

This report gives an account of our findings with this group of workmen.

FINDINGS

Placement Technique

It was obvious that most users either never knew, or had forgotten, that a particular fitting technique is recommended by the manufacturer for optimum attenuation. Very few followed specified placement techniques.

I   Pre-molded Plug Type Defenders

In the case of most ear plugs, printed directions on the package instruct the user to pull the pinna up and back with the contralateral arm, while the user inserts the plug with the other hand. This fitting procedure is virtually impossible to follow when wearing a hard hat. In reality, most of the users preferred to push the plug in with one hand only, without straightening the ear canal. Consequently, the plug was often not lodged far enough inside in the ear canal. In other cases, it was marginally adequate but became unseated with talking or chewing. If all the flanges of a plug are not inside the ear canal, sound leaks will occur and reduce attenuation.

2   Foam Type Plugs

This type of plug should be rolled to form a thin cylinder, the tapered end of which is then inserted into the ear canal, where the plug expands to the shape of the ear canal to form an effective acoustic seal. It should be held in place for 1 minute to allow it to expand. Only few workmen rolled them into a sufficiently small cylinder and almost none held it in place for one minute. In one case, the plug was inserted, not length wise, but sideways. If these plugs are not inserted sufficiently deep into the ear canal and held in place to expand inside the canal, they too can be worked loose with talking and chewing.

3   Custom Molded Plugs

These are difficult to fit properly, and frequently were worn too superficially, a common finding also with hearing aid molds, with which they have some similarities.

4   Pre-molded Plugs on a Band

In the case of pre-molded plugs on a band, positioning of the band under the chin, over the head, or behind the head will result in different attenuation values. Furthermore, orientation of the plug is marked by an arrow, indicating which end is forward. Few workers were aware of these fitting instructions.

5   Muffs

An advantage of ear muffs, whether on a band or on a helmet, is that fitting technique is usually easier than for plugs. Nevertheless, for an adequate seal, the muff must be properly positioned over the ears and a good, leak free contact made with the surface of the head (Fig. 1a). Such was not always the case. Occasionally, the muff was positioned sideways or upside down, with obvious leaks present (Fig.1b). In the case of muffs attached to a helmet, the indentation on the top of the muff was

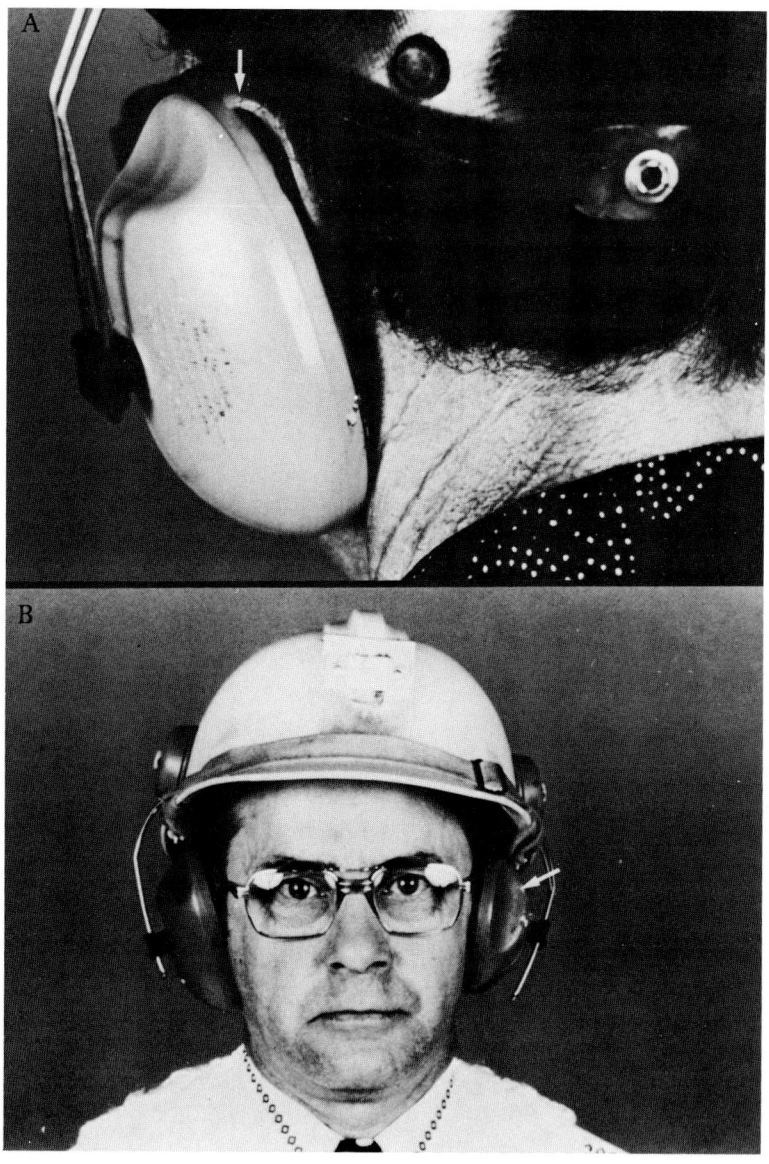

Figure 1a. Incorrectly placed cup, resting on pinna, rather than covering it
Figure 1b. Cups incorrectly orientated with superior recess facing forward.

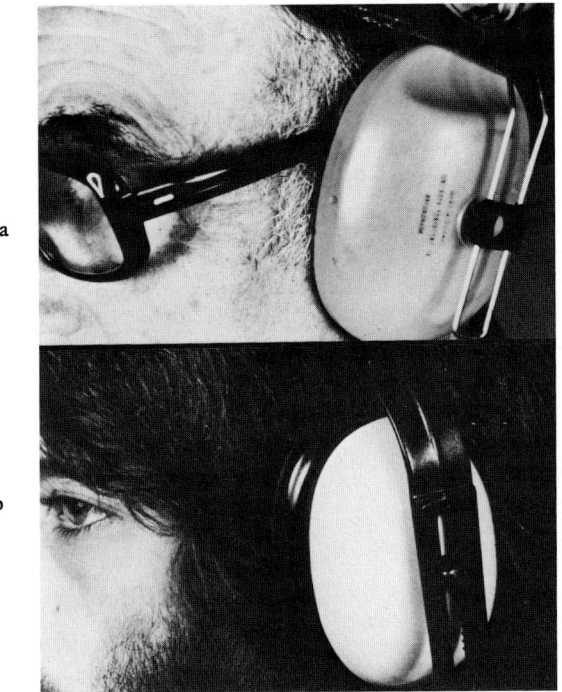

Figure 3a.   Safety glasses side temple produce break in seal.
Figure 3b.   Long hair prevents adequate seal.

takes time to accommodate the "plugged" feeling. One worker was a reluctant plug user because he frequently required medical assistance to remove one of his ear plugs. His ear canals were of unequal size and he had been given plugs which fitted his smaller ear. Consequently, the plug for the other ear was too small and slipped too far into his ear canal for easy removal.

Our clinical impressions regarding the importance of sizing when selecting insert type protectors have been substantiated in a study by Smith et al[14]. Using KEMAR they demonstrated that even skilled technicians found it very difficult to measure ear canal sizes accurately enough with available instruments; even small differences between measured ear canal diameter and insert size affect the sound pressure level in the ear canal in high noise levels. They also found that individuals, on their own, select inserts smaller than their ear canal size, which has also been commented upon by Royster[15].

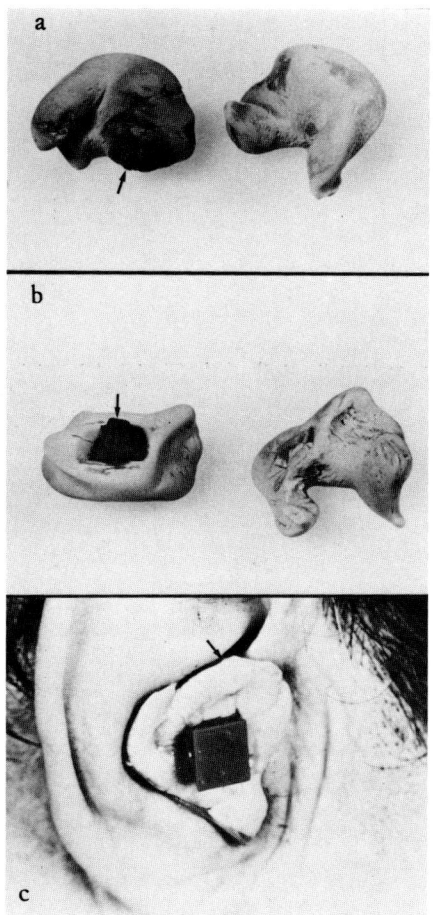

Figure 4a.   Worn off sealer on custom molded plug.
Figure 4b.   Mold deformed by use; handle compressed into mold.
Figure 4c.   Custom molded plug with edges obviously cut off.

Maintenance Problems

Poor physical condition of hearing protectors was yet another significant difference between practice and the laboratory. The physical properties of protectors change with time and hostile environment, some more than others. Yet there was little evidence of any maintenance programmes in many industries.

I   Pre-molded Plugs

Although pre-molded plugs were usually found to be in good condition, their size and shape can be altered. Rubber plugs can become flattened so that they no longer provide an effective seal. In severe cold, they can crack and shrink in very short periods of time. Royster[15] has commented on problems with some type of VR51's; others have commented upon the effect of ozone on plastic. Plug replacement programmes are an essential part of a hearing conservation programme but are not frequently found.

2   Custom-molded Plugs

Custom-molded plugs were invariably found to be in poor condition. Frequently, the sealer had cracked or worn off (Fig. 4a) or the original shape of the mold had become obliterated with repeated use (Fig. 4b). In other cases, cleansing of the mold with particularly caustic agents had eroded it out of shape.

3   Muffs

The major difficulty noted with muff defenders was the poor condition of many seals. They are either foam or liquid filled and serve to ensure a good contact between the uneven head contour and the muff. If this contact is not achieved attenuation is minimal. The seals receive the most wear and tear in daily use, are designed to be changed, and are relatively inexpensive and simple to replace. However, permanent indentations were visible on seals from eyeglass temples, safety gear or the seals had poor resilience due to old age (Fig. 5), or were frankly broken - all evidence of poor maintenance. The plastic of the seals is subject to the same environmental hazards as plugs, and may alter with age. Sometimes the foam liners were missing from the cups of the ear muffs and had not been replaced. Regular muff maintenance programmes are essential, but uncommon.

An even more serious problem noted with many of the muffs was poor head band tension; unless the muff is clamped against the head with sufficient force, serious sound leaks can occur. Because the pressure against the head produces discomfort, the bands had occasionally been bent out of shape. In other cases, the bands had lost their tension due to repeated use.

What is disturbing about these kinds of maintenance problems is that they are not obvious on cursory inspection to health and safety personnel. The worker himself must be motivated and on the alert to correct them.

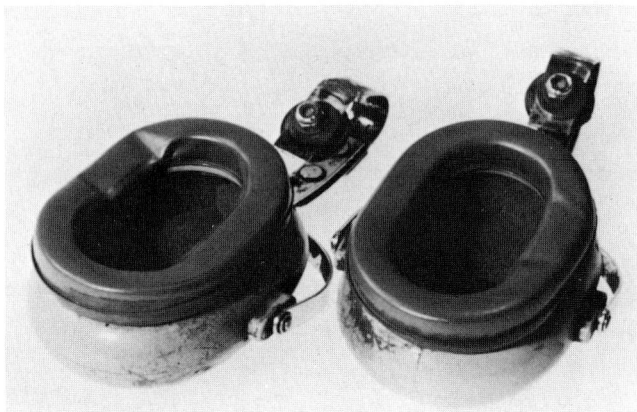

Figure 5. Aged earmuff seals permanently deformed by safety glasses.

Hygiene

Although there seems to be little documented evidence of the incidence of ear infections due to the use of dirty hearing protectors, a number of workers reported that they had infections or irritated ear canals from using the wax or foam insert-type ear plug. Although these protectors are disposable, many of the workers re-used them. These protectors have to be molded and if the hands of the user are dirty or greasy, dirt may be transferred to the ear canal by the protector. In industries where dirt and grease are common, the economics of using disposable plugs are questionable because of the number that have to be used if they are discarded each time they are removed.

A common complaint about disposable mineral fiber inserts was that frequently they shredded when removal was attempted and medical assistance was required. On occasion some of the material remained in the canal resulting in infection. However, this plug is now available with a plastic sheath, avoiding this problem.

In other cases, because of the individuals concern for good hygiene, the protectors had been cleaned with particularly corrosive agents, ruining the protector itself. This finding was particularly true for the custom-molded protectors.

Very few workers had sufficient practical knowledge about the proper care of hearing protectors.

Deliberate Abuse

A significant proportion of the hearing protectors inspected had been deliberately altered by the user himself, for a variety of reasons. One of the most commonly given was to reduce discomfort. Perspiration, pressure, and pain all precipitated purposeful changes. Difficulty hearing others speak or inability to hear sounds vital to the work process were two other causes. In other cases, the occlusion effect prompted modifications; reports of voice quality change, the sound of footsteps on pavement, difficulty in speaking and even dizziness were not uncommon. In one case, the workman altered his hearing protectors because he found the silence with them on deafening.

1   Molded Plugs

Any number of alterations are possible with pre-molded plugs. Plugs were seen with flanges cut off or holes drilled into them. In the case of some plugs on bands, the plugs had been removed and only the tips of the band inserted in the ear canal, so it would appear that safety regulations were being adhered to!

2   Custom-molded

This type of protector is especially amenable to tampering. Many were found with canal and/or external portions clipped down for comfort (Fig. 4c). The concept of custom fitting lent itself admirably to this type of protector abuse.

3   Muffs

Although muffs are fairly difficult to abuse deliberately, some had been; holes had been drilled between the cups and seals in order to hear better. In one plant it was standard practice to drill initials into the cups of the muffs for ease of identification; others drilled holes for ventilation (Fig. 6). Some users had deliberately bent the bands out of shape to reduce pressure discomfort.

Multiple Safety Gear

A significant problem for many workmen is the need to use several items

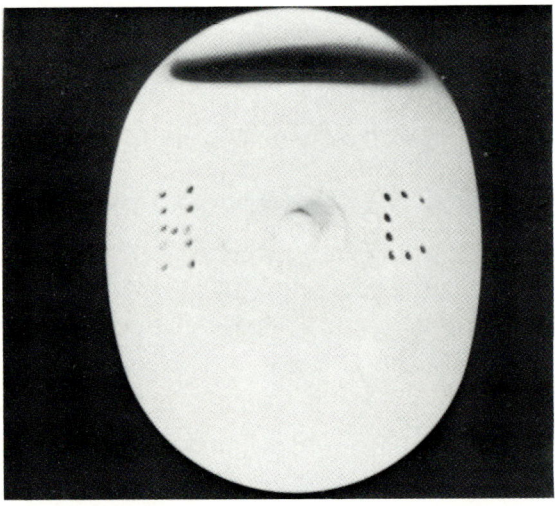

Figure 6.   Initials drilled into earmuff cups.

of safety gear simultaneously, especially when muff-type protectors are mandatory (as they often are in high noise level areas). They are difficult to use with a welding shield and some workers report pain at the temples when using muffs and safety glasses together. Some workers reported them too bulky for use in their workspace, in conjunction with all their other safety equipment. Muffs attached to hard hats bounce on the heads of heavy equipment operators, who were unaware of the existence of underchin retention straps.

The use of ear plugs is an obvious solution to the multiple safety gear problem but many of the workers reported that they did not like to use them because it was too time consuming to take them off to hear other speakers or when the noise level was reduced. Plugs on a band were reported to be a good compromise, combining the advantages of both types of hearing protectors; they are as easy to don and doff, but not as cumbersome as muffs. The ease of taking muffs off was a frequently cited advantage over plugs but it is also a disadvantage from a hearing conservation point of view. Safety personnel reported that it was often noted that workmen only slipped the muffs on when supervisory staff came to inspect and slipped them off at other times because of discomfort. Yet many industries prefer to issue muffs because it is supposedly

HOW EAR PROTECTORS FAIL

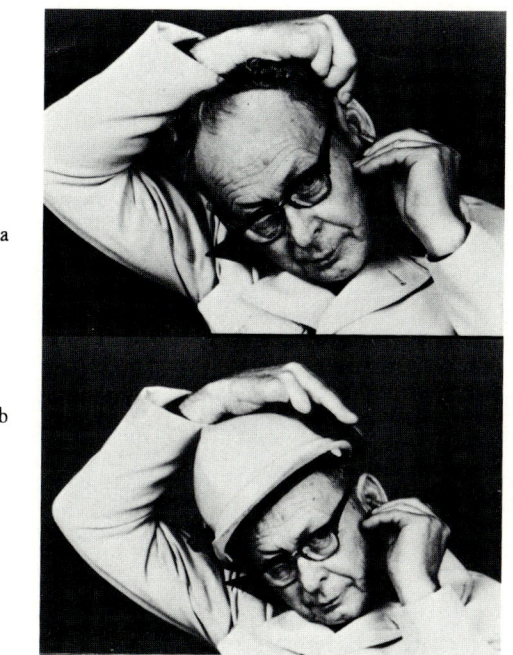

Figure 7a. Correct insertion of plug; pinna pulled up and back by contra lateral band.
Figure 7b. Above manoeuvre impossible while wearing hard hat.

simpler to monitor muff use because of their obvious visibility.

Individuals' Problems

Ultimately the choice of the most appropriate protector depends on the individual himself. Work environment, working conditions, physical characteristics and other peculiarities have to be taken into account when selecting a hearing protector for a specific person. In our sample of workers a number of unique problems and solutions were encountered.

One worker, because he had arthritis of the shoulder, could not raise his arm high enough to insert his ear plugs correctly when he was using his hard hat (Fig. 7). Another concerned worker designed and paid for his own hearing protector because he needed to hear other speakers but wanted protection against noise. The protector he designed was a custom molded plug with a considerable amount of narrow diameter tubing coiled inside.

Despite his enthusiasm and ingenuity however, he simply succeeded in producing a hearing protector with very poor attenuation characteristics; he increased his already present high frequency loss by about 20 dB and achieved almost no protection from low frequency noise - the opposite of his stated goal. Despite the best of intentions, this man would be considered a hearing conservation failure.

In another case, there was some confusion as to the purpose of a hearing aid earmold. A new hearing aid user was counselled to use his hearing aid earmold in one ear and a plug in the other for hearing protection but little attention was paid to the fact that hearing aids should not be used in high noise and dirt areas. Hearing aids cannot be ignored in populations with significant hearing loss.

CONCLUSION

Many workers who brought and fitted their own hearing protectors were found to be misusing and/or abusing their devices. The discrepancy between optimum and realistic attenuation of hearing protectors can undoubtedly be related to patterns of use which should be a major area of concern for those responsible for implementing effective hearing conservation programs. Getting the protector into proper use is obviously the bottom line and weak link in many hearing conservation programs.

Often workers are unaware of straightforward solutions to their problems. Many were very enthusiastic about protecting their hearing but did not know how to keep the protector effective.

More effort is required to give the worker as full an understanding as possible for how and why hearing protectors should be used. It is also clear that such knowledge must periodically be reinforced. Otherwise, assuming the sample of workers seen to be representative, users tend to develop their own protocols of hearing protector usage. More education and heightened motivation of the users is vital if hearing protectors are to be an effective part of any Hearing Conservation Program. To implement this, instruction in protector maintenance and fitting must be given to safety and health personnel, and routine maintenance programmes implemented as an integral part of the hearing conservation programme.

ACKNOWLEDGEMENTS

The authors wish to thank the staff of the Division of Audiology for assistance in the data colleciton, the workmen who so generously contributed their time and experience, and the Workmen's Compensation Board of Ontario whose support and co-operation made this report possible.

REFERENCES
1. CSA Standard Z94.2-1974. Hearing Protectors Canadian Standards Association, 178 Rexdale Blvd., Rexdale, Ontario, Canada.

2. ASD STD-1, Method for the measurement of real ear protection of hearing protectors and physical attenuation of ear muffs. Acoust. Soc. Amer., N.Y., 1975

3. Tobias, J.V., Measurers' choices in standard and non standard testing of hearing protector effectiveness. Personal Hearing Protection in Industry, ed. P.W. Alberti, Raven Press, New York, 1981, Croome Helms, London, 1981.

4. List of Personal Hearing Protectors and Attenuation Data. NIOSH technical information HEW (NIOSH), 1975.

5. Flugrath, J.M., Wolfe, B.N., The effectiveness of selected ear muff type hearing protectors. Sound Vibration 5, 25-27, 1971.

6. Peterson, P.G., Gross, E.E., Handbook of Noise Measurement. General Radio, Concord, Mass., 1974.

7. Padilla, M., Earplug performance in industrial field conditions. Sound Vibration 10, 33-36, 1976.

8. Regan, D.E., Real ear attenuation of personal ear protector devices worn in industry. Audiol Hearing Educ 3, 16-18, 1977.

9. Edwards, R.G., Hauser, W.P., Moiseev, N.A., et al: Effectiveness of earplugs as worn in the workplace. Sound Vibration 12, 12-22, 1978.

10. Alberti, P.W., Riko, K., Abel, S.M., Kristensen, R., The effectiveness of hearing protectors in practice. J. Otolaryngol. 8, 354-359, 1979.

11. Abel, S.M., Alberti, P.W. and Riko, K., User fitting of hearing protectors: attenuation results. P.W. Alberti, ed, loc. cit.

12. Industrial Noise Manual (2nd Ed.). American Industrial Hygiene Ass., 1966.

13. Personal Hearing Protective Devices - Fitting, Care and Use. US Army, Environmental Hygiene Agency, Aberdeen Proving Ground, Maryland 21010, 1975.

14. Smith, C.R., Barton, T.E., Patterson, L.E., Mozo, B.T., Camp, R.T., Insert hearing protector effects on SPL's in a simulated external ear canal: preliminary reports using KEMAR. Ear Hear $\underline{1}$, 26-32, 1980.

15. Royster, L.Y., and Susan Holder, Personal hearing protection & problems associated with the hearing protection phase of the hearing conservation programs, in P.W. Alberti, ed, loc cit.

22 THE EFFECTS OF HEARING PROTECTION ON THE PERCEPTION OF WARNING SOUNDS

P. A. Wilkins and A. M. Martin

INTRODUCTION

The perception of warning sounds can be vital to the safety of workers in industry. Auditory warnings may be generated by devices such as sirens and bells with the intention of alerting people to imminent danger. In addition, many sounds incidental to a process may act as a warning either due to its specific context or due to a change in its character. These incidental as distinct from intentional warning sounds may be associated with potentially dangerous events such as a malfunctioning piece of machinery, an approaching fork-lift truck, an impending roof fall in a coal mine ("roof talk"), or the loosening of a die key in drop forging ("the ringing of the keys").

A number of surveys have indicated that approximately a half of the workers who have to wear hearing protectors think that the protectors make it more difficult to hear warning sounds[1-6]. This attitude disrupts the implementation of hearing protection programmes, and has caused concern to legislators who are considering making the wearing of ear defenders mandatory under specific conditions of noise exposure. If the hearing protectors do impair the wearer's ability to perceive warning sounds they would expose the person to dangers potentially more serious than hearing damage due to excessive noise exposure. There is therefore an urgent requirement for a comprehensive assessment of the basis, if any, of this attitude.

A consideration of the sensory processes involved in the perception of a warning sound in the presence of noise suggests the conceptual model shown in Figure 1. This model incorporates not only the audibility of the

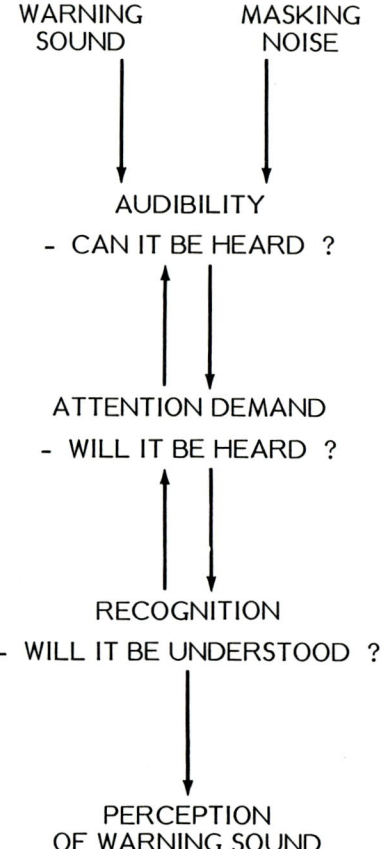

Figure 1.   Conceptual model of the perception of a warning sound.

sound, but also its attention demand (whether it will be heard when it is unexpected) and its recognition (whether when heard its meaning will be understood). A review of the literature relevant to each of these components of the model has been performed as part of a continuing programme of research on this topic[7].

Five studies have investigated the effects of wearing hearing protection on the first component of the model, the detection of sounds in noise[8-12]. These do not cover an adequate range of conditions, but suggest that in general the protectors may not have any large effect on the audibility of warning sounds. Since the protectors attenuate the signal and noise equally, the signal-to-noise ratio which governs the detection of the signal remains essentially unchanged.

There have, however, been no directly relevant studies which have examined the effect of hearing protectors on the wearer's ability to perceive a warning sound when it is largely unexpected, and when it must be recognized amongst other environmental sounds. These latter two components of the conceptual model represent the conditions under which an auditory warning normally occurs in industry, and must therefore be incorporated into an assessment of the effectiveness of a sound as a warning.

A series of experiments have been conducted to investigate the psycho-acoustical basis of the effects of wearing hearing protectors on the perception of warning sounds in the context of the conceptual model[13-15]. All the experiments were performed in an anechoic room with the signal and noise mixed electronically and presented via a single loudspeaker located at a distance of 2 m directly in front of the subject. The subjects all had hearing levels better than 20 dB HL re ISO 389:1975 at test frequencies over the range 0.5 to 6 kHz in both ears.

THE EFFECTS OF HEARING PROTECTION ON THE DETECTION OF WARNING SOUNDS

Two experiments were undertaken to measure the masked thresholds of several typical intentional warning sounds in different noise environments with the subjects' ears unoccluded and wearing different types of hearing protectors. Sixteen subjects participated in each experiment. The masked thresholds were measured using a standard manual audiometric technique (a "staircase" variant of the method of limits), with signals presented at 2 dB intervals.

Experiment 1 investigated the audibility of two warning sounds, a siren and a bell, which were tape recorded and presented in short bursts of duration 1 to 3 seconds with rise and fall times of 50 ms. The signals were presented in the presence of broad-band random noise at one of two

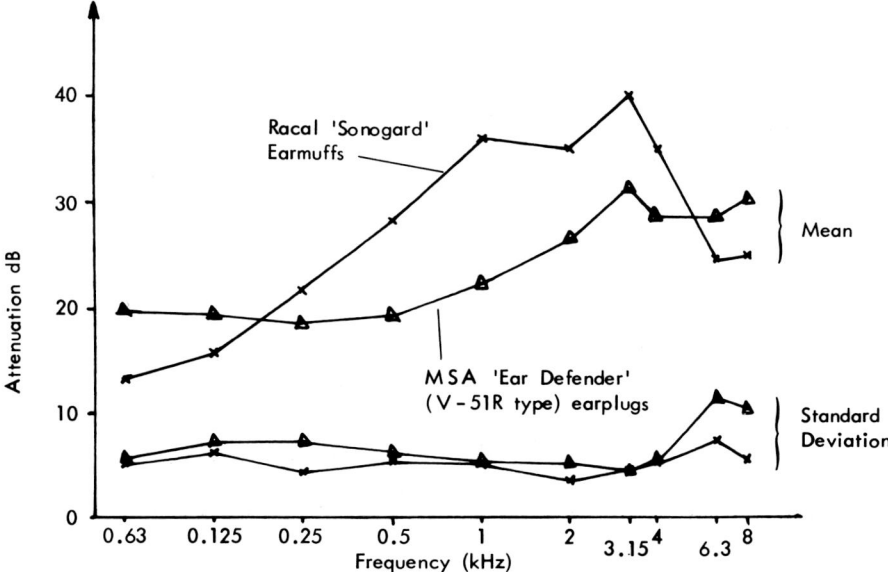

Figure 2. Attenuation of the hearing protectors employed, based on measurements at the ISVR in accordance with the British standard BS5108 (1974).

sound pressure levels: 75 and 95 dB(C). The hearing protectors employed were Racal (formerly Amplivox) "Sonogard" earmuffs, MSA "Ear Defenders" (Type V51R) earplugs, and an electronic simulation of the attenuation provided by the earmuffs. The attenuation of these protectors is shown in Figure 2.

Experiment 2 assessed the masked thresholds of four warning sounds: a siren, a two-tone "high-low" warning sound, and the "high" and "low" components separately as intermittent signals. These sounds all had temporal variations which are characteristic of intentional warning sounds (Figure 3). The complex frequency and amplitude modulations of the "wailing" siren are evident in this figure, and are in contrast with the steady siren used in experiment 1. Two broad-band noise spectra, the random noise of experiment 1 and a tape recorded workshop noise environment, were used (Figure 4). Both noise spectra were at the single level of 90 dB(C). Two ear conditions, the subjects' ears unoccluded and wearing the earmuffs were investigated.

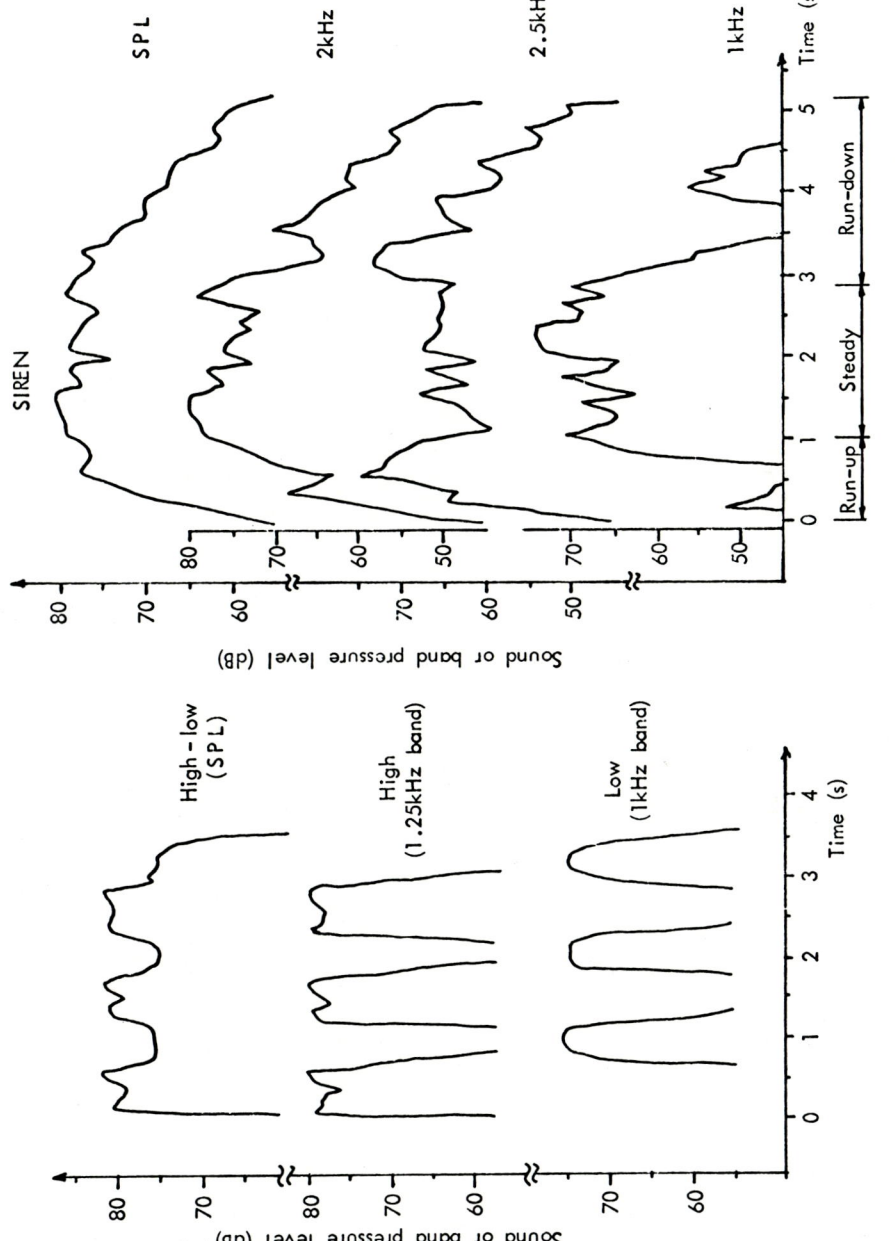

Figure 3. Time histories of the warning sounds investigated in experiment 2.

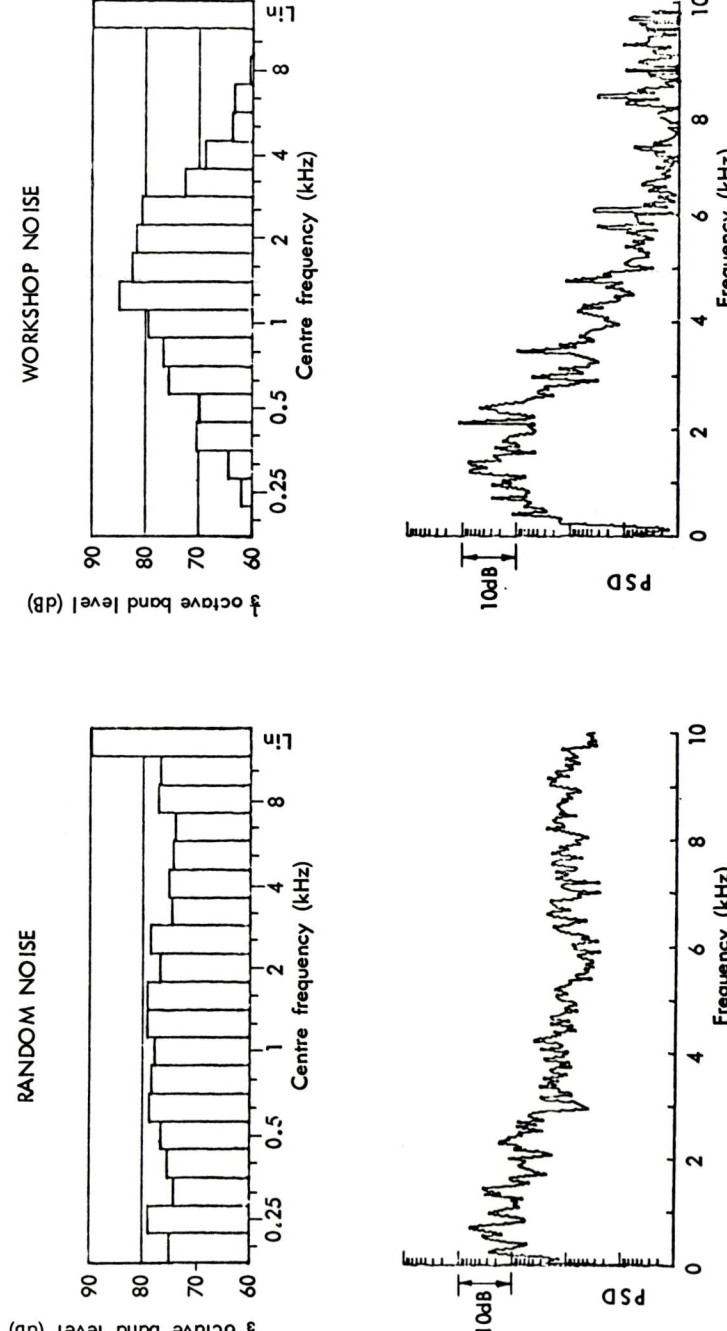

Figure 4. One-third octave band and power spectral density (PSD) spectra of the ambient noises investigated in experiment 2.

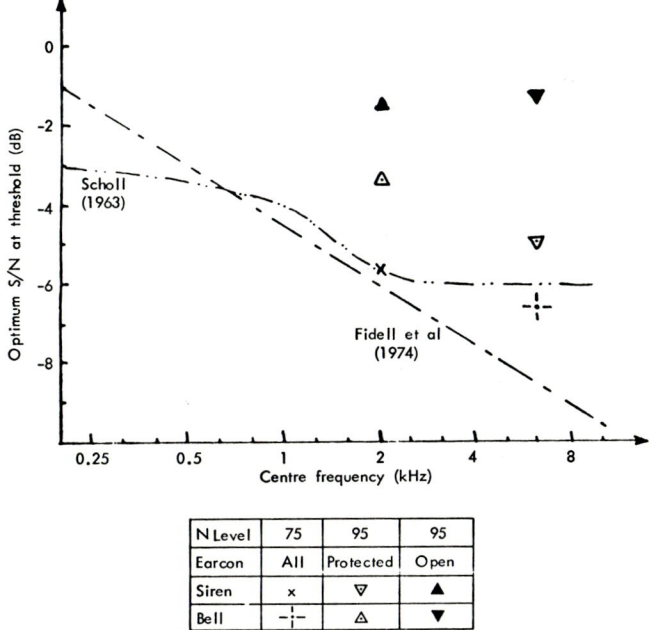

Figure 5. Optimum one-third octave band signal-to-noise ratio at masked threshold for experiment 1[7]. Data compared with the detection criteria of Scholl[16] and Fidell et al[17].

Both experiments employed randomized block factorial designs, with the order of ear conditions and warning sound-noise conditions separately balanced for first order carry-over effects.

Results

The mean masked thresholds are summarised in Figures 5 and 6 in relation to criteria for the prediction of the masked threshold of complex sounds. The prediction method is based on integrated sound energy measures (L_1) of the signal and noise in one-third octave bands[16,17]. The detectability of the sounds is assessed on the basis of the frequency band with the highest signal-to-noise ratio.

The results show that the wearing of hearing protection did not have any large effect on the detection of the warning sound under any of the noise conditions. The largest difference between mean occluded and unocclud-

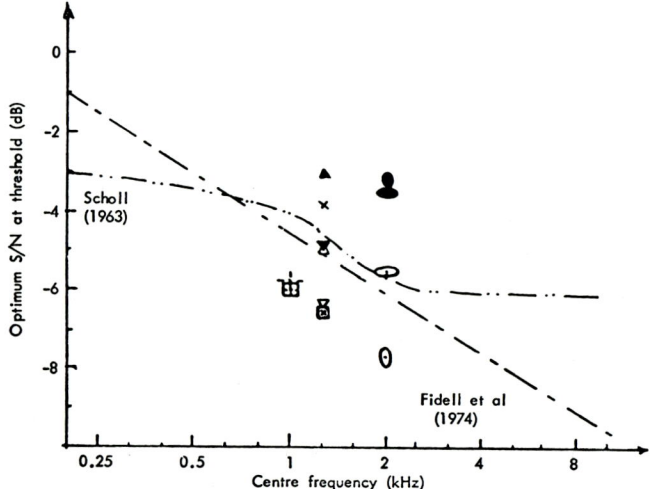

Figure 6.   Optimum one-third octave band signal-to-noise ratio at masked threshold for experiment 2. Data compared with the detection criteria of Scholl[16] and Fidell et al[17].

ed ear conditions is 4.5 dB for the wailing siren in the workshop noise in experiment 2.

Separate analyses of variance of the data of the two experiments indicated that the only significant differences between ear conditions were for the unoccluded condition and the three protected conditions in the 95 dB(C) noise in experiment 1, and between the unoccluded and occluded conditions for the siren and high-low sounds only in experiment 2. The wearing of hearing protection in the high noise conditions for which they are normally required, improved the audibility of these sounds by an average of approximately 3 dB over the masked thresholds with ears unoccluded. In relation to the predicted S/N at threshold, the results suggest that this difference is due to less efficient detection (higher S/N at threshold) in the high noise condition with ears unoccluded.

Discussion

The results of the two experiments indicate that there are no large effects of wearing hearing protection on the audibility of warning sounds in noise. They are therefore in general agreement with the five previous studies and extend the scope of the conclusion to a variety of typical intentional warning sounds, noise spectra and intensities and hearing protectors[8-12].

The results of both experiments indicate that in general there is a small but significant relative improvement in detection when wearing hearing protection in the high noise conditions. This effect can be attributed to a broadening of the auditory filter which occurs at progressively higher noise intensities, and would degrade the signal-to-noise ratio of tonal stimuli in broad-band noise[18,19]. By reducing the intensity of both the signal and noise the hearing protection would therefore provide a relative improvement in the detection of warning sounds by restoring the S/N to that occurring at lower intensities. It appears however, that this non-linear growth in masking may not occur for intermittent warning sounds such as the "high" and "low" sounds in experiment 2.

A similar small improvement in the perception of speech when wearing hearing protection in noise levels above approximately 85 dBA has been reported,[20] however the measure employed was that of the intelligibility of the speech material, and the effect may therefore be due to changes in either the detection or recognition of the sounds.

THE EFFECTS OF HEARING PROTECTION ON THE ATTENTION DEMAND OF WARNING SOUNDS

Previous studies have indicated that inattention may elevate the masked threshold of warning sounds by an average of up to 9 dB[21,22]. Counter to this there is, however, a widespread attitude that the perception of important sounds remains unaffected by lack of attention. Typical of this school of thought is the statement by Durlach and Colburn that "the fact that nature did not provide us with earlids is probably due to .... the use of the acoustical channel for warning signals, a function to which it is exceptionally well matched"[23].

Experiment 3 therefore investigated the effects of hearing protectors on the ability of subjects to perceive a warning sound when it is largely unexpected. To simulate in the laboratory the inattention which typically occurs in industrial situations, uncertainty as to the time of occurrence of the warning sound and an additional loading task were provided to ensure that the subject's attention was directed away from continuously listening for the sound. This <u>effective response</u> (ER) condition provides a measure of the effectiveness of the sound as a warning. It is compared with the baseline measure obtained under <u>detection response</u> (DR) conditions where the sound is deliberately listened for and its time of occurrence is known. The detection response function is measured prior to and after the assessment of the effective response (DR1 and DR2 respectively), to assess its variation across each effective response condition.

The warning sound is presented at different intensities using the method of constant stimuli to provide measures of the probability of a warning being perceived under different signal-to-noise ratio conditions[24]. This is more appropriate than the single metric "elevation of threshold" obtained in the earlier studies of the effectiveness of warning sounds[21,22].

The temporal uncertainty during the effective response condition was created by presenting the signal at five different levels in random order at random time intervals. The mean inter-signal interval was 93s, which resulted from a random choice of times from a rectangular distribution over the range 20-160s, and corresponds to 20 presentations of the sound over a 31 minute period. The provision of temporal uncertainty on its own is typical of the studies of vigilance which model the watch-keeping task of deliberately listening for infrequent sounds. To assess the relative importance of the loading task both the vigil and a task condition were investigated.

The loading task used was a modified version of a television tennis game. The subject controlled a "bat" and attempted to direct a "ball" through the moving "hole" on the right of the screen. Points for or against the subject were scored plus or minus one point starting from zero, and a set was won or lost when the score reached plus or minus seven, respectively. Subjects were instructed to try to win by as many sets as possible. They were encouraged in their performance at the task by continuous feedback of the points score by the marker at the bottom of the screen, and at both the task and responding to the warning sound by a financial bonus awarded at the end of the experiment on the basis of their overall performance.

The warning sound and noise employed were the wailing siren and the broad-band random noise of experiment 2, with the noise at an intensity of 75 dB(C).

The experiment had a 5 x 3 x 2 x 2 x 12 split-plot factorial design. The treatments were the five signal levels, L1 to L5 at 5 dB intervals; the three response conditions, the effective response condition ER and the two detection response conditions DR1 and DR2; the two task conditions, the ER condition occurring either as a VIGIL or with the TASK; the two ear conditions, the subject either having OPEN ears or wearing the MUFFS; and the twelve subjects.

Measures of the number of responses, the response times and the performance at the loading task were obtained. The data was collected with each subject participating in four experimental sessions which covered the four combinations of task and ear conditions. The order of sessions and the order of sound presentations within sessions were suitably randomized.

Results

The mean numbers of correct responses across subjects as a function of signal level for the detection response and effective response conditions are presented in Figure 7. The curves show the typical sigmoid shape of psychometric functions, rising from a chance rate at the lowest signal

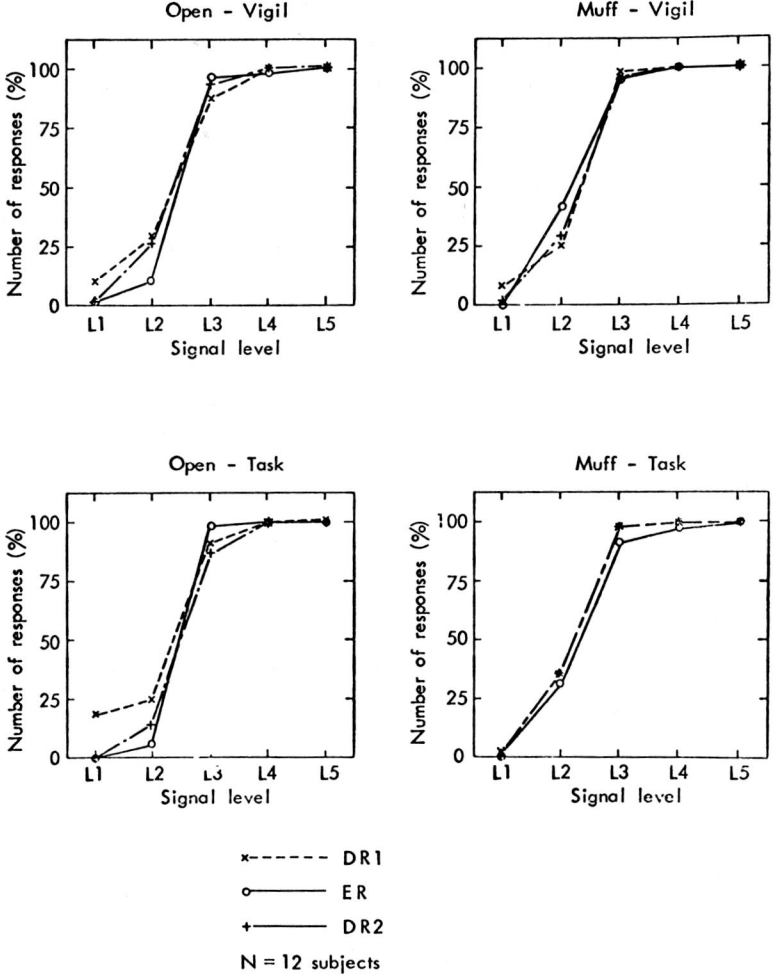

Figure 7. Number of responses averaged across subjects in experiment 3.

level (L1), to 100% response rates at the highest signal level (L5). Examination of the data indicates that there were no large consistent differences in the response rates due either to the response condition, or the task and ear condition combinations.

The data were statistically analysed using the two response differences:

detection response difference $\quad$ DRD = $DR_1 - DR_2$

and

effective response difference $\quad$ ERD = DR - ER

where

DR_1 = pre-test detection response rate
DR_2 = post-test detection response rate
ER = effective response rate
DR = ½($DR_1 + DR_2$)

The only significant effects of the hearing protectors occurred at levels L2 and L3 with the siren close to its masked threshold. These suggest a 21% advantage in terms of ERD at L2 when wearing the earmuffs. However, as the detection response (DR) rate at this level is only 26%, the sound under these conditions would never constitute a reliable warning. At the next higher level L3, with a DR of 94% there is however a 10% relative disadvantage when wearing the earmuffs.

Discussion

The results of this experiment suggest that neither inattention, nor the combination of inattention and the wearing of earmuffs, will necessarily reduce the probability of the perception of an unexpected but important sound. There was some suggestion that with the signal just above its masked threshold there was an impairment in its perception when wearing the earmuffs. However this effect is too inconsistent to permit any definite conclusion.

These results may however be specific to the siren warning sound which is very distinct, and is familiar to most people as a warning. The results suggest that for an appropriately chosen warning sound there is normally sufficient spare attentional capacity for the warning to be perceived.

The absence of any effect due to inattention is in contrast with the previous studies which have reported an elevation of threshold[21,22]. This may be due to methodological differences, including the use of a method of ascending limits, and inappropriate motivation of the respective subjects in both these previous studies, which could have produced the elevation of threshold as an artefact.

THE EFFECTS OF HEARING PROTECTION ON THE COMBINED RECOGNITION AND ATTENTION DEMAND OF WARNING SOUNDS

In typical industrial situations auditory warnings occur in the context of other meaningful sounds, and must be recognized as warnings to be effective. Given the proper choice and use of a warning sound for a particular situation, it is unlikely that problems will occur with its recognition per se. However it is possible that the need to distinguish the warning sound from other irrelevant sounds may impair its effectiveness by reducing its attention demand. That is, there may be an interaction between the second and third components of the model of the perceptual process (Figure 1).

The ability of subjects to perceive warning sounds which are largely unexpected and must be recognized amongst meaningful irrelevant sounds, and the effects of their wearing hearing protection, was therefore investigated in experiment 4. The methodology was essentially the same as that employed in experiment 3^{25}. However, during the measure of the effective response rate to the warning sound, four other irrelevant sounds were also presented at one of five levels at random time intervals (mean inter-stimulus interval = 19s, mean inter-signal interval = 95s), with these sounds at their respective levels occurring in a randomized order throughout the experimental session. The subjects' ability to recognize the warning sound amongt the irrelevant sounds was also assessed when the sounds were listened for deliberately, termed the recognition response (RR).

The intentional warning sound and the noise employed were the same as those investigated in experiment 3. Four tape recorded workshop sounds were used: the sounds of the grinder, a diesel engine, a lathe and a drill. The temporal variation of the estimated audible components of the five sounds above the noise is shown in Figure 8. Typical narrow band analyses

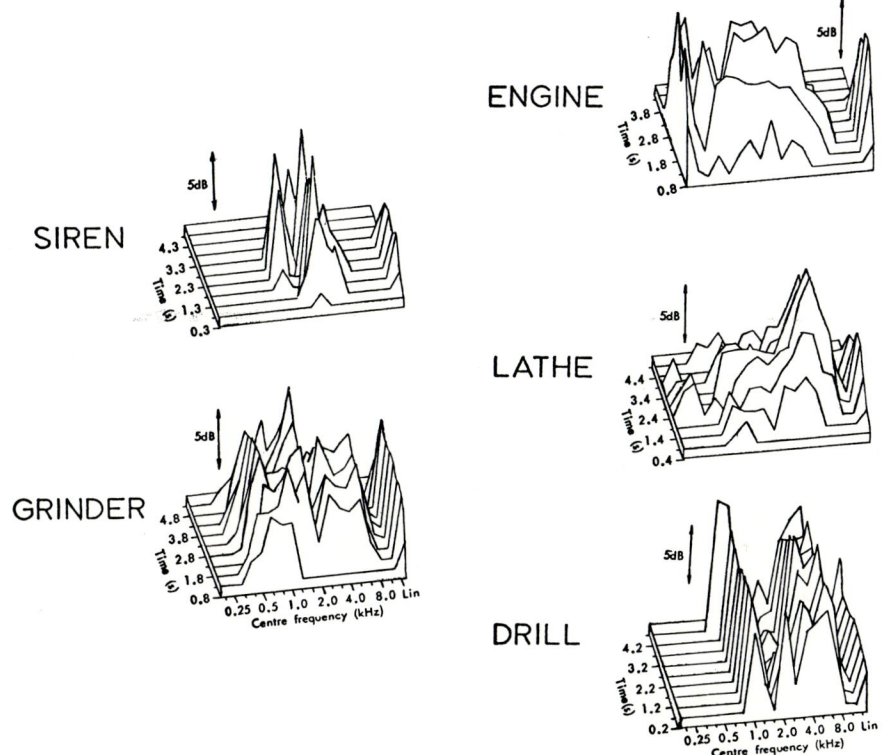

Figure 8. One-third octave band signal-to-noise ratios of the sounds in experiment 4. The three-dimensional displays show the variation in S/N and frequency with time based on 0.1s integration periods every 0.5s.

of the sounds are presented in Figure 9.

The effectiveness of both the siren and the grinder sounds as warnings were evaluated separately. Either sound acted as a warning in the context of the remaining four sounds in the set. The grinder typifies incidental warning sounds which are associated with malfunctioning machinery or other unexpected and potentially dangerous events.

The experiment had a 5 x 4 x 2 x 2 x 16 split-plot factorial design. The treatments were the five signal levels L1 to L5; the four response conditions DR1, DR2, RR and ER; the two ear conditions with the subjects either havings ears unoccluded or wearing earmuffs; the two

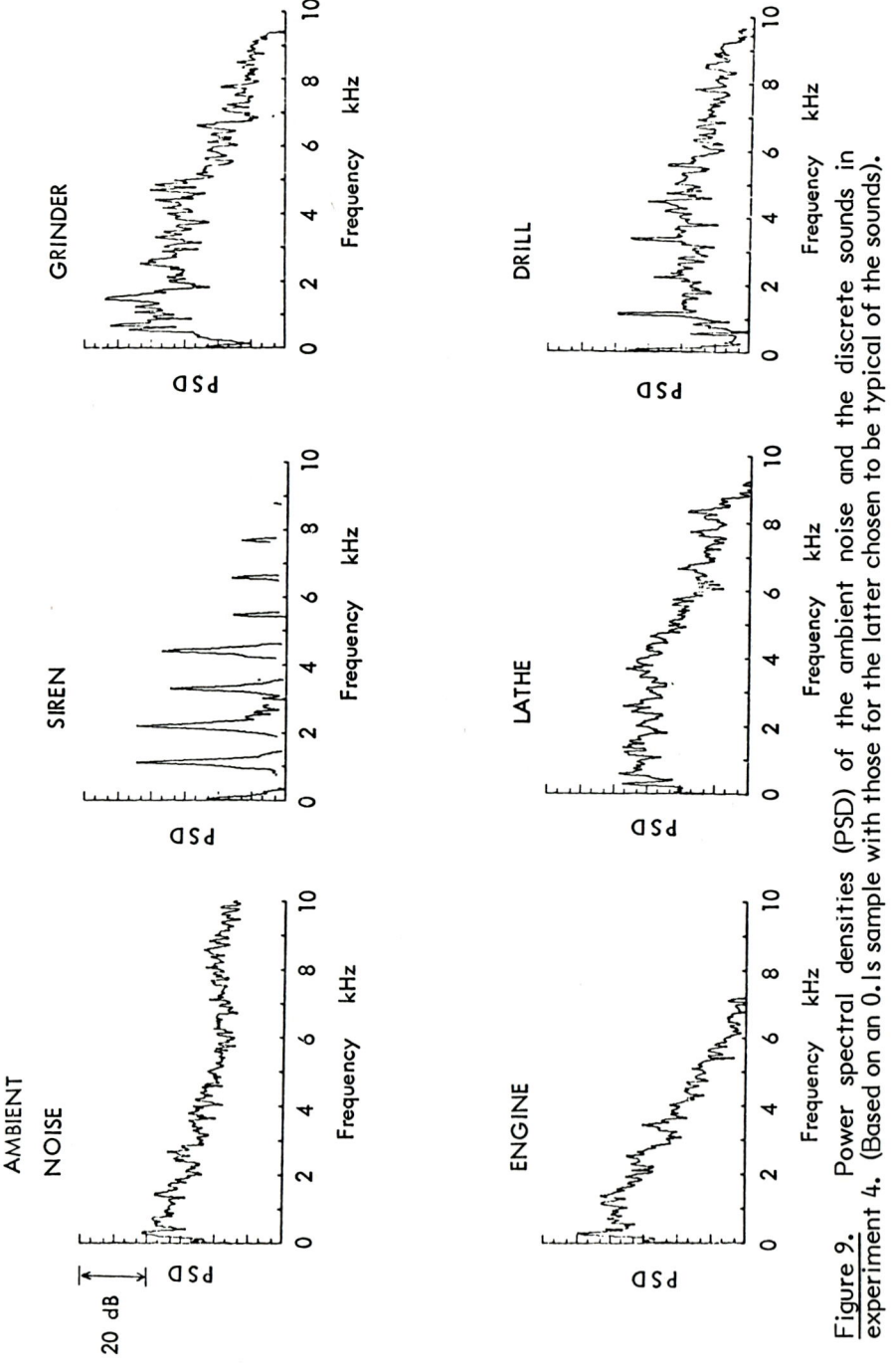

Figure 9. Power spectral densities (PSD) of the ambient noise and the discrete sounds in experiment 4. (Based on an 0.1s sample with those for the latter chosen to be typical of the sounds).

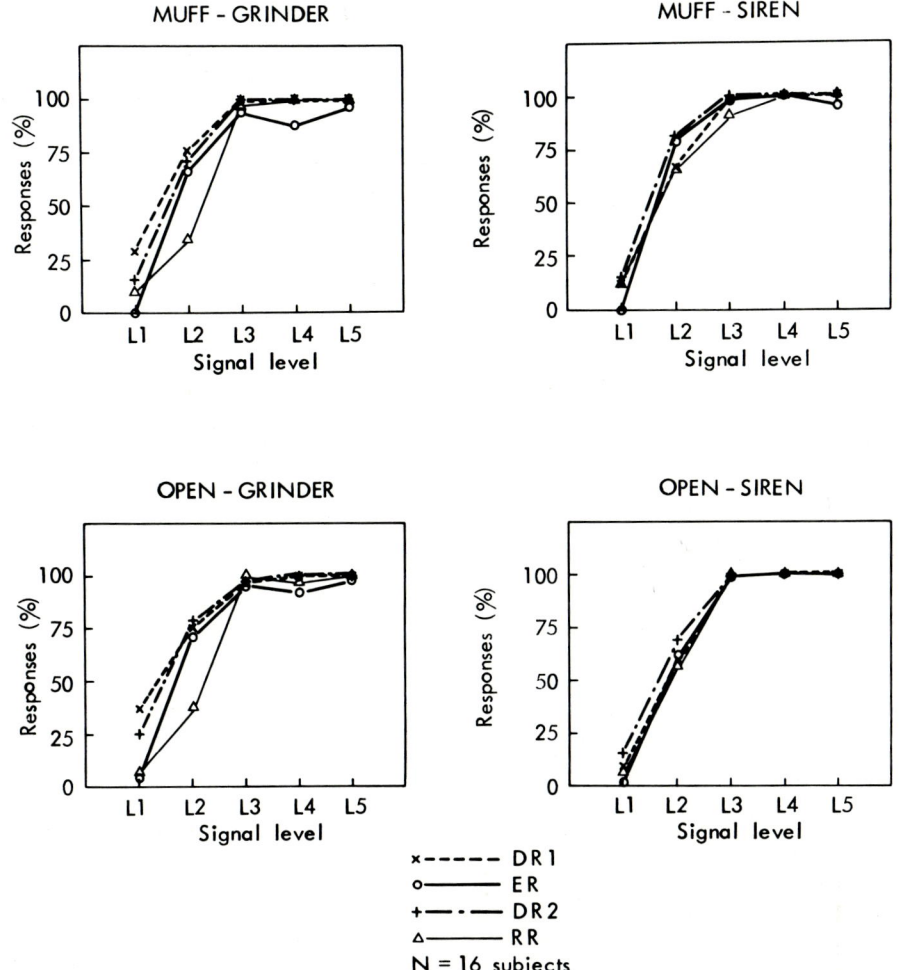

Figure 10. Number of responses averaged across subjects in experiment 4.

target sounds either the siren or the grinder; and the sixteen subjects.

Results

The mean numbers of correct responses across subjects as a function of the signal level are presented in Figure 10. These indicate that there were different trends apparent for the two target sounds in both the recognition and effective response conditions.

The statistical analysis of the data employed the two response differences DRD and ERD, and in addition the

recognition response difference RRD = DR - RR

where

RR = recognition response rate.

The RRD data indicates that the grinder was significantly less well recognized than detected at level L2 (response rates of 36% and 76% respectively), whilst the siren was reliably recognized at all levels. The siren also in general acted as an effective warning in terms of ERD under the combined conditions of recognition and inattention. By contrast the grinder was significantly less well perceived under the effective than the detection response conditions. This effect was relatively consistent across the five signal levels, however, there was a non-significant trend for the ERD of the grinder to be larger when the subjects wore the earmuffs than with ears unoccluded (mean values over the levels L2 to L5 of 8% and 4%, respectively).

Discussion

The siren in general acted as a reliable warning, which indicates that the addition of the requirements of recognition between experiments 3 and 4 did not influence its effectiveness as a warning. This conclusion is in agreement with a smaller study in which the effectiveness of four intentional warning sounds was evaluated with each in turn occurring in conjunction with four irrelevant workshop sounds[26]. The absence of any systematic trends for failures in the perception of the four warning sounds suggests that the conclusion from the present study may be applicable to a wide range of intentional warning sounds. The small but significant proportion of failures in the perception of the grinder as a warning at levels L3 to L5 is not due to the recognition requirement per se, as at these levels the sounds were recognized with almost complete reliability. It is therefore likely that at these levels the warning effectiveness of the grinder was reduced due to its acoustical similarity to the other machinery sounds, an interpretation which is supported by the difficulty in its recognition at level L2, and the larger number of confused responses made to the irrelevant sounds with the grinder as the target sound. Alternatively, it is possible that the grinder was not an entirely reliable warning because it was not sufficiently distinct relative to the ambient noise. It is of particular note that this effect is evident at levels up to approximately 17 dB above the masked threshold of the sound, which suggests that the failures in perception may not be overcome by simply increasing the intensity of the signal.

Whilst there was no large effect of wearing the earmuffs on the perception of either warning sound, the results suggest a possible small further degradation in the effectiveness of the grinder sound. The most likely cause of such an effect would be an interaction of the reduction in loudness of the signal due to the attenuation of the protectors and the pre-existing difficulty in the perception of the grinder due to the recognition requirement.

THE ROLE OF SOUND CHARACTERISTICS AND HEARING PROTECTION IN THE COMBINED RECOGNITION AND ATTENTION DEMAND OF WARNING SOUNDS

The results of experiment 4 indicated a significant difference between the effectiveness of the two warning sounds, and a non-significant trend for the wearing of hearing protection to further impair the effectiveness of the grinder sound. Experiment 5 was therefore conducted to assess whether these differences can be attributed to the acoustical characteristics of the two sounds. In particular, it was postulated that the siren acted as an effective warning because its tonal character (see Figure 9) put it in sharp contrast with the other irrelevant sounds and the ambient noise, whereas the grinder was less distinctive in terms of both these contrast factors (C_S and C_N respectively). The experiment was designed to assess the relative importance of these two contrast factors.

The methodology and experimental design were essentially the same as those employed in the preceeding experiment[27]. The set of sounds investigated consisted of three pure tones (at frequencies of 0.8, 2 and 5 kHz) and a one-third octave band of noise (centred at 2 kHz). As target sounds, the noise band is distinctive from the other irrelevant sound but

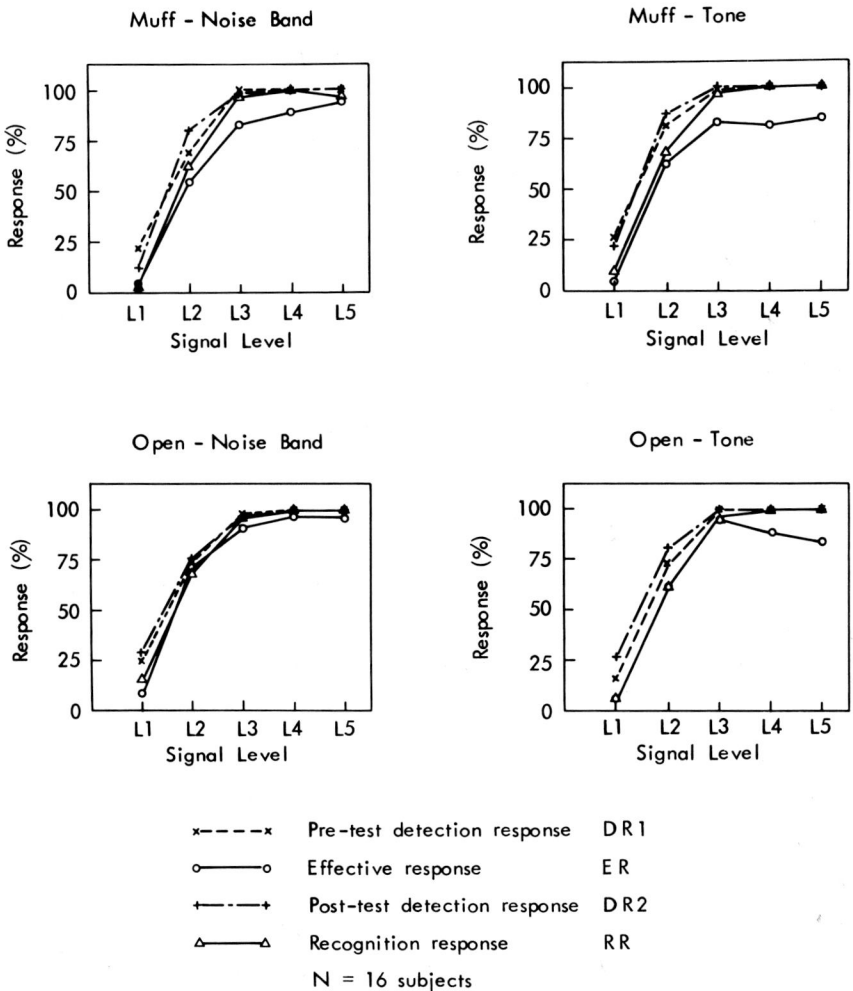

Figure 11. Number of responses averaged across subjects in experiment 5.

similar in character to the ambient noise (high C_S/low C_N) whereas the tone of frequency 2 kHz is similar to the other two tones but distinctive from the ambient noise (low C_S/high C_N).

Results

The resulting psychometric functions are presented in Figure 11. Both warning sounds were significantly less well recognized than they were detected at levels L1 and L2 close to their respective masked thresholds (mean RRD = 13%). Under the combined conditions of recognition and inattention the tone was significantly less effective than the noise band (mean ERD = 16% and 10% respectively). This effect was consistent across the signal levels investigated.

Both target sounds were significantly less well perceived when the subjects wore the earmuffs, than when they had their ears unoccluded (mean ERD = 16% and 10%, respectively). There was a non-significant trend for the adverse effect of wearing the earmuffs to be largest at levels L2, L3 and L4.

Discussion

The failures in perception of both the tone and the noise band target sounds indicate that the contrast with both the other irrelevant sounds (C_S) and the ambient noise (C_N) are important to the effectiveness of an auditory warning (Table 1). Although either factor would be sufficient to account for the failures in the perception of the grinder in experiment 4, the greater potency of C_S and the similar pattern of confused responses for the grinder and the tone suggests that the predominant factor was the low contrast of the grinder sound with the other machinery sounds. This would imply that there was an interaction of inattention and the recognition requirement (the second and third components of the conceptual model in Figure 1), since difficulties in recognition per se cannot account for the effects observed at levels L3 to L5.

The target sounds used in this experiment were acoustically simple relative to the siren and the grinder, as they did not vary with time in intensity or spectral content. The results of the two experiments suggest that such simple sounds are less effective as warnings than more complex sounds. As such, the relatively large failure rates in perception of these simple sounds should be taken as upper limits on the likely ineffectiveness of inappropriately selected warning sounds.

The results indicate a small additional reduction in the effectiveness of both sounds as warnings when the subjects were wearing the earmuffs.

Table 1: Results of experiments 4 and 5 in terms of the contrast factors C_S and C_N. The percentages shown are the overall mean effective response differences (ERD).

C_S \ C_N	High C_N	Low C_N
High C_S	Siren 3%	Noise band 10%
Low C_S	Tone 16%	Grinder 10%

C_S = contrast with irrelevant sounds
C_N = contrast with ambient noise

The adverse effect therefore appears to be associated with warning sounds which are already difficult to perceive because of low contrast with either (or both) the other irrelevant sounds or the ambient noise. The most likely explanation of the reduced effectiveness of the warning sounds is their reduced loudness due to the acoustic attenuation provided by the hearing protectors. This interpretation is supported by the significant regression between the mean effective response difference measure and the estimated loudness of the signal at the different presentation levels with and without the earmuffs shown in Figure 12[28]. The correlation is primarily due to the occluded ear condition, and suggests that the loudness of the sound was a predominant factor at intensities less than the loudness equivalent of a tone at approximately 40 dB in quiet. This suggests that the effectiveness of such warning sounds is unchanged when hearing protection is worn and the intensity of the signal is greater than approximately the masked threshold plus 15 dB. It is therefore likely that, although presenting a warning sound at an intensity more than 15 dB above its masked threshold will not ensure that it is entirely effective, it will minimize the adverse affects of wearing hearing protection on its perception.

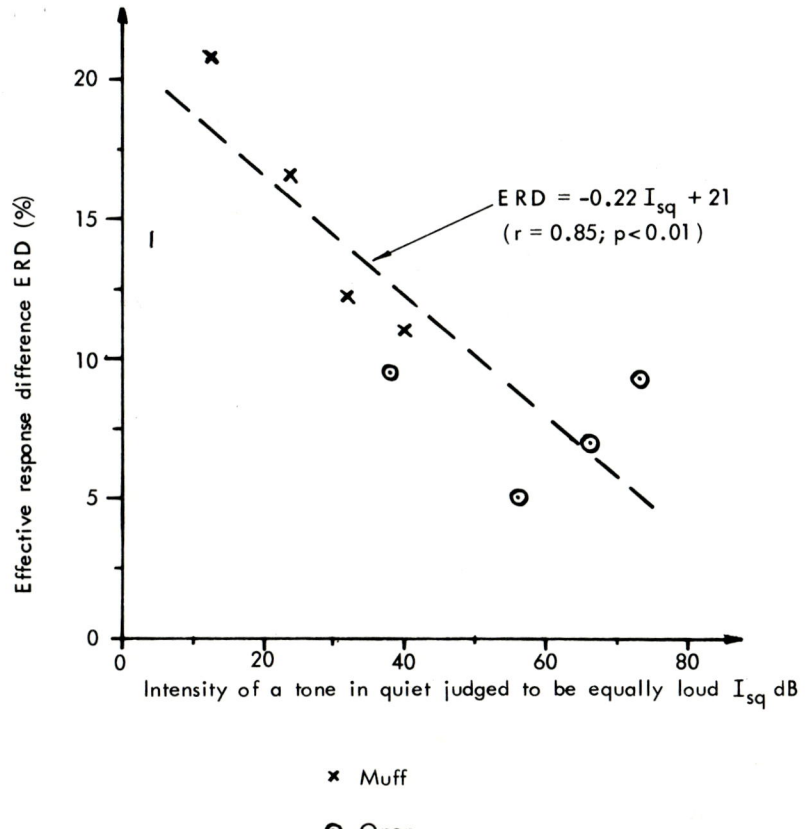

Figure 12. Relationship between the effectiveness of the warning sounds in experiment 5 with their estimated loudness[28] at the presentation levels L2 to L5 with ears unoccluded and wearing the earmuffs[28].

GENERAL DISCUSSION

The conceptual model of the perception of a warning sound provides a useful framework for the investigation of the psychoacoustical basis of the effects of wearing hearing protection. In particular it suggests the use of the detectability of the warning sound as a baseline measure for assessments of its effectiveness under conditions of inattention and recognition.

The evaluation of the probabilities that a warning sound will be perceived at different signal-to-noise ratios indicates that under realistic conditions a sound may not be 100% effective as a warning. This is most likely to occur for inappropriately selected intentional warning sounds, and incidental warning sounds which are not sufficiently distinct from other environmental sounds and from the ambient noise.

The results emphasise that the widely accepted safety margin which requires a warning sound to be at a level at least 15 dB above its masked threshold,[7] need not in fact provide an entirely reliable warning. The psychometric functions can be converted to indicate the signal level above masked threshold required to achieve a specified probability of perception of a warning sound. This is shown in Table 2 for the "worst-case" data of Figure 11. Whilst an auditory warning may be detected and recognized with 100% reliability at a level approximately 12 dB above its masked threshold, it is evident that it may be difficult to achieve greater than approximately 90% reliability in conditions typical of their occurrence in industry, even when the intensity of the sound is further increased.

Table 2: Signal levels above masked threshold (dB) required to attain a specified proportion of correctly perceived warning sounds (1)

Response condition	Probability of Perception							
	50	60	70	80	90	95	99	100
Detection	0	1	2	3	5	7	8	12
Recognition	1	2	3	5	6	7	11	12
Effective-ears open	1	2	3	5	7	>18	>18	>18
- muffs.	2	3	5	7	>18	>18	>18	>18

(1) Based on average data for the two warning sounds investigated in experiment 5. Values shown are the levels above masked threshold (dB) and were obtained by linear interpolation of the data shown in figure 11.

The largest effect of wearing hearing protection observed was an increase in the failures in perception from one in ten to one in six signals. It is evident in Table 2 that this adverse effect might in principle be compensated for by a 1 to 2 dB increase in signal levels over intermediate S/N, but that at high S/N the effectiveness of the warnings may never reach the 90% reliability achieved with ears unoccluded.

Implications for the Selection and Use of Hearing Protection
Whilst it appears that the wearing of hearing protectors only affects adversely the perception of warning sounds which are already difficult to perceive with ears unoccluded, it is possible that an additional 6% of failures in their perception could have serious consequences for the safety of the wearer.

It is not possible to predict accurately the risks associated with this reduction in the effectiveness of warning sounds. Existing accident data does however indicate the likely proportions of various categories of accidents, as shown in Figure 13[29]. It is evident that the incidence of serious or disabling injuries is only the pinnacle of much larger numbers of minor accidents. Extension of the pyramid to include the ratios between the number of times that:

(i) a warning sound occurs but is not perceived due to the wearing of hearing protection. (The ratio shown is based approximately on the rate of perceptual failures of 6% due to the earmuffs in experiment 5),

(ii) the warning sound is not perceived and the warning is not communicated by any other means (Y),

(iii) the warning is not perceived and a critical incident occurs (X).

Estimates of the ratios X and Y of 10:1 suggest that for every one million occurrences of warning sounds amongst people wearing hearing protection, one disabling injury and ten minor injuries would be precipitated by the use of the protectors. Whilst a risk of this order may appear to be small, it could represent a significant number of accidents in terms of the total number of occurrences of both intentional and incidental warning sounds in industry each year.

(a)		(b)
1	Disabling and serious injuries	1
10	Minor injuries	10
30	Property-damage accidents	30
600	Accidents with no visible injury or damage (critical incidents)	600
	Warning not perceived	600X
	Warning sound not perceived due to the wearing of hearing protection	600XY
	Occurrence of warning sound whilst wearing hearing protection	10,000XY

Figure 13. Relative occurrence of different categories of accidents and incidents in industry.
(a) General accident rate in industry (after Bamber)[29]
(b) Estimated rates associated with the failure to perceive a warning sound due to the wearing of hearing protection.

To the extent that the failures in the perception of the warning sounds observed in this study are due to the reduction in loudness of the signals, it is possible that the use of lower attenuation protectors would alleviate this problem. This therefore provides some support for the view that hearing protectors should provide adequate but not excessive attenuation[30,31]. The argument against over-protection is strengthened when account is taken of possible limitations on the audibility of warning sounds due to absolute threshold requirements. It also supports the development and evaluation of amplitude sensitive hearing protection for use in variable noise environments. These can adjust the attenuation provided by electronic means to ensure that excessive attenuation does not occur during the quieter periods of an intermittent noise exposure[32-34].

Absolute threshold limitations may also be critical when hearing protection is worn in conjunction with a temporary or permanent threshold shift. Particular problems may therefore arise with the inconsistent use of hearing protectors in high noise environments, or their use by people with an existing noise-induced hearing loss.

Implications for the Specification and Use of Warning Sounds

Adverse effects of wearing hearing protection were only observed in this study for warning sounds which did not constitute entirely reliable warnings under normal unoccluded ear conditions. Thus where action is contemplated to counter the possible risks associated with the use of hearing protectors, it should be co-ordinated with a review of the general effectiveness of the warning sounds concerned.

In the selection of intentional warning sounds it is important to ensure that they are distinctive from other environmental sounds and from the ambient noise. The commonly adopted procedure of listening to a range of warning sounds in a quiet environment and then selecting one for use in a noisy condition where the occurrence of the sound is largely unexpected, is clearly inappropriate. Until further experimentation provides a basis from which to predict the relative effectiveness of different warning sounds in particular noise environments, a measure of this can only be obtained by conducting trials under realistic conditions. This general approach is already embodied in a German Standard[35]. In addition to ensuring the salience of the warning sound, it can be noted that the intensity of the sound should be approximately 15 to 25 dB above its masked threshold. At intensities greater than this there is unlikely to be any increase in the effectiveness of the warning, but there is the possiblity of causing undue annoyance or startle.

In situations where the perception of a warning sound is of vital importance, consideration should be given to employing warning systems which use suitable visual or vibro-tactile signals to complement the auditory warning.

In general it is not possible to alter the acoustic characteristics of incidental warning sounds such as the "ringing of the keys" or the sound of malfunctioning machinery. In occupational situations where such sounds may be important to safety, special consideration must therefore be given to the potential risks associated with the wearing of hearing protection. Whilst the "risk pyramid" shown in Figure 13 indicates the possible consequences of failures in the perception of warning sounds due to the use of hearing protection, it should be noted that this represents a risk additional to that which may already exist due to the inherent ineffectiveness of such warning sounds. In specific instances it should be possible to surmount this limitation on the use of hearing protection by developing warning systems which automatically recognize the incidental warning sound and then communicate the warning by a more effective means.

CONCLUSION

The wearing of hearing protection may impair the perception of inappropriately selected intentional warning sounds, and many incidental warning sounds when they occur under conditions typical of the industrial environment. The widespread attitude that such an impairment does occur when protectors are worn may however arise from a misconception of how auditory warnings are detected in noise, and how they are perceived when they are largely unexpected and must be recognized amongst other environmental sounds. The results therefore suggest an important role for the education component of any hearing conservation programme to inform properly the potential wearer of the possible risks associated with the use of the hearing protection.

There is also a clear need for further research to assess the particular problems of people with an existing noise-induced hearing loss when wearing protection, and the extent to which the adverse effects observed in this study can be compensated for by experience gained in a structured training programme. A deeper understanding of the recognition of complex sounds is also required to enable predictions of the effectiveness of specific warning sounds in particular noise environments.

ACKNOWLEDGEMENT

The authors wish to thank the Health and Safety Executive for their support during the latter part of this study.

REFERENCES
1.   Maas, R.B., Hearing protection in industry. Nursing Outlook 9, 281-283, 1961.

2.   Sugden, D.B., Some notes on the provision of personal hearing protection for fettlers in an iron foundry. Ann. Occup. Hyg. 10, 263-268, 1967.

3.   Lambert, D.R., Preliminary study of the effects of ear protectors on recognition of shipboard machinery sounds. Tech. Note 1464, Naval Undersea Centre, San Diego, 1975.

4.   National Coal Board. National Coal Board Medical Service Annual Report, 1974-1975.

5.   Karmy, S.J., Coles, R.R.A., Hearing protection - Factors affecting its use. In Man and Noise. Eds. G. Rossi and M. Vigone, Edizioni Minerva Medica, Torino, 1976.

6.   Robertson, R.M., Maxwell, D.W., Williams, C.E., The landing signal officer. Auditory aspects. NAMRL Rep. 1255, Naval Aerospace Medical Research Laboratory, Florida, 1978.

7.   Wilkins, P.A., Martin, A.M., The effect of hearing protectors on the perception of warning and indicator sounds - A general review. Tech. Rep. 98, Institute of Sound and Vibration Research, 1978.

8.   Houston, R.C., Walker, R.T., The evaluation of auditory warning signals for aircraft. Aero-Med. Lab. Report AF-TR-5762, 1949.

9.   Ceypek, T., Chrusciel, R., Kuzniarz, J., Lepkowski, A., Szymczyk, K., Detectability and acoustic signals in industrial noise (Polish). Proc. XXVII Conf. Otolaryngology (1968), 29-32, 1970.

10.   Casey, W.D., Effect of wearing hearing protection on the detection of warning or indicator sounds in noise. Unpub. B.Sc. Thesis, Univ. of Southampton, 1975.

11.   Talamo, J.D.C., Effects of cab noise environment on the hearing perception of agricultural tractor drivers. Appl. Acoust. 12, 125-137,

1979.

12. Levin, G., Perception of acoustic signals when wearing hearing protectors (German). Die Berufsgenossenschaft, No. 12, 471-474, 1976.

13. Wilkins, P.A., Martin, A.M., The effects of hearing protectors on the masked thresholds of acoustic warning signals. Unpub. Presented at 9th Int. Cong. Acoustics, Madrid, 1977.

14. Wilkins, P.A., Martin, A.M., The effects of hearing protection on the attention demand of warning sounds. Scand. Audiol., 10, 37-43, 1981.

15. Wilkins, P.A., Martin, A.M., The effects of hearing protection on the recognition and attention demand of warning signals. In prep., 1980.

16. Scholl, H., Uber ein objectives verfahren zur ermittlung von horschwellen und mithorschwellen. Frequenz 17, 125-133, 1963.

17. Fidell, S., Pearsons, K.S., Bennett, R.L., Prediction of aural detectability of noise signals. Hum. Factors 16, 373-383, 1974.

18. Reed, C.M., Bilger, R.C., A comparative study of S/N_o and E/N_o. J. acoust. Soc. Amer. 53, 1039-1044, 1973.

19. Weber, D.L., Growth of masking and the auditory filter. J. acoust. Soc. Amer. 62, 424-429, 1977.

20. Martin, A.M., Howell, K., Lower, M.C., Hearing protection and communication in noise. In Disorders of Auditory Function II. Ed. S.D.G. Stephens, Academic Press, London, 1976.

21. Kreezer, G.L., Attention value of audio and visual warning signals. WADC Tech. Rep. 58-521, Wright-Patterson Air Force Base, Ohio, 1959.

22. Potter, R.C., Fidell, S.A., Myles, M.M., Keast, D.N., Effectiveness of audible warning devices on emergency vehicles. Report No. DOT-TSC-77-38. U.S. Dept. of Transportation, Washington, 1977.

23. Durlach, N.I., Colburn, H.S., Binaural phenomenon. In Handbook of Perception, vol. IV Hearing. Eds. E.C. Carterette and M.P. Friedman. Academic Press, New York, 1978.

24. Wilkins, P.A., Martin, A.M., The role of attention in sound perception. Proc. Inst. of Acoustics 4, 15.01.1 - 15.01.4, 1978.

25. Wilkins, P.A., Martin, A.M., The role of recognition in the perception of unattended auditory stimuli. In Disorders of Auditory Function III. Ed. I.G. Taylor, Academic Press, London (in press) 1980.

26. Whatson, M.E.C., The relative effectiveness of warning sounds. Unpub. B.Sc. Thesis, University of Southampton, 1979.

27. Wilkins, P.A., Martin, A.M., The role of recognition and sound characteristics in the perception of unattended auditory stimuli. Paper presented at the Short Papers Meeting of the British Society of Audiology, Cambridge, 1979.

28. MaCrae, J.H., The general form of the loudness function. Inf. Rep. 51, Nat. Acoust. Lab., Australian Dept. Health, 1977.

29. Bamber, L., Accident costing in industry. Health and Safety at Work, 2, 32-34. 1979.

30. Else, D., Hearing protectors. Unpub. Ph.D. Thesis. University of Aston in Birmingham, 1976.

31. Lepor, M., Lambert, D.R., A special purpose ear protector: Preliminary development. Tech. Note 1741, Naval Undersea Centre, San Diego, 1977.

32. Murphy, J.N., Sacks, H.K., Durkin, J., Summers, C.R., Progress in noise abatement. Mining Cong. J. 58, 59-63, 1972.

33. Michael, P.L., Saperstein, L.W., Prout, J.H., A study of roof warning signals and the use of personal hearing protection in underground coal mines. U.S. Bureau of Mines Final Report. Grant No. G0133026, 1973.

34. Bumm, P., Berg, M., Gerät zur spracherkennung bei gleichreitegem lärmschutz. Arch. Oto-Rhino-Laryng. 215, 293-299, 1977.

35. DIN 33 404 Danger signal for work places; acoustic danger signals. 1977.

23 Speech Intelligibility in Noise With and Without Ear Protectors

Sharon M. Abel, Peter W. Alberti, Caroline Haythornthwaite, and Krista Riko

INTRODUCTION

It is generally agreed that exposure to intense sound may result in a loss of hearing, either temporary or permanent.[1] In industrial settings ear defenders have been chosen as one method of hearing conservation which is both effective and inexpensive. The practicality of this solution, however, has been challenged by many workmen, who complain that protectors used on the job prevent them from hearing warning signals and understanding instructions.

The complaints levelled at personal hearing protection programs are in contrast to published data indicating that the wearing of ear defenders does not interfere with speech intelligibility. Kryter,[2] for example, studied the perception of monosyllables in noise in college students with normal hearing. The results showed that as the signal-to-noise ratio was varied from -15 to +10 dB intelligibility scores increased substantially from 0 to 80% correct. The presence of an ear plug had no effect for noise less than 80 dBA. For higher levels, there was a gain of about 10% in discrimination.

Studies of subjects with hearing impairment show substantial differences compared with that of normal observers. Coles and Rice,[3] for example, found that subjects with severe high tone losses performed more poorly both with and without and ear plug when listening to speech in quiet. The explanation typically given is that in the listener who already has noise-induced deafness, the protector puts the level of speech below the already raised thresholds in the high frequency region.

The effect of combining a white noise background and the wearing of a muff in subjects with high tone loss was examined by Lindeman.[4] For levels of speech and noise of 80 and 90 dBA, the results showed a decrease in performance significantly correlated with an increase in hearing loss. In the presence of a slight impairment, the muff produced some improvement in speech perception.

The present experiments are an extension of the work described above. Our purpose was to define some of the relevant subject and environmental factors that influence speech intelligibility in noise, with and without protectors. In particular, we were interested in assessing changes in performance that occur with variation in age, type of hearing loss, the spectrum and relative level of the noise background, and the attenuation characteristics of the protector. Of special concern in this study was the extent to which non-fluency with the spoken language provides an additional handicap for the hard-of-hearing.[6,7] Census data indicate that at least 1/4 of the workforce in Ontario have acquired English as a second language.[5] The question we asked was the extent to which poor comprehension of instructions in English would interact with a hearing disability in interfering with communication in the industrial setting.

DESIGN AND METHODS

The design and methods have been described elsewhere.[6] Briefly, there were three main groups of subjects defined by the configuration of the audiogram: (1) normal, according to conventional audiometric tests; (2) bilateral noise-induced high frequency loss (i.e. 5 to 25 dB at 500 Hz with a slope in loss of 35 to 65 dB between 500 and 4000 Hz); and (3) bilateral flat loss (i.e. 30 to 50 dB at 500 Hz and 45 to 65 dB at 4000 Hz.

For each of these three categories of hearing, we tested a group of 12 subjects who were fluent in English and a group comprised of 12 subjects who had learned English as a second language and were poorly conversant. The effect of age was investigated in a limited way. For both fluent and non-fluent subjects with high frequency loss, we tested subjects in two age ranges: 35-50 years and 51-65 years. In all, there were 8 categories of subject.

Each subject was presented with and attempted to repeat 12 lists of 25 monosyllabic words. Each of the 12 lists was presented under one of 12 listening conditions. We varied the background noise (quiet, white noise or taped crowd noise of 85 dBA), the amplitude of speech (80 or 90 dBA) and the presence of ear protection. Combinations of levels of these three variables gave the 12 listening conditions. Both the order of conditions and lists used for each condition were randomized across the 12 subjects in each group.

Over replications of the design, various ear protectors were tested:
1   the MSA Comfo-500 muff for each of the eight subject categories
2   the EAR plug for six of the eight categories (excluding normal, non-fluent, and flat loss, non-fluent subjects)
3   the Willson Sound Silencer plug for the four fluent groups.

For one of the 8 categories, high frequency loss and fluent in English, we also replicated the experiment with the No-Noise muff on helmet, Willson Sound Ban occluder and Proppo-plast Swedish wool. For each replication a different set of subjects was used. Exclusions of categories was due to the unavailability of sufficient individuals to match the criteria.

Free-field hearing thresholds were obtained for each subject both with and without the protector which had been specified for the particular replication. Measurements were made at 10 one-third octave band noises with centre frequency ranging from 125 to 10,000 Hz. The difference in the measurement at each frequency gave the attenuation measurement. Protectors were always fitted by an audiologist to ensure the best possible attenuation.

The experiments were performed in an IAC booth. The ambient level of the booth met ANSI standards. The taped speech was presented over a single 12 inch diameter conical loudspeaker (Madsen Electronics, Model FF73) placed free-standing on the floor at a distance of 80 inches directly in front of the subject. Noise was presented through two 6 inch diameter conical loudspeakers (Madsen Electronics, Model FF72) mounted on the sidewalks of the booth at a distance of 54 inches from the subjects' ears and approximately 11 inches above the head.

RESULTS

Attenuation

The attenuation data obtained for the Comfo-500 muffs are presented in Figure 1 for each of eight experimental groups. The abscissa gives the centre frequency of the narrowband noise tested and the ordinate shows the mean attenuation score for the 12 subjects in the group. Generally, the muff gave poor low frequency attenuation. The value increased to 20 to 30 dB at 2000 to 4000 Hz and then decreased. In the region of 2000 to 4000 Hz subjects with high frequency loss in the 51-65 age range got significantly less attenuation than both those in the younger group and normal subjects. Subjects with flat loss appear to do best.

Figures 2 and 3 show the attenuation data for the EAR sponge insert plug and Willson Sound Silencer. Low frequency attenuation appeared to be better with the plugs than the muff, about 15 dB at 125 Hz and 35 to 40 dB in the region of 4000 Hz. The various groups tested were fairly similar for both plugs. The exception was the normal fluent group who get significantly more attenuation at 8000 Hz.

A comparison of attenuation scores across the six protectors for groups of subjects with high frequency loss and fluent in English are presented in Figure 4. Data for the two muffs are in the left panel, and for the four plugs in the right panel. Pairwise statistical comparisons between the various protectors indicate that the No Noise muff on helmet provides significantly more attenuation than the Comfo-500 for frequencies ranging from 125 to 8000 Hz. The plugs are fairly similar in this range, although differences are observed at selected frequencies. Comparing across muffs and plugs, we find that the No Noise and EAR provide the best protection overall, with no significant differences between them. The Willson Sound Silencer gives significantly lower attenuation scores

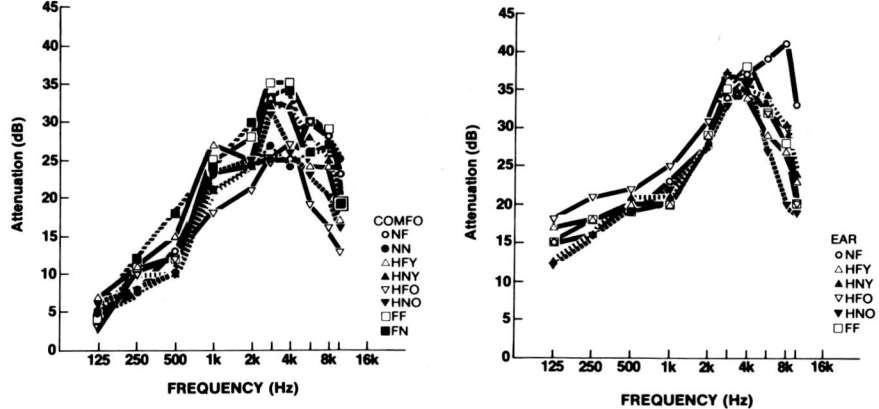

Figure 1.   The attenuation of the Comfo-500 muff: Effects of hearing, fluency and age.

Figure 2.   The attenuation of the EAR plug: Effects of hearing, fluency and age.

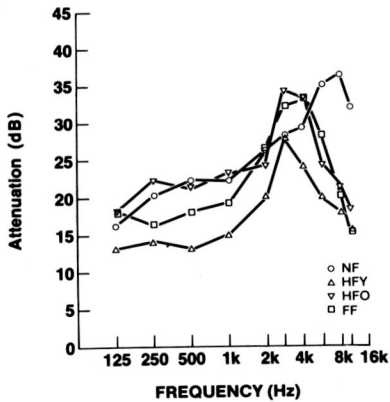

Figure 3.   The attenuation of the Willson Sound Silencer plug: Effects of hearing and age.

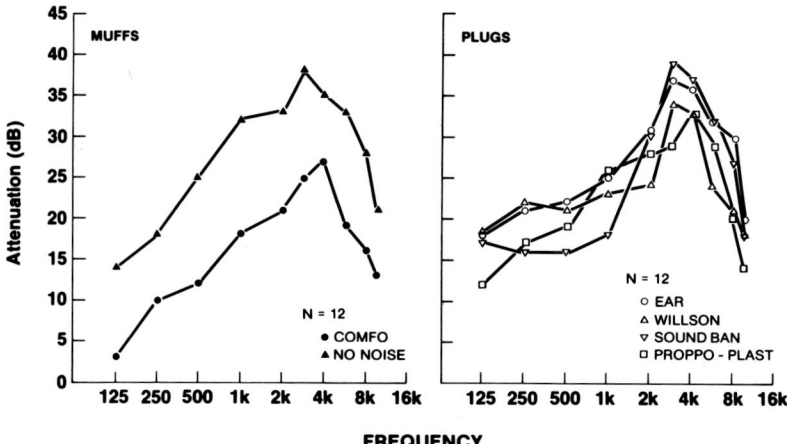

Figure 4. A comparison of the attenuation of six types of muffs and plugs in fluent subjects with high frequency loss, aged 51-65 years.

than the No Noise muff at 1,2,6 an 8 kHz.

Speech Intelligibility

The results for speech intelligibility are given in Figures 5-8 for the Comfo-500 muff replication. Figure 5 shows the data for subjects with normal hearing and fluent in English. The percentage of words correctly repeated is plotted against the noise background: quiet, white or taped crowd noise. Each data point is the average percent correct for the 12 subjects in the group. For the left panel the speech was presented at 90 dBA and for the right panel at 80 dBA. In each panel, the scores for unprotected and protected listening are compared.

The figure shows three results:
a) listening in quiet is easier than listening in noise and crowd noise is a more effective masker than white noise
b) in white noise or crowd noise intelligibility decreases significantly with a 10 dB drop in the level of speech
c) for any combination of noise background and amplitude of speech, the protector has no effect on intelligibility

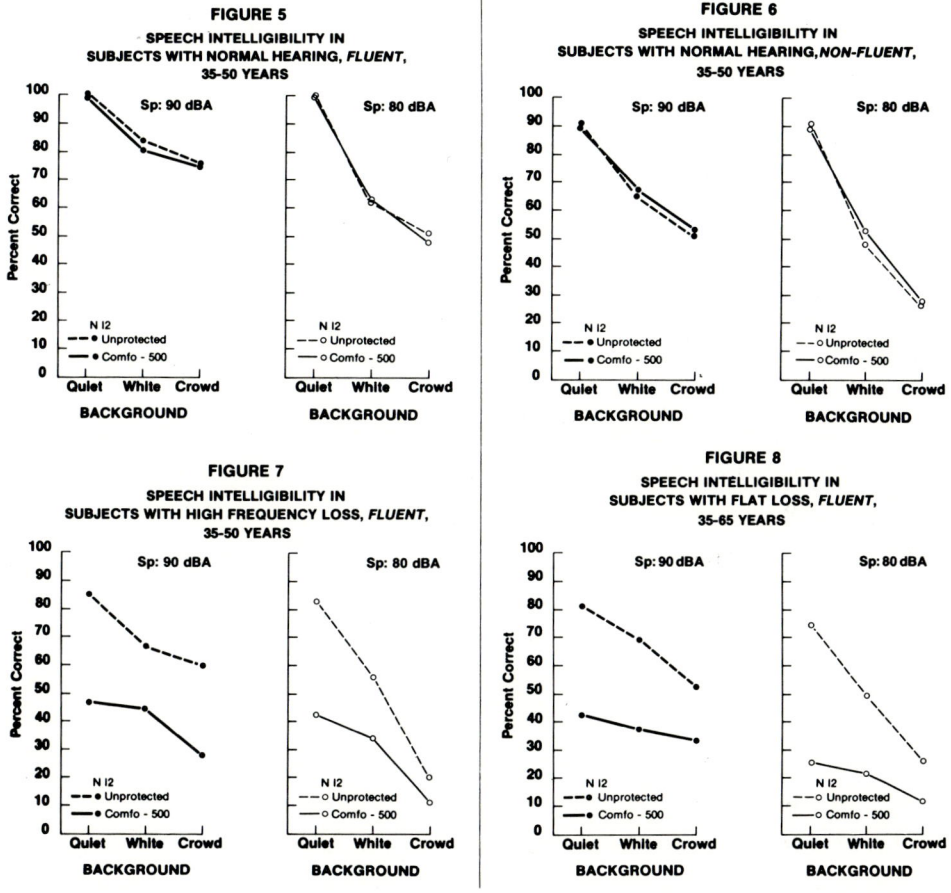

Figure 5. Speech intelligibility in fluent subjects with normal hearing, aged 35-50 years.

Figure 6. Speech intelligibility in non-fluent subjects with normal hearing, aged 35-50 years.

Figure 7. Speech intelligibility in fluent subjects with high frequency loss, aged 35-50 years.

Figure 8. Speech intelligibility in fluent subjects with flat loss, aged 35-65 years.

The data for non-fluent, normal hearing subjects are shown in Figure 6 for comparison. The overall pattern of results is the same, but the average score for each condition has decreased by 10 to 15%.

Figure 7 shows the results for subjects with a noise-induced high frequency hearing loss, who are fluent in English. The picture is considerably different. Again listening is easier in quiet than in noise, and intelligibility decreases with the lower speech to noise ratio. However, unlike normal hearing subjects, those with high frequency loss show a substantial protector effect. In quiet, there is a drop of 40% when the muff is worn.

The results for fluent subjects with a flat loss (i.e. low tone as well as high tone hearing loss) are shown in Figure 8. The decrement in performance compared with the high frequency group is especially evident for protected listening in the low signal-to-noise ratio condition.

An analysis of variance, comparing the data (the difference between protected and unprotected scores) for all eight groups using the Comfo-500 muff indicates that hearing configuration, fluency and background are all significant main effects. Older subjects tend to do better than younger subjects but the effect was not consistent. In addition, there are significant interactions between hearing configuration and background, hearing configuration and signal-to-noise ratio and background and signal-to-noise ratio. Essentially this means that the size of the effect of one variable depends on the particular level of the other. Fluency does not interact significantly. This means that it acts like an attenuator and the effect is a relatively constant drop of about 10 to 15% no matter what the values of the other variables.

A comparison of the data obtained for Comfo-500 muff, EAR plug and Willson Sound Silencer showed that the trends observed as function of the signal level, noise background, hearing loss configuration and fluency were virtually identical for the three protectors. Figure 9 shows the data for all six protectors taken on different samples of fluent subjects with high frequency loss and 51-65 years of age. The data for these groups should

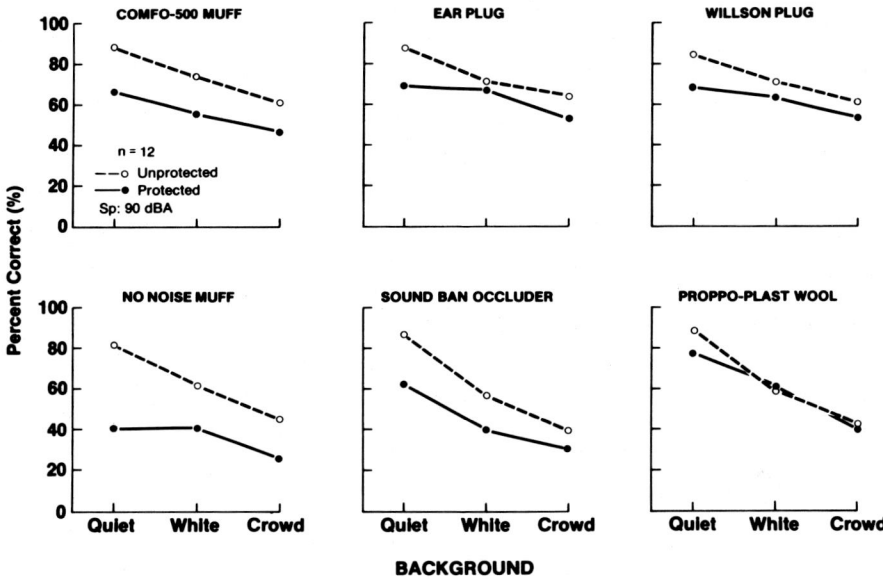

Figure 9. Speech intelligibility in fluent subjects with high frequency loss, aged 51-65 years. A comparison of six protectors.

not be different in the unprotected listening conditions. Since some significant differences were observed, we evaluated the effect of the protector by comparing difference scores (protected-unprotected) between groups. Statistical tests indicated that in general the wearing of the No Noise muff on helmet resulted in a greater change in speech perception than any other protector when the speech was at 90 dBA. For the low signal-to-noise ratio, there was no consistent trend. The Proppoplast Swedish wool produced the least amount of change, and the least amount of attenuation.

The Effect of Attenuation on Speech Perception

Although group trends appear to indicate that changes observed in speech perception are independent of the particular protector chosen, one may ask whether, individual by individual, there is a correlation between the

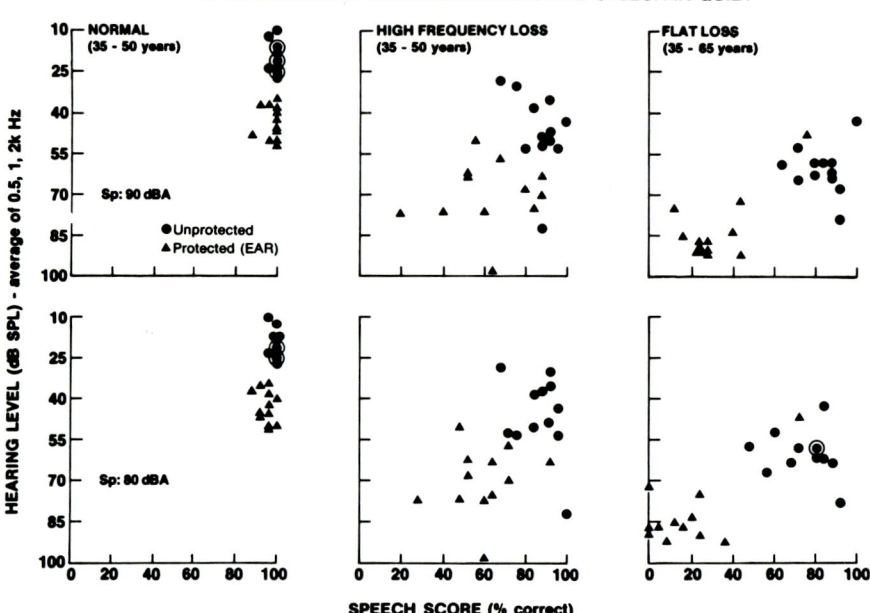

Figure 10. The relationship between hearing and speech in quiet for subjects with normal hearing, high frequency loss and flat loss.

level of hearing with and without the protector and the intelligibility score.

Scattergrams plotting the average free-field hearing threshold for 500, 1000 and 2000 Hz unprotected and protected against the percentage of words correctly repeated are shown in Figure 10 for the EAR plug. In the upper three panels the speech was presented in quiet at 90 dBA and in the lower panels, in quiet at 80 dBA. A comparison across hearing categories shows striking differences. For normal subjects the attenuation provided by the protector does not affect speech intelligibility. For the groups with hearing loss attenuation causes both a decrement in intelligibility and an increase in the variability of results across subjects. Subjects with

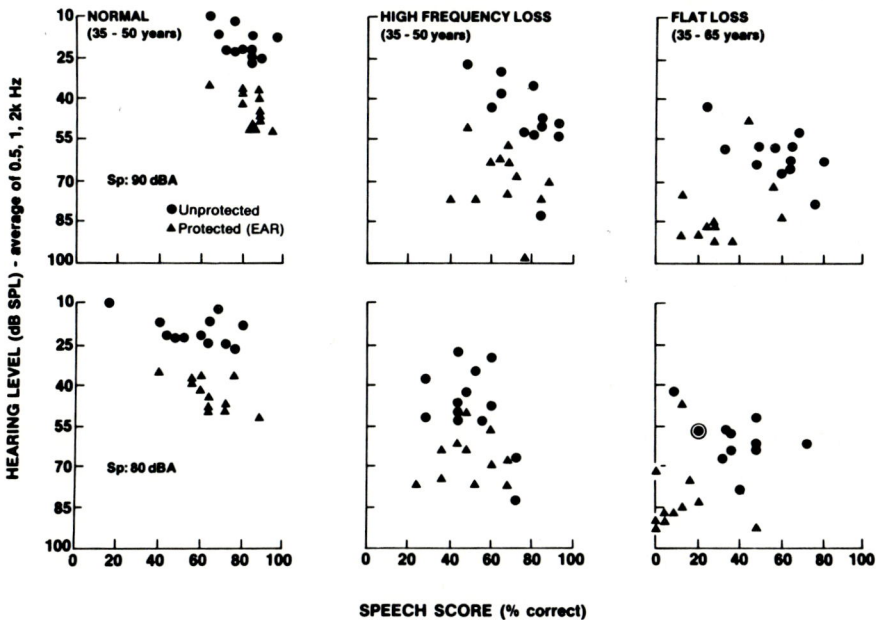

Figure 11. The relationship between hearing and speech in white noise for subjects with normal hearing, high frequency loss and flat loss.

flat loss are particularly devastated by the protector. Their intelligibility scores are close to zero.

Figure 11 shows the relation between hearing threshold and speech intelligibility in white noise. The trends are identical to those in Figure 10 but exaggerated. Normal hearing subjects exhibit much more variability in both the unprotected and protected listening conditions.

DISCUSSION

The research described above was a study of the perception of speech in a background of noise. Our aim was the delineation of those conditions or stimulus variables which might contribute to a change in the intelligibility of speech as it would be heard in an industrial setting. In particular we were interested in the effects of three subjects variables: the frequency configuration of hearing loss, the listener's fluency in English and age; and two environmental variables: energy spectrum of the noise background and the ratio of intensities for speech and noise. Measurements were made of both the attenuation of narrowband signals for a number of hearing protective devices in common usage and the ability to repeat lists of words presented free-field in a sound proof booth, with and without the protector worn. The protectors chosen for study were the MSA Comfo-500 muff, the No-Noise muff on helmet, the EAR sponge plug, the Willson Sound Silencer plug, the Willson Sound Ban occluder and Proppo-plast Swedish wool.

The attenuation data indicate that there are consistent differences between muffs and plugs: low frequency attenuation in the region of 125 to 500 Hz is significantly better for the plugs. Within protector type, the amount of attenuation is generally independent of the subject variables chosen for study, i.e. hearing configuration, fluency and age. There were some anomalies. For both the EAR and Willson plugs, subjects with normal hearing and fluent in English showed a shift of the peak attenuation to 8000 Hz as compared with the peak at 4000 Hz observed for the hearing impaired groups. Statistical comparisons indicated that overall across frequency and subject group, the No-Noise muff and EAR plug provided the best protection.

An important focus of interest defined at the outset was the restriction in communication that might be imposed on the workman wearing a hearing protector. The evidence available at the time the investigation was initiated indicated that speech intelligibility in noise did not change significantly, and indeed in some instances actually improved when a hearing protector was worn. These data were contrary to reports by workmen that protectors prevented the hearing of warning signals and instructions.

The results of the present investigation show quite clearly that the effect of wearing a protector interacts (in the statistical sense) with the hearing configuration. In normal hearing subjects, the percentage of words correctly repeated does not change when either a muff or plug is worn. This holds true for both listening in quiet and in noise, and for the two levels of signal-to-noise ratio investigated. By contrast, subjects with hearing impairment show a substantial protector effect. This appears to be greater in quiet than in noise, a finding which may be an artifact of proximity to the "floor" (0% correct) for unprotected listening in noise, especially for the lower signal-to-noise ratio.

The findings described above are in line with the results of current investigations of the perception of warning signals. Wilkins and Martin,[8] for example, presented observers with a siren or bell mixed with random noise of 75 or 95 dB SPL and delivered over a loudspeaker in an anechoic room. Measuring the change in masked threshold for the signal, they found a slight advantage of 3 or 4 dB with the protector. All their subjects had normal hearing. The effect of a moderately severe bilateral sensori-neural hearing loss on such measurements has been demonstrated by Forshaw.[9] The wearing of a Canadian Forces standard issue ear muff did not affect detection in noise for pure-tones of 500, 1k, 2k and 6k Hz. However, a tone of 3000 Hz could not be heard. Again normal observers showed an advantage with the muffs.

The other significant main variables for the present study were noise background, and fluency with the language spoken. With regard to background, subjects in each of the hearing configuration by fluency groups produced significantly lower scores when listening in noise than in quiet, for both unprotected and protected listening. Further, crowd noise was a more effective masker than white noise. Significant interactions were noted between hearing configuration and background, hearing configuration and signal-to-noise ratio and background and signal-to-noise ratio. The results confirm the earlier findings of Suter[9] for the perception of speech in babble noise. Her study showed a significant interaction between hearing loss and speech-to-noise ratio for unprotected listening.

In examining the difference between protected and unprotected listening, we found no consistent significant difference due to age. Comparisons were made between subjects with high frequency loss in the 35 to 50 and 51 to 65 year age groups, and for both fluent and non-fluent subjects. On the other hand fluency with the language spoken was a significant main effect but did not interact with the other variables. Non-fluency produced a drop of about 10 to 15% for any combination of listening conditions. By contrast signal-to-noise ratio interacted significantly but was not on its own a potent factor. This might indicate that the levels chosen were not spread apart significantly.

Although the results showed clear differences in the attenuation provided by the various protectors there were no substantial differences in the overall pattern of results for speech intelligibility. Significance tests indicated that the No-Noise muff on helmet ranked highest in effect and the Proppo-plast wool lowest.

In order to establish the exact nature of the relationship between hearing level and speech intelligibility, we considered pairs of data points for individuals. The hearing level scores were based on the average free-field hearing thresholds at 500, 1k and 2k Hz. The correlation of the two measures was not significant for either protected or unprotected listening. This may be due to the non-linearity of the trend. For normal subjects, increasing attenuation score showed no relation to intelligibility score. Speech perception was constant. In hearing impaired listeners, an increasing value for attenuation was related to a lowering of the intelligibility score and in addition to a greater dispersion of the result across subjects. The trend was exaggerated for listening in noise as compared with quiet and for subjects with flat loss as compared with high frequency loss.

The practical implications of this study is that when a hearing conservation program based upon the use of personal protective devices is introduced into a plant or industry where there are already hearing impaired workers, real communication problems may be introduced. These may be minimized by the use of hearing protectors which provide the minimum necessary attenuation rather than the maximum. Consideration should also be given to the introduction of visual means of communication with a de-emphasis of purely verbal communication. The same is true when there are workers not fluent in the primary language of the plant.

ACKNOWLEDGEMENT

Supported by grants from the Ontario Ministry of Health, DM 318, and the Ontario Ministry of Labour, 004/R. The cooperation and support of the Workmen's Compensation Board of Ontario is gratefully acknowledged.

REFERENCES

1. Henderson, D., Hamernik, R.P., Dosanjh, D.S., and Mills, J.H., Effects of Noise on Hearing. Raven Press, New York, 1976.

2. Kryter, K.D.; Effects of ear protective devices on the intelligibility of speech in noise. J. Acoust. Soc. Am., 18, 413-417, 1946.

3. Coles, R.R.A., Rice, C.G., Earplugs and impaired hearing. J. Sound Vibr., 8, 521-523, 1965.

4. Lindeman, H.E.; Speech intelligibility and the use of hearing protectors. Audiology, 15, 348-356, 1976.

5. Canada Year Book, 1975. An Annual review of economic, social and political developments in Canada. Information Division, Statistics Canada.

6. Abel, S.M., Alberti, P.W., Riko, K., Speech intelligibility with ear protectors. J. Otolarnygol., 9, 256-265, 1980.

7. Gat, I.B., R.W. Keith, An Effect of Linguistic Experience. Audiology, 17, 339-345, 1978.

8. Wilkins, P.A., Martin, A.M., The effect of hearing protectors on the masked thresholds of acoustic warning signals. Proc. 9th International Congress on Acoustics, Madrid, 1977.

9. Forshaw, S.E., Listening for machinery malfunctions in noise while wearing ear muffs. DCIEM Technical Report No. 77X43, August, 1977.

10. Suter, A.H., The ability of mildly hearing-impaired individuals to discriminate speech in noise. Aerospace Medical Research Laboratory, Wright-Patterson Air Force Base, Ohio, January 1978, EPA 550/9-78-100.

Personal Hearing Protection in Industry, edited by P. W. Alberti, Raven Press, New York ©

24 Hearing Protector Problems in Military Operations

S. E. Foreshaw and J. I. Cruchley

INTRODUCTION

In 1955, the U.S. Armed Services asked the National Academy of Science - National Research Council Committee on Hearing, Bioacoustics, and Biomechanics (CHABA) for advice with respect to damage-risk criteria and noise-exposure contours[1]. The resulting recommendations enabled the U.S. Air Force to prepare its initial regulation on hearing conservation[2], and formed the basis for the introduction of a hearing conservation program in the Canadian Forces (CF)[3].

The purpose of a military hearing conservation program is to promote operational effectiveness and conserve manpower resources[4]. The environment of the CF contains most of the sources of noise to which the civilian community or the industrial worker may be exposed and, in addition, extremely intense noises that emanate from weapons systems and special military vehicles.

The impulse-noise level (peak) produced by the Carl Gustav 84mm Medium Anti-Tank Weapon is 185 dB at the gunner's ear; the peak levels at crew positions around the M109 155mm Self-Propelled Howitzer range from 166 to 179 dB at powder-charge No. 6; and the peak level produced by the 7.62mm FN rifle at the firer's right ear is 161 dB. The A-weighted sound pressure levels in the passenger sections of the M113-A1 Armoured Personnel Carrier and the CH-147 Chinook Medium Transport Helicopter are 115 and 110 dBA respectively[5]. A hearing conservation program becomes essential for the welfare of military personnel operating in such intense noise levels.

CANADIAN FORCES HEARING CONSERVATION PROGRAM

The CF Hearing Conservation Program utilizes all available means to protect the hearing of service personnel. The objectives of the program are:

(a) The reduction, wherever possible, of noise levels through the modification of equipment, change of its location, or restriction of time spent by personnel in high noise-level areas.

(b) The education at all levels regarding the effect of noise on hearing and the procedures to be followed to prevent noise-induced hearing loss.

(c) The identification and clear marking of hazardous noise areas and sources.

(d) The identification of the hearing risk to individuals by recording their hearing threshold levels upon enlistment and at periodic intervals throughout their service careers, with emphasis on those individuals frequently employed in noisy environments.

(e) The protection of affected individuals from more serious hearing loss by controlling further exposure to hazardous levels of noise.

(f) The provision of approved hearing protection devices to personnel working temporarily or permanently in noise-hazardous areas.

Guidelines for the control of noise exposure, when hearing conservation recommendations based on detailed octave-band data are not available, are as follows:

(a) Ear plugs or earmuffs should be worn by personnel exposed to noise for more than two hours per day when the A-weighted sound pressure level is between 90 and 100 dBA.

(b) Ear plugs or earmuffs should be worn for any exposure of any duration when the A-weighted sound pressure level is between 101 and 130 dBA.

(c) Ear plugs and earmuffs should be worn for any exposure to steady-state noise above 130 dBA. At this level, exposures must necessarily be restricted in frequency and duration.

(d) Ear plugs or earmuffs should be worn for any exposure to weapon impulse noise. In addition, special restrictions apply in the case of surface-to-air guided missiles, anti-tank weapons, tank guns, Howitzers, recoilless rifles, mortars, etc.

It is realized that in any group of individuals exposed to the same average (and acceptable) noise environments, a small percentage will develop relatively large hearing losses. A few individuals are susceptible to noise-induced hearing loss, and at present there are no simple and reliable tests available to identify such persons at the time of enlistment.

The problem of controlling noise-induced hearing loss in some branches of the CF is further complicated by the nature of the operations conducted. Although studies suggest that personnel engaged in intensive operational exercises can be protected to a reasonable level of hearing-loss risk from most current in-service weapons[6,7], relatively large percentages of combat arms personnel (artillery, infantry, armoured corps) do sustain significant permanent hearing loss, for reasons to be discussed later.

For the purpose of medical assessment, hearing levels are classified by the CF as shown in Table I. It can be seen that hearing sensitivity deteriorates progressively from category H1 to H2, H3 and H4.

Table I Canadian Forces Hearing Standards

Category	Hearing Standard
H1	Hearing level not greater than 30 dB between 500 and 6000 Hz in both ears.
H2	Hearing level not greater than 30 dB between 500 and 3000 Hz in both ears.
H3	Hearing level not greater than 30 dB between 500 and 2000 Hz in the better ear.
H4	Hearing level not greater than 50 dB between 500 and 2000 Hz in the better ear.

The percentages of CF personnel within these categories, in age groups from 21 to 25, 31 to 35, and 41 to 45 years are shown in Table II as a function of three career classifications: infantry, artillery, and for

Table II Percentage Distribution of Hearing Categories in Three Canadian Forces Career Classifications

	21-25 Years				31-35 Years				41-45 Years			
	H1	H2	H3	H4	H1	H2	H3	H4	H1	H2	H3	H4
A.	86.0	11.7	2.3		67.0	21.0	11.5	0.5	53.3	25.7	19.2	1.8
B.	86.6	10.7	2.7		63.4	27.6	9.0		47.7	27.3	23.0	2.0
C.	94.4	5.4	0.2		83.7	13.3	2.8	0.2	69.7	22.9	7.0	0.4

A. Infantry   B. Artillery   C. Pilots

comparative purposes, pilots. The population sizes of these classifications are 8006, 1932 and 2639 respectively[8].

As would be expected, an increasing proportion of the personnel in the three career classifications drops from H1 to H2, H3 or H4 in successive age groups.

The rate of hearing deterioration is high among individuals in the infantry and artillery confirming that they experience exposure to hazardous levels of noise during their military career.

In the pilots, the onset of hearing loss due to noise exposure and/or presbycusis occurs at a slightly faster rate than is observed in people not exposed to occupational noise[9]. Many military pilots must operate in moderately high levels of steady-state noise. However, aircrew are generally aware that their flying careers can be jeopardized if their hearing category drops below an acceptable level. Not only must an effective sound-attenuating flight helmet or headset be worn in intense steady-state noise environments to hear the auditory signals essential for flight and operational effectiveness, but the majority of flight personnel are also sufficiently motivated to attempt to preserve their hearing. In situations where such motivation is lacking, hearing protection is not always worn conscientiously.

At the same time, it is a gross oversimplification of the problems faced by the infantry and artillery to attribute the rate of hearing loss experienced by these groups solely to a lack of individual motivation. In many training and combat situations, standard hearing protection devices are simply not compatible with other equipment or activities.

HEARING PROTECTION REQUIREMENTS

Foremost, a hearing protection device for use in the combat arms must provide the maximum possible protection from the intense noise levels encountered around weapons and in fighting vehicles. At the same time, the device must be comfortable, relatively easy to don and doff, sufficiently robust to withstand the rigours of field use, and should not present any extraordinary hygiene problems to the wearer.

At first glance, it would appear that a relatively large volume liquid-sealed circumaural earmuff would best meet these requirements. In many environments, however, personnel must wear combat helmets or hard hats for head protection, and/or other protective items such as safety or anti-glare spectacles, respirators, toques and other cold-weather head garments.

At present, a number of NATO combat helmets do not allow the user to wear standard large volume earmuffs. Considerable effort has gone into the design of muffs and helmets that are mutually compatible, but in practice these combinations have tended to result either in uncomfortably snug fits or poor fitting helmets[10].

Compatibility with helmets requires that the sprung headband of an earmuff (normally worn over the top of the head) be replaced by a non-sprung fabric and/or sprung headband worn behind the nape of the neck.

As with the kits that attach earmuffs to hardhats, the resulting force that is applied to the circumaural region of the wearer's head through the earmuff seal is appreciably lessened, relative to that provided by the sprung headband worn over the head, thereby reducing the low-frequency attenuation of the muff[11,12].

Further, to fit under the rim of a combat helmet, an earmuff cup must have either a relatively small volume, thus reducing the low-frequency attenuation[13], or have most of its volume below the helmet rim, pushing the center of gravity of the cup outwards and causing an incompatibility problem with weapon sights[14].

Spectacles, respirators, etc. worn between the earmuff and the wearer's head, produce leakage paths beneath the earmuff seals, compromising the effectiveness of the earmuffs in attenuating sound (see Table III[15]).

Some form of ear plug might prove to be an acceptable alternative to the earmuff in certain combat arms situations. It must be remembered however that there are also problems with ear plugs. In order that a plug provide effective protection against noise, it must fit reasonably tightly in the ear canal, which causes some discomfort. Furthermore, it must be inserted into the canal with reasonable care if an air-tight seal is to be achieved and maintained.

Perhaps the most acceptable and effective plug is the type consisting of a polymer foam cylinder approximately one-half inch in diameter and three-quarter inches in length. The device must be compresssed by rolling it into as small as possible a diameter before inserting it into the ear canal. After insertion, the plug must be held in place with the fingertip until the foam has expanded to its original dimensions, otherwise it will tend to dislodge itself from the ear canal. Typical manufacturer's instructions suggest that the ear plug should be held in place about 60 seconds while this expansion takes place. If the plug is not compressed sufficiently or held in place long enough, problems will be encountered in inserting the plug into the ear canal and maintaining it there. Persons with very small

Table III Reduction in Sound Attenuation, in Decibels, of the SSC 258L Earmuffs, when Worn with Glasses with Various Size of Skull Temples or Temple Straps

		TEST FREQUENCY (Hz)								
Cross Sectional Shape and Dimensions of Skull Temple or Temple Strap, at the Point Where it Disturbs the Earmuff Seal		125	250	500	1000	2000	3000	4000	6000	8000
Standard Rim Glasses	Shape: Rectangular with rounded edges	6.8	6.0	6.6	5.9	5.5	3.5	5.6	8.2	7.1
	Width: .425 in.									
	Thickness: .141 in.									
Standard Pattern Aviation Spectacles	Shape: Oval	4.0	3.0	5.0	4.0	ns	ns	ns	ns	ns
	Width: .070 in.									
	Thickness: .070 in.									
Canadian Forces Combat Spectacles	Shape: Rectangular with rounded edges	ns	ns	ns	ns	ns	ns	ns	ns	ns
	Width: .260 in.									
	Thickness: .026 in.									

The reductions in sound attenuation shown above are statistically significant (p 0.01). Reductions shown as "not significant" (ns) indicate a probability of p 0.05.

diameter ear canals (including most females) may also experience difficulty in any event. Indeed, many women cannot be adequately fitted with "universal-size" triple flange ear plugs and require a small or extra-small size in plugs that are available in multiple sizes. If the foam ear plug is inserted too far into the ear canal, the wearer may have added difficulty in removing it. In some cases, tweezers have been required to remove impacted plugs.

The attenuation provided by this type of ear plug when reasonably well fitted in the ear canal exceeds the low-frequency protection provided by the standard multi-flange plugs. Moreover, most wearers find the foam type ear plugs to be more comfortable, particularly for long periods of wear, than other ear plugs.

In spite of these apparent advantages, the foam-type ear plug is not being considered as a direct replacement for the current standard issue plugs in the CF. The plugs soil very easily and in work situations where wearer's hands are continually soiled, dirt and grease will be transported to the ear canals by the porous plugs. Although the foam plugs can be cleaned with mild soap and water, this procedure is not really practical in many military work and operational environments.

The risk of increased incidences of otitis externa due to the porous nature of the foam material used in this type of ear plug has been a concern in the CF. As a result, a small study was carried out in which over 60 long-range patrol-aircraft crew members were randomly divided into three groups: the first continued to wear the standard multi-flange ear plugs currently in use in the CF, the second wore the foam plugs which were washed after each wearing, and the third also wore the foam plugs, but washed them only once per week[16].

The study continued for eight weeks during which three swabs of skin scrapings were taken from the subjects' ear canals (prior to the start of the study and at the end of the fourth and eighth weeks) for bacterial culture and fungal examination. Also, most of the participants were examined by a medical officer at the termination of the study to determine the presence or absence of overt signs of otitis externa.

The results of the study indicated (a) no fungal infections, and (b) no clinically significant bacterial infections, although 25 percent of the participants did have positive cultures on at least one sample. There was no difference, however, in the rate of positive cultures among the three groups. The Flight Surgeon conducting the study concluded that although the foam-type ear plug did not constitute any greater hygiene problem than did the standard issue ear plug, the foam plug should be discarded after every flight, as intended by the manufacturer.

Current CF policy with respect to ear plugs is that a range of standard devices ("universal-size" triple-flange plugs and the two smallest of a multi-size plug) be available to meet most ear-plug noise-protection requirements. However, in noise environments requiring greater protection than that afforded by the standard plugs, or where the standard-issue ear plugs are not providing satisfactory protection, the foam-type plug is available as an alternative.

LISTENING TO SPEECH AND OTHER SIGNALS WHILE WEARING HEARING PROTECTION

A crucial question is the effect of wearing a hearing protection device upon the reception of speech and other auditory signals. Kryter[17], the first of many to investigate the problem, concluded that in the acoustic conditions encountered in many industrial and military environments (i.e., noise levels that mask (elevate) the threshold of hearing for speech by 80 dB or more), the use of ear plugs should not decrease speech intelligibility.

More recently, Howell and Martin[18] have shown that wearing hearing protection can have varying effects upon speech reception, depending on the type of protection worn and the nosie conditions. Below 70 dB, for example, a person wearing earmuffs or plugs is likely to experience a reduction in received speech intelligibility, due to the fact that the less intense segments of speech are reduced to inaudible levels. Above 85 dB, however, wearing a hearing protector while listening to speech from a loudspeaker will not cause a reduction in speech intelligibility, and in fact, may result in an improvement in intelligibility to the extent that the hearing protector reduces distortion because of overloading in the auditory system. Aural harmonics are produced in the cochlea at levels above about 65 dB, and this distortion increases with increasing sound pressure level.

On the other hand, when a hearing protection device is worn by a talker in noise, his vocal effort is reduced, thereby decreasing the signal-to-noise ratio and intelligibility of his transmitted speech. This happens because a normal-hearing talker unconsciously regulates the intensity of his own voice according to the acoustic environment; wearing a protector reduces the environmental sound reaching the cochlea. When protectors are worn by both talker and listener, the composite effect is an overall reduction in intelligibility.

Howell and Martin further showed that the intelligibility of received speech in noise is two or three per cent less when wearing earmuffs than when wearing standard ear plugs. They speculate that since the attenuation provided by the earmuffs is greater than that provided by most ear plugs in the 1000- to 4000-Hz frequency range, earmuffs attenuate relatively more of the energy contained in the consonant sounds (crucial for speech discrimination) than do ear plugs. Anecdotal evidence suggests that wearers of the foam-type ear plug likewise have relatively greater difficulty in hearing and understanding speech in certain noise conditions.

Hearing sounds while wearing earmuffs is of particular concern to personnel who work in ships' engine and boiler rooms. Unless the propulsion and auxiliary machinery controls are located in sound-treated areas, individuals standing watch at these stations are exposed to levels of noise that can exceed 95 to 100 dBA. It is generally believed by the technicians who work in these areas that the attenuation provided by an effective earmuff or plug will adversely affect their ability to detect by ear those cues that indicate real or potential machinery malfunction. Hence, there is considerable reluctance to wear such protection.

Normal hearing observers are probably not handicapped by earmuffs, however, at least for such tasks as detecting pure tones in engine and boiler room noise above 85 dBA[19]. Indeed, at some frequencies, their performance may improve with muffs. However, individuals with bilateral hearing losses will be adversely affected by earmuffs if the attenuation of the muffs reduces the level of the signal below their threshold of audibility.

SPECIAL HEARING PROTECTION DEVICES

To be effective on the battlefield, a soldier must know where the enemy is and what he is doing. For an infantryman, this means seeing him or hearing him. Vision is often limited by terrain, by vegetation, or in the absence of a night-vision aid, by low ambient light levels. In such circumstances, a soldier can hear further than he can see, if he is not deafened. Earmuffs or ear plugs in this situation would immediately give their wearer a 30 to 40 dB conductive hearing loss. In impulse-noise environments such as firing ranges, where the steady-state background noise is otherwise at a relatively low level, voice commands and instructions cannot always be heard when hearing protection is worn. Rather than doff and don earmuffs or plugs CF gunners prefer to cover their ears with their hands, but this presupposes that both hands are free and that the blasts from adjacent weapons are not a problem.

An ideal device in these situations should give the wearer the maximum protection possible against high intensity noise, and yet permit low-level sounds to be heard at normal sensation levels. Additionally, the device should be compatible with other protective equipment (e.g., combat helmet, respirator) and weapon and communications systems.

An ear plug has been developed that meets these requirements: the Gunfender (Gundefender) amplitude sensitive ear plug[20]. The device is a modified V-51R ear plug with a 0.025-inch diameter opening into the wearer's external ear canal. The combined opening and ear-canal volume act as a Helmholtz resonator for sound of low intensity. That is, there is no attenuation below the cut-off frequency of the system (in this case, 1000 Hz), and attenuation above the cut-off frequency increases at a rate of 12 dB per octave to a maximum of about 20 dB. As a result, speech intelligibility is unaffected by the ear plug[21,22].

Low-intensity sounds are thus passed through the ear-plug opening with laminar-flow (low-loss) characteristics. At high intensities, however, the flow becomes turbulent, resulting in increased energy dissipation. Above about 110 dB, the Gunfender is as effective as a standard ear plug in reducing the temporary threshold shift that otherwise occurs from exposure to high intensity impulse noise[23].

It is noted, however, that the Gunfender does not protect the wearer from high level steady-state noise. Indeed, at about 850 Hz, the device has an attenuation of about -8 dB. A soldier relying on ear plugs for protection from noise should therefore be issued with two types: standard ear plugs for riding in an armoured vehicle or helicopter, and amplitude sensitive plugs for firing his weapon.

Because of the earmuff/combat-helmet incompatibility discussed previously, noise attenuating helmets are being considered for certain artillery and infantry operations. A requirement for such a helmet arose with the introduction into the CF of portable guided missile systems. During missile firing, the system operator and the launch safety officer are exposed to peak sound pressure levels of at least 180 dB.

In the training environment, it is possible that the instructor and safety officer can be exposed to at least 10 launches per day. It is clear that they must have the most effective hearing protection possible. At the same time, both crewmen require helmets that will provide ballistic protection. Also, the safety officer must maintain radio contact with his command post, and must be able to pass on firing instructions to the operator. The operator, in turn, must hear these instructions clearly

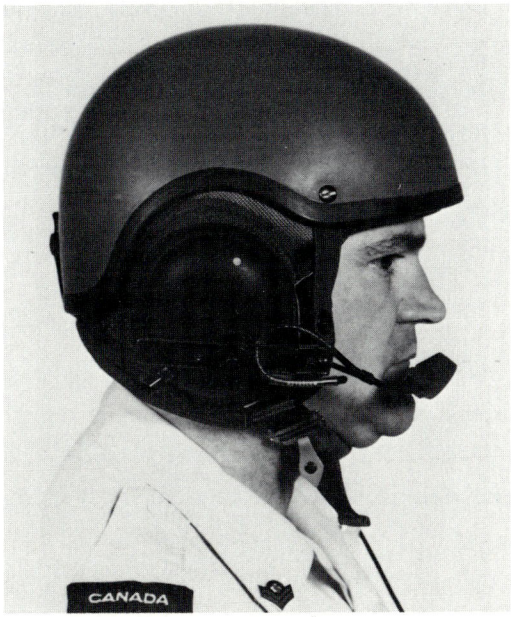

Figure 1. Prototype Artilleryman's helmet, including noise excluding ear cups/phones and a boom mounted noise cancelling microphone.

without removing his hearing protection.

A prototype DH-178 Artilleryman's Helmet (Figure 1) was built by the Gentex Corporation to CF specifications to meet this requirement. The helmet is basically the U.S. Army DH-132 Combat Vehicle Crewman's helmet, consisting of an outer ballistic/fragmentation protection shell, an inner liner, noise excluding ear cups/phones, a visor, and a boom-mounted noise cancelling microphone (only on the Safety Officer's helmet).

In addition, the right ear cup of the helmet is fitted with a miniature microphone and amplifier (sound intensifier) which permits the wearer to hear ambient sounds up to about 85 dBA at normal loudness, but limits ambient sounds above this level. A switch to turn the system "off" when the helmet is not being worn is located on the left ear cup.

The prototype helmets have undergone field evaluation with certain weapon-system instructors and students at the Combat Arms School at CF

Base Gagetown, and have received generally positive acceptance. Although most personnel were not required to wear the helmet continuously for more than about 30 minutes, the users have reported the helmet to be not too bulky or heavy, and if fitted properly, to be reasonably comfortable. One respondent complained that perspiration was a problem and suggested that some type of ventilation would be necessary in hot weather.

About 20 per cent of the users had high-frequency hearing losses in excess of 30 dB. Neither this group nor the remainder (with normal hearing) reported difficulties in understanding speech through the helmet's amplifier. Speech intelligibility testing of the prototype helmet by the US Army indicates that in quiet, there is no significant difference in speech reception scores when the helmet is worn in the passive and in the active mode (i.e., microphone amplifier turned "off" and "on"), and in a free field (no helmet). It is noted, however, that the non-linear characteristics of the amplifier contribute to degraded speech intelligibility when used in moderately intense noise environments[24]. More recent versions of the helmet contain separate channels for the two ears to facilitate auditory localization, amplifiers with improved frequency and overload characteristics, and a suspension inner liner to increase wearer comfort.

The difficulty remains of protecting infantrymen from the intense levels of acoustic energy produced by portable anti-armour weapons. Given that the electronic components of an "active" earmuff may not be sufficiently robust to withstand the rigours of the combat arms training and operational environment, the best compromise may be a specially-designed "passive" earmuff/helmet combination.

In the future, however, we do foresee the need for "active" noise-reduction/signal-enhancement devices that will enable sonar operators, for example, to more effectively detect and discriminate auditory-display signals in a background of fixed or rotary-wing aircraft noise. The technology required to implement such systems will undoubtedly have wide application in the industrial noise environment.

REFERENCES

1. Kryter, K.D., Ward, W.D., Miller, J.D., Eldredge, D.H. Hazardous exposure to intermittent and steady-state noise. J. Acoust. Soc. Amer. 39, 451-464, 1966.

2. U.S. Air Force, Medical Service. Hazardous Noise Exposure. AF Regulation No. 160-3, Washington, D.C., 1956.

3. Neely, K.K., Hearing Conservation for the Armed Forces. Med. Ser. J. Canada. 15, 235-247, 1959.

4. Canadian Forces Medical Order 40-01. Hearing Conservation Program. Ottawa, 1976.

5. Forshaw, S.E., Coffey, C.G., Strong, R.A., A survey of noise hazards at the Combat Arms School, CFB Gagetown. DCIEM Report No. 814. Defence and Civil Institute of Environmental Medicine, Toronto, 1972.

6. Forrest, M.R., Protection given by ear muffs against Howitzer noise. Report APRE No. 6/77. Army Personnel Research Establishment, Farnborough, England, 1977.

7. Hodge, D.C., Price, G.R., Dukes, N.L., Murff, S.J. Effects of artillery noise on the hearing of protected crew personnel. Technical Memorandum 17-79. US Army Human Engineering Laboratory, Aberdeen Proving Ground, Maryland, 1979.

8. Forshaw, S.E., Noise problems in combat arms operations. Proceedings of TTCP Action Group WAG-3 Seminar on Man and Crew-Portable Unguided Anti-Armour Weapons. Aberdeen Proving Ground, Maryland, 1974.

9. Passchier-Vermeer, W., Steady-state and fluctuating noise: its effects on the hearing of people. Proceedings of a conference on Occupational Hearing Loss held at the National Physics Laboratory, Teddington, England. Academic Press, London, 1971.

10. Forrest, M.R., Effect of wearing a combat helmet or spectacles on gunfire noise attenuation of ear muffs. Report APRE No. 39/76. Army Personnel Research Establishment, Farnborough, England, 1976.

11. Cruchley, J.I., Acoustic evaluation of four earmuff kits for use with hard hats (U). RESTRICTED. DCIEM Report 79X14. Defence and Civil Institute of Environmental Medicine, Toronto, 1979.

12. Couture, C.D., Acoustic properties of headgear: XXXVI. The Safety Supply Company 285 Earmuffs and The Bilsom Military NFM-1 Earmuffs (U). DCIEM Technical Memorandum No. 76-x-66. RESTRICTED. Defence and Civil Institute of Environmental Medicine, Toronto, 1976.

13. Di Mattia, A.L., A practical ear enclosure with selectively coupled volume. J. Aud. Eng., 15, 295-298, 1976.

14. Forrest, M.R., Hearing protection - infantry requirements. Report APRE No. 5/78. Army Personnel Research Establishment, Farnborough, England, 1978.

15. Forshaw, S.E., Stairs, E.D., The effects of wearing standard rim glasses on the attenuation characteristics of the SSC 258 earmuffs (U). DCIEM Report No. 73-R-961. RESTRICTED. Defence and Civil Institute of Environmental Medicine, Toronto, 1973.

16. Kearns, J.A., Personal Communication, 1978.

17. Kryter, K.R., Effects of ear protection devices on the intelligibility of speech in noise. J. Acoust. Soc. Amer., 18, 413-417, 1946.

18. Howell, K., Martin, A.M., An investigation of the effects of hearing protection on vocal communication in noise. J. Sound and Vib., 41, 181-196, 1975.

19. Forshaw, S.E., Listening for machinery malfunctions in noise while wearing ear muffs. DCIEM Report No. 77X43. Defence and Civil Institute of Environmental Medicine, Toronto, 1977.

20. Forrest, M.R., Coles, R.R.A., Problems of communication and ear protection in the Royal Marines. J. Roy. Naval Med. Ser., 56, 162-169, 1970.

21. Mosko, J.D., Fletcher, J.L., Evaluation of the Gunfender earplug: Temporary threshold shift and speech intelligibility. J. Acoust. Soc. Amer. 49, 1732-1733, 1971.

22. Forshaw, S.E., Goodfellow, G.L., Sound reception and attenuation characteristics of the Cosmocord Limited ERDEfender Mk I Earmuff and the Sonex Gunfender (Gundefender) amplitude sensitive ear plug (U). DRET Technical Memorandum No. 767. RESTRICTED. Defence and Civil Institute of Environmental Medicine, Toronto. 1971.

23. Hughes, W.P., An assessment of the effectiveness of amplitude sensitive ear plugs - Gunfenders - against high intensity impulse noise from the 120 mm Bat anti-tank weapon. APRE Technical Memorandum 40/72. Army Personnel Research Establishment, Farnborough, England, 1972.

24. Patterson, J.H., Nelson, W.R., Marrow, R.H., Hargett, C.E., Camp, R.T., Medical evaluation of sound attenuation and electroacoustics of a prototype DH-178 Protective Helmet. USAARL Report No. 78-12. US Army Aeromedical Research Laboratory, Fort Rucker, Alabama, 1978.

25 Practical Problems of Hearing Protector Use in Canadian Mines

M. Savich

INTRODUCTION

Miners are exposed to high levels of noise and become temporarily or permanently deafened. Because of the high incidence of hearing loss, major steps have been taken to introduce hearing conservation programmes into Canadian Mines. The occupational hazards in the working environment due to noise and vibration should be kept within limits[1] by:

a)   technical measures

b)   supplementary administrative measures, where the technical measures alone do not provide sufficient protection.

Often the noise level cannot be reasonably reduced at its source or by the use of acoustical materials and noise barriers. In such cases, some form of ear protection should be considered for noise exposed workmen. The major benefit of noise control by means of hearing protector usage in Canadian mines are as follows:

1.   reduced risk of hearing loss
2.   more pleasant working conditions.

In Canadian mines, fifty percent of noise exposed workers use ear muffs, forty percent ear plugs and three percent ear muffs and ear plugs. The remaining seven percent do not use ear protection equipment, or use it temporarily. As foam ear plugs are the only ones in general use in Canadian mines, but many different types of muffs are in service, a research study was conducted to investigate the efficiency of ear muffs under working conditions.

Results obtained under the three general headings, factory procedures, laboratory tests and underground performance were computed and compared. Simple methods and simple equipment were used during these studies.

Ear protectors must comply with the following basic requirements:
1. Achieve high attenuation of ambient noise. The best ear protectors do not attenuate more than 25 to 30 dB and theoretical attenuation is limited to about 50 dB because noise can by-pass the ear-protector by pick-up and by bone conduction[2]. Used by themselves, ear plugs provide more attenuation at low frequencies than do ear muffs. Ear plugs and ear muffs can be worn at the same time to provide greater attenuation. The attenuation offered by the combination is less than the sum of the individual attenuations, a phenomenon which has not yet been explained.
2. Be comfortable. An uncomfortable ear protector becomes intolerable after prolonged use.
3. Avoid harmful side effects; such as skin disorders.

TECHNICAL AND ATTENUATION DATA FOR EAR MUFFS

Technical and attenuation data on ear muffs is given in Tables 1 and 2. Cushion areas, cup volumes and weight vary visibly. Cups are covered by foam on the inside for two reasons: to increase attenuation because uncovered cups permit entry of sound; and to prevent the formation of standing waves. Several attempts have been made in the laboratory to increase attenuation using metal ear muffs, adding one or more Helmholtz resonators, or by using soft hollow cushions filled with wax[3]. An older example is the NRC type ear muff developed at the National Research Council, Ottawa, by Shaw and Thiessen[4]. This device when properly fitted may be worn for many hours without discomfort[5]. Constant technical progress in ear muff design is evident by all manufacturers.

Comfort: One of the Main Requirements of Ear Muffs
The comfort provided by ear muffs depends both upon the ear cushion seal against the head and the overall design of the muff. The pressure of ear cushion seals against the head is a direct consequence of the clamping

Table I Characteristics of Muffs Tested

Ear Muff No.	Filled Cushion	Cross-sectional Dimensions (cm)						Area of cushion (cm²)	Volume of cup (cm³)	Weight (g)				wt	Total Weight of Ear Muff (g)
		A	B	C	D	E	F			Cup	Cushion	Foam	Fibre-Glass		
1 A	Foam	9.7	9.7	6.5	4.3	1.1	4.2	48.0	180	49.86	13.67	7.61	-	71.14	185
2 B	Air	9.5	9.5	6.5	4.2	0.8	4.8	40.0	159	73.45	11.44	3.90	-	88.79	284
3 C	Foam	10.7	8.0	6.7	4.0	1.0	3.6	35.6	117	51.13	5.79	0.59	2.46	59.97	188
4 F	Foam	10.5	8.0	6.8	4.1	0.9	3.8	28.5	131	45.30	4.49	1.11	-	50.90	182
5 E	Foam	10.6	8.0	6.8	4.2	1.0	3.8	28.0	131	42.80	4.43	1.27	-	48.50	151
6 F	Foam	9.8	8.3	6.5	3.9	1.0	4.5	43.1	158	63.40	10.47	8.07	-	81.94	291
7 G	Fluid	11.0	8.3	6.3	3.6	0.7	4.4	38.7	167	68.64	56.29	2.90	-	127.83	335
8 H	Foam	11.0	8.3	6.4	3.7	0.8	4.4	42.5	164	57.02	19.87	4.91	-	81.80	274
9 I	Foam	9.4	6.9	6.9	4.6	1.0	4.4	26.7	171	73.94	8.92	3.21	-	86.07	278
10 J	Foam	9.4	6.9	6.9	4.6	0.9	4.4	24.5	171	76.26	9.05	3.34	-	88.65	275
11 K	Foam	11.0	8.2	6.5	4.2	1.0	3.6	42.2	141	52.92	15.92	2.48	-	71.32	295
Arithmetic Mean		10.24	8.2	6.62	4.13	0.93	4.17	36.16	153.6	59.50	14.58	3.58	2.46	80.12	248
Std. Dev.		0.68	0.86	0.21	0.32	0.12	0.4	7.98	20.4	12.16	14.61	2.46	-	29.25	60.5

force, adjustment, softness and weight.

1. Clamping force (Head force): The clamping force is the force exerted by an ear muff on the skin and it is the most important element of discomfort. The clamping force against the sides of the head varies between 500 and 1000 g wt[6]. Pressure limits have not yet been important aspect. The clamping force varies and depends on the bizygomatic diameter of the head.

2. Adjustment: Ear Muff adjustment is necessary to adjust to the shape and dimensions of a worker's head. To fulfil the criterion of a tight fit, the muffs should have the capability of moving the support up and down so as to be parallel with the wearer's ears. To make allowances for each person's unique head shape, they should also be rotational on a pivot point. An effective seal inside the cup prevents acoustical leakage around the bearing surface. A poor linkage between the helmet and the cups hinders clamping force and comfort. Poor mounting and asymmetry of ear muffs is caused by two things; inadequate data for hole locations on helmets and the poor mounting of ear muffs on helmets in mines.

A good solution is to use separate ear muffs with a spring worn behind the head (back-band with strap) and a support strap in conjunction with a safety helmet. This head-strap is adjustable over the head to avoid discomfort caused by the pull of gravity on the ear cups. It also helps maintain the ear cups in position.

3. Softness: Softness is a prime consideration for ear cushions. Apart from the vital aspect of comfort, an effective noise seal depends upon the cushion being soft enough to assume the contours of the head and to fit snugly around the frames of glasses or eyeglass adapters. New materials for cushion seals perform the function of adapters. The No. 3 ear muff, model C, has foam filled cushions with covering material of soft, supple plastic film. Some ear cups have special cushions with replaceable snap in/out foam over a liquid sealing ring to afford even pressure without gaps, even when wearing eye glasses.

Table 2 Attenuation Characteristics (in dB)* and Technical Data of Ear Muffs Acquired for Testing

No.	Ear Muff	Band	Characteristic	125	250	500	1k	2k	3k	4k	6k	8k
1	A	B	Measured	9.70	16.10	24.90	33.90	34.10	36.00	41.00	33.80	31.50
			Std. Dev.	3.20	2.50	2.80	5.10	2.90	5.60	5.70	6.60	5.90
2	B	H	Measured	5.00	13.00	22.00	31.00	31.00	41.00	36.00	28.00	21.00
			Std. Dev.	–	–	–	–	–	–	–	–	–
3	C	H	Measured	10.00	16.00	30.00	34.00	37.00	41.00	45.00	39.00	34.00
			Std. Dev.	–	–	–	–	–	–	–	–	–
4	D	H	Measured	11.50	16.50	26.50	36.50	38.00	38.50	44.50	39.50	–
			Std. Dev.	–	–	–	–	–	–	–	–	–
5	E	B	Measured	13.40	17.30	28.60	41.80	40.70	45.20	42.70	32.60	29.30
			Std. Dev.	3.30	3.90	3.00	3.40	5.60	4.60	5.30	4.10	4.70
6	F	B	Measured	17.00	18.00	29.00	36.00	38.00	44.00	44.00	43.00	43.00
			Std. Dev.	2.60	2.60	3.10	3.20	4.10	7.20	4.60	4.70	5.70
7	G	T	Measured	18.00	23.00	33.00	44.00	44.00	47.00	45.00	42.00	39.00
			Std. Dev.	–	–	–	–	–	–	–	–	–
8	H	T	Measured	18.00	23.00	33.00	44.00	44.00	47.00	45.00	42.00	39.00
			Std. Dev.	–	–	–	–	–	–	–	–	–
9	I	H	Measured	12.00	17.00	30.00	35.00	35.00	36.00	37.00	32.00	30.00
			Std. Dev.	2.50	3.00	4.60	5.60	4.50	4.30	4.20	4.10	2.90
10	J	B	Measured	10.00	17.00	28.00	37.00	36.00	44.00	39.00	32.00	30.00
			Std. Dev.	2.00	2.60	4.30	5.40	4.50	5.60	3.80	5.40	4.90
11	K	B	Measured	15.00	17.00	26.00	43.00	36.00	38.00	38.00	33.00	34.00
			Std. Dev.	5.20	3.90	8.80	3.60	4.90	6.60	6.80	1.30	5.30
			Arithmetic Mean of all Ear Muffs	12.16	17.09	27.80	37.22	36.98	41.07	41.22	35.49	33.53
			Std. Dev.	3.86	2.47	3.09	4.31	3.58	3.90	3.49	5.00	7.36

B: Behind Head; H: Attached to hard hat; T: Band on top of head

* Attenuation characteristic measured in accordance with American National Standard Specification Z.24.22-1957 (from Factory Data).

4. Weight: The weight of ear muffs greatly affects comfort because the force of gravity adds to the irritants already present. The total weight of a pair of muffs varies between 151 g and 335 g (Table 1). For comfort the weight of an ear muff must be limited to approximately 200 grams[7].

Table 3: Comfort Test of Ear Muffs using industrial elimination

#	Ear muff/age	# of Subject 2	5	10	15	16	17	19	21	22	23	24	25	26	27	
		24	29	30	40	42	42	46	49	52	52	55	57	59	60	
1	A	X	Y	X	X	X	X	Y	Y	O	Y	X	Y	O	Y	40
2	B	Y	O	O	O	O	Y	Y	X	O	Y	O	Y	Y	O	83
3	C	X	Y	Y	X	Y	Y	Y	X	X	X	X	X	Y	Y	40
4	D	O	O	Y	Y	O	X	X	Y	X	Y	O	Y	O	X	43
5	E	X	O	X	X	X	X	X	X	X	Y	Y	Y	X	X	38
6	F	O	O	X	Y	Y	X	X	X	X	O	Y	Y	Y	Y	56
7	G	X	X	X	X	Y	Y	Y	Y	Y	O	O	Y	Y	Y	54
8	H	X	X	X	X	Y	Y	Y	Y	Y	O	O	Y	Y	Y	54
9	I	O	X	X	X	O	Y	Y	X	Y	Y	O	Y	O	Y	67
10	J	Y	O	X	X	Y	X	Y	Y	O	Y	O	X	Y	X	56
11	K	Y	X	X	X	Y	X	O	Y	Y	O	X	Y	O	Y	56
		43	56	24	27	49	22	33	25	33	52	56	34	62	36	562

Note:

Evaluation   X Satisfactory (1)
                  Y Good (2)   83 Maximum   Industrial
                  O Very Good (3)   elimination

Tests of Comfort

Ear muffs must be sufficiently comfortable to be worn for long periods of time, perhaps up to 8 or 10 hours a day. The comfort of ear muffs can be quantified, although, such a test has yet to be generally accepted. Women were eliminated from the tests because so few are employed in mining industries[8]. A subjective evaluation was undertaken (Table 3). Subjects were asked to classify comfort as 1) satisfactory; 2) good; and 3) very good. The experiment was designed so that the differences among age (rows) and qualitative evaluation (columns) represented a major source of variation. Such an arrangement is known as a Latin square[9]. We used the method of industrial elimination in the parallel entries. Full details are given elsewhere[10].

The data obtained from fourteen reliable subjects (mean age is 45.5 ± 3.09 years) showed a significant difference between muffs. In the analysis, larger cushion areas (Tables 1 and 3) seemed to be a significant feature in determining comfort.

Head Size Survey
The variety of size, shape, and contour of the human head poses a difficult problem for manufacturers of ear muffs. The major reason for making the bizygomatic diameter survey was to evaluate the clamping force required in ear muff design. A measurement of maximum distance between the bony structures (zygomatic arches) forward of the ears was carried out on 27 men. Statistical analysis of the samples showed that small, but significant differences existed between ethnic groups (Table 4). Subjects came from the United Kingdom, Continental Europe and Asia, and were classified accordingly. The number of people of non-Caucasian origin is large, 26 percent of the population.

In the literature, the volume of bizygomatic diameter data which has been published of Caucasian ethnic origin is relatively small. Comparison of results from Table 4, with other surveys from the literature, showed minor differences of no practical importance[11,12,13,14]. Bizygomatic diameter surveys indicate that differences in head size may be sufficient to affect clamping force in some instances and give low attenuation or discomfort.

The ANSI S3.19-1974 standard recommends separating ear cups 14.35 cm. (medium head width), when measuring the clamping force.

Table 4 Bizygomatic Diameter Surveys

No.	Population	No. of persons	Means D (cm)	Means Age (years)
1	Caucasian	20	14.47 ± 0.17	38.70 ± 2.55
2	Non-Caucasian	7	14.13 ± 0.26	43.29 ± 4.43
3	Canadian[+]	16	14.43 ± 0.16	38.94 ± 3.07
4	Non-Canadian[+]	11	14.23 ± 0.26	41.27 ± 3.18
5	U.K.[++]	13	14.17 ± 0.13	37.38 ± 2.90
6	Cont. Europe[++]	10	14.17 ± 0.28	45.20 ± 4.13
7	Slavic[++]	5	15.00 ± 0.50	44.80 ± 4.55
8	Asia[+++]	7	14.13 ± 0.26	43.29 ± 4.43
9	Age 19-39	13	14.05 ± 0.15	30.00 ± 1.48
10	Age 40-60	14	14.44 ± 0.19	49.07 ± 1.85
	Canadian	27	14.35 ± 0.14	39.89 ± 2.21

+   16 Canadian-born versus 11 non-Canadian-born

++ U.K. origin, Cont. Europe origin, Slavic origin in Cont. Europe.

+++ Including Hungary and Finland.

LABORATORY TESTS OF EAR MUFFS

Measurements of ear muff attenuations have been made using two methods:

1. Psychophysical method using human heads by static range-of-movement:
    a) Movement of the joint of the neck in normal position. Subject used glasses and adapters.
    b) Movement of the joint of the neck, flexion, (dorsal and ventral) and neck rotation (right and left). Subject used glasses.
2. Physical method using apparatus for determining the efficiency of cup cushions.

These tests were made to provide performance data for eleven models of ear muffs under testing procedures established in the Elliot Lake

Laboratory (Table I).

Psychophysical Method

The ear muff attenuations was measured as a transmission loss, the difference between the noise level outside the ear muff (measured 0.1 m from the side of the head) and that inside the ear muff[15]. This method can be expected to give slightly different results than the American Standards Association's standard method[16,17].

Equipment The test signals were produced with a Bruel and Kjaer random noise generator, type 1402. The high powered loudspeaker was placed 1 m from the subject. Microphones were suspended at the subject's ear: one under the cup and one over the cup, 1.3 m above the floor, and located in the centre of the room.

The basic system for measuring soundpressure levels with a sound level meter consists of the following:
1.   Transducer: a) A 1 in., type 4145, B and K microphone was used over the cup. b) A 1/4 in., type 4135, B and K microphone was used under the cup.
2.   Preamplifier: a) A type 2619, B and K preamplifier was used over the cup. b) A type 2615, B and K preamplifier was used under the cup.
3.   Sound level meter: a) Impulse precision sound level meter, type 2209, B and K. An octave filter, type 1613, B and K, was connected to an impulse precision sound level meter. b) A precision sound level meter, type 2203, B and K. An octave filter, type 1613, B and K, was connected to a prescision sound level meter.

The calibrator was a pistonphone, type 4220, B and K, and the sound level calibrator was a type 4230, B and K.

Subject Selection and Test Room

Two subjects for these tests were selected from the laboratory personnel. Subject 1 (age 35) with long hair, had a mezzocephalic head with a bizygomatic diameter of 13.6 (significantly smaller than average), and subject 2 (age 54) short haired, had a brachycephalic head with a bizygomatic diameter of 16.5 (significantly larger than average).

The tests were conducted in an empty semi-reverberant room held at constant temperature, 4.25 m long, 4 m wide and 2.5 m high. The walls, ceiling and floor were constructed of wood and there was one window and one door in the room. Maximum ambient noise levels at the position of the subject were 35 dBA.

Test Procedure:
Each of the subjects was taught the correct fitting procedures for the eleven models. The device was first positioned by the experimenter and then adjusted by the subject for a final orientation for each test.

Attenuation Measurements: Measurements of variation in sound pressure levels for a constant test signal level were made on both the left and right sides of the head. The ear muff attenuation was determined at the following frequencies: 125, 250, 1000, 2000, 4000 and 8000 Hz and at the dBA weighting network using the factory attenuations given in Table 2. Average noise levels of the test signals was calculated, and the noise reduction ratings for eleven ear muffs were determined. There were 7 tests on both ears of two subjects, thus 28 sets of measurements in all. One ear muff had 4 extra tests.

Effect of Glasses and Adapters on Attenuation of Ear Muffs
During this test the listener's neck joint was in normal position. The raw data of the attenuation tests of ear muffs are summarized in a graph (with frequency in hertz). Total noise was estimated from the octave-band noise levels. Approximate agreement with the total noise measured indicates a reasonably constant condition during the period of measurement.

Measurements of ear muff attenuations were made in the current series of tests with: (a) ear muffs; (b) ear muffs and glasses; and (c) ear muffs, glasses and adapter. Muffs/ eyeglass adapters were specially designed for people wearing glasses in conjunction with hearing protectors.

The detailed results are presented elsewhere[10], but summarized, show the following:
1. Attenuation for subject 2 with large head and short hair was higher than attenuation for subject 1 with small head and long hair, except in four measurements.

Table 5 Comparison of manufacturers' data and field test performance of muffs

Ear Muff No.	1	2	3	4	5	6	7	8	9	10	11
Noise Reduction (dBA)[+]	34.2	31.1	36.8	37.5	39.9	38.0	43.6	43.6	35.0	36.3	36.4
Attenuation (dBA)[*]	27.3	29.7	30.0	30.0	31.5	27.0	29.9	34.8	31.6	32.1	27.3
Difference (dBA)	6.9	1.4	6.8	7.6	8.4	11.0	13.7	8.8	3.4	4.2	9.1
Order of Performance [**]	5	1	4	6	7	10	11	8	2	3	9

NOTE: [+] from manufacturers literature

     [*] from Table 6

    [**] 1 = best; 11 = worst

Only No. 2 ear muff came close to the factory attenuation value.
The largest attenuation was displayed by ear muff No. 8.

2. Ear muffs No. 2, No. 5, and No. 8 had almost equal attenuations for both subjects.
3. The largest attenuation difference for both subjects occurred with the No. 6 ear muff, apparently due to subject 1's long hair. Substantial differences were also found with ear muffs No. 2, 7 9 and 10.
4. With the use of glasses and their adapters, attenuation decreased. The adapters are not effective sound barriers.
5. Most ear muffs show a lower attenuation than those given by the factory specification as shown in Table 5.

Effect of Movement of Joint of the Neck, Flexion and Neck Rotation on Attenuation of Ear Muffs

This test was similar to the previous one. The object of this test was to see the stability of ear muffs on heads in motion, and to measure air leaks when wearing glasses. The left hemisphere was tested with glasses and the right hemisphere was tested without them. The detailed results are presented elsewhere, but in summary, they show:

1. There are no great differences in attenuation when the neck moves;
2. The test performed on subject 1 (D = 13.6 cm) showed that the amount of hair trapped between the ear muff cushion and the head had a significant effect on ear muff attenuation.
3. The largest difference in attenuation between two subjects is once again with the No. 6 ear muff (left side 16 dBA, and right side 18.06 dBA).
4. The greatest attenuation occurred with the No. 10 ear muff on both subjects (34.21 dBA).
5. On the average, with both subjects, glasses decreased attenuation by 1.42 dBA.

Cushion Seals and Clamping Force

Manufacturers' specified attenuations were attained only on ear muffs No. 2 and No. 10 when worn on a large head with short hair, subject 2. The hair length had the largest effect on ear muff attenuation even if the ear muff has cushion seals that retain softness. With the use of glasses and adapters attenuation decreased substantially on small as well as large heads. Eye-glass adapters do not have the characteristics attributed to them in the literature[18]. The cause is simple: new materials for cushion seals perform the function of adapters.

Attenuation mainly depends upon two factors: clamping force and cushion seals. An increase in clamping force results in an increased attenuation.

PHYSICAL METHOD

Ear muff attenuation was measured as the difference between the outputs of the microphone uncovered and the cup covered microphone. For this test the apparatus to determine the efficiency of cup cushions under different clamping forces was made in the Elliot Lake Laboratory.

Instrumentation

The sound field of a pure tone at 500 Hz, 1000 Hz, 3000 Hz and 8000 Hz, was generated by a Hewlett-Packard test oscillator, model 650A. A loudspeaker was placed 1 m from the centre of the apparatus taken in horizontal and vertical directions. The microphones, preamplifier and sound level meter were as described earlier.

Apparatus Full details of the apparatus are given elsewhere[10]. Accoustical isolation of the apparatus was greater than 60 dB in any test frequency band in the range of interest.

Test Procedure

The ear cup was spread and placed on the plane plexiglass surface. A steelyard's rubber pin was pressed against the ear cup and a clamping force was selected. Loss of attenuation by an ear cup under a constant clamping force and different test signal level was examined.

Ear Muff Attenuation

The algebraic difference in sound pressure levels, in the dBA weighting network, at each test frequency signal, with and without the ear cup in place on the plexiglass, is considered to be the attenuation of the device. For a discussion of results, the clamping force at 450 g wt for one cup was used as a basic level (ANSI S 3.19-1974).

The ear muffs could be divided into three main groups:

Group	Ear Muff	Minimum Force (g wt)	Attenuation Behaviour
1	No. 4, No. 5, No. 8 No. 9, and No. 10	150 to 350	Steady at all frequencies and clamping forces above min.
2	No. 1, No. 3, and No. 6	350 to 550	Steady at some frequencies and clamping forces
3	No. 2, No. 7, and No. 11	550	Variable at all frequencies and clamping forces

In general, the attenuation values of ear cups are dependent upon two factors:
1. Clamping (head band) force (g wt), and
2. Design of the ear cup cushion.

Both factors were taken into consideration in this test. It was evident that attenuation is a function of size of air paths as shown by poor contact. An air path causes different losses of attenuation at various frequency test signals as well as different losses among the various ear muffs.

A greater attenuation is obtained when an ear cup is exposed to horizontal sound, than when it is exposed to vertical sound. According to acoustical laws, the opposite should be expected. Shaw came to the same conclusion and this phenomenon is yet to be explained[19].

This test explained the following:
1. Ear muffs with a small cushion area start serving their purpose more quickly because the force per square centimeter is larger;
2. A clamping force larger than 900 g wt, in the first and second groups, does not cause an increase in attenuation;
3. Attenuation characteristics (ANSI Z 24.22-1957) of ear muffs

show a correlation with physical tests. They cannot be completely compared because their values differ, dB versus dBA.

Based on the extensive literature and the physical tests performed, the apparatus for determining the efficiency of cup cushions can be used effectively to apply theory in the design of ear muffs.

EAR MUFF ATTENUATION TESTS IN MINES

A study was undertaken to measure ear muff attenuation in mines. A series of nine ear muffs was tested under uniform conditions in mines.

Objective of the Study

The only certain means for evaluating the efficiency of the hearing protection program, equipment, training and supervision, is to measure, periodically, the hearing thresholds of all miners exposed to noise[20]. However, this method does not detect problems until some hearing loss has occurred.

Because of this a new method, the "Noise Dosimeter Vest", has been developed in the Elliot Lake Laboratory to provide an assessment of attenuation efficiencies of ear muffs in use. It is fully described elsewhere[10].

Experimental Method

The Noise Dosimeter Vest provides a technical solution for the determination of the noise exposure index and the attenuation of ear muffs. It does so under the most difficult working conditions (i.e., single platform (giraffe), the load-haul-dump (LHD) vehicle, etc.). These tests require only two dosimeters and a stop watch. The dosimeters have small microphones and provide accurate short time readings of the noise exposure index. A pocket-sized calculator designed for sound amplitude analysis is also necessary (dBA, L_{eq}, L_{max} and time duration of the sampling period).

The surveyor must measure the distance between the bony structures just forward of the ears (bizygomatic diameter) using an outside caliper. On the basis of bizygomatic diameter measurements, the clamping force can be evaluated. An apparatus was designed in the Elliot Lake Laboratory for the immediate measurement of clamping force at the mines. Evaluations are done on the spot and the worker is immediately informed about the noise exposure index level and ear muff attenuation data. If the attenuation is unsatisfactory, the cause should be investigated.

Participants

In this study one man at each of three working sites was chosen:
1. Jumbo (Three Drills) operator
2. Drill Hydrofore operator
3. Jaw Crusher operator

Of particular importance were the following items:
- the miner is informed of the test's objective.
- the miner is asked to adjust his own ear muffs to his particular liking, and to make qualitative evaluations of comfort before and after the test.
- if a miner wishes to withdraw at any time and for any reason, he may do so.

It was explained that all testing would be conducted under the full support of miners and supervisory personnel.

Results

The results of the study indicate poor attenuation of ear muffs in underground mining conditions. As a result of analyzing the data obtained, three major findings are presented below.

1. Jumbo (Three Drills) Operator: While working, the jumbo operator used only ear plugs. The miner was of the opinion that his ear muffs were inefficient and wore them only because regulations required it. The ear muff was No. 6, model F, with hat mounting, that did not properly cover the ears, and which provided a mean attenuation of only 8.6 dB.

The noise levels are high (115 dBA) and that the ear muffs supplied do not offer adequate protection. For all ear muffs, one of the factors contributing to the low attenuation found was this man's extremely small head size. The ear muffs with adequate attenuation were Nos. 1, 2, 5 and 10. The jumbo operator judged ear muffs which are worn behind the head (Nos. 6 and 11) to be uncomfortable.

2.   Hydrofore Drill Operator: Hydraulic drills are used increasingly on jumbo machines, replacing the heavy pneumatic rock drills (21). A hydrofore drill (hydraulic-electric fan) has no air exhaust noise and thus produces low noise levels at low frequencies. Because the attenuation of ear muffs is better at high frequencies, it should be expected that their efficiency would be very high. Test results demonstrate that good attenuations were obtained by ear muffs Nos. 5, 6 and 10 (25, 25 and 18 dB, respectively) with band passing behind the head. The other ear muffs did not provide satisfactory attenuations.

3.   Jaw Crusher Operator: Generally speaking, ear muffs should be used where the ambient sound levels exceed 105 dBA. Below this value, ear plugs give good protection. Because ear muffs are practical for intermittent noise (and because infection can result from the use of ear plugs), usually only ear muffs are used to protect from lower noise levels in all areas of mines.

Test results from eight ear muffs show sufficient attenuation, to 90 dBA and below. Only ear muff No. 9 had a very low attenuation (8.3 dBA). Once again, extremely good attenuation was provided by three muffs: No. 5 (18.8 dBA), No. 6 (23.8 dBA) and No. 10 (23.1 dBA). The full results are published elsewhere (10).

Clamping Force and Comfort

On the average, ear muffs have poor attenuation (15 dBA). The efficiency of an ear muff is determined by its clamping force and its fit over the ear. If the clamping force is decreased, attenuation also decreases. Clamping force will vary in each case because of different head sizes. A good fit over the ear is an important factor for noise attenuation, and it is inter-related with comfort. From the tests performed it is evident that comfort and attenuation affect one another.

Characteristically, ear muffs mounted on the hat have different comfort evaluations and different attenuation results. In all cases, hats cause these discrepancies. There are numerous other causes: poor mounting due to insufficient instructions, varying head dimensions and ear heights, improper fitting, interference by hair or eye-glasses, improper wearing of ear muffs, etc. Because of this the value of a measured attenuation in use does not equal the value obtained by an approximate method for calculating noise reduction and factory attenuation[22,23]. Results of the factory noise reduction can be easily compared with EPA's (The Environmental Protection Agency, U.S.A.) proposed labelling of hearing protection products[24].

Clamping force studies were made with eleven ear muffs. The mean value was 1256 ± 77 (g wt) (Standard error is ± 77 (g wt)). In various references in the literature it can be found that a clamping force can vary between 500 and 1000 grams (6). Many manufacturers' catalogues contain no information about clamping forces. Only the Mark IV, MSA, specifications claim that the head pressure (clamping force) is 1191 (g wt) at 14.2 cm (25). According to the calculated mean, this would correspond to $1256 - 77 = 1179$ (g wt) at 13.4 cm. The data in the literature differ from practical data. Manufacturers have increased clamping forces in their products thus creating discomfort for the wearer. They did this because they are well aware that too small a pressure results in the creation of air leaks.

Discussion

To verify the value of the tests and poor ear muff attenuation, ten tests were made on the No. 4 ear muff - D, which is used extensively in Canadian mines. Test results are shown in Table 6.

To find the reason for the poor attenuation, we used the same ear muff on

Table 6 Attenuation of ear muff 'D' in a local Elliot Lake mine

No. / Occupation	Ear Muff	Bizygo-matic Diam.	Equivalent Continuous Sound Level - L_{eqs} (dBA)						Average Attenuation (dBA)	Remarks
			Left Muff			Right Muff				
			Over	Under	Diff.	Over	Under	Diff.		
1 Jackleg (Driller)	D	14.70	114.60	98.2	16.4	114.9	105.00	9.90	13.15	Long hair
2 Jackleg (Driller)	D	14.00	111.80	93.20	18.60	112.70	94.60	18.10	18.35	Ideal condition
3 Jackleg (Helper)	D	13.80	112.60	108.00	4.60	114.30	98.80	15.50	10.05	Long hair
4 Rock Bolter (Helper)	D	13.60	114.60	106.20	8.40	115.20	104.90	10.30	9.35	
5 Slusherman	D	13.70	93.60	80.40	13.20	94.40	86.10	8.30	10.75	Lack spring pressure
6 Slusherman	D	14.00	96.80	80.00	16.80	97.50	80.00	17.50	17.50	
7 JC800 Scooptram	D	14.20	102.00	89.50	12.50	101.00	91.40	9.60	11.05	New liner
8 ST8 Scooptram	D	13.30	101.7	91.6	10.10	101.50	89.8	11.70	10.90	
Mean		13.91	105.96	93.39	12.58	106.44	93.83	12.61	12.59	
Std. Dev.		0.42	8.43	10.47	4.73	8.69	8.83	3.85	3.38	
9 2-Boom Jumbo*	D	14.00	107.20	80.00	27.20	106.60	80.00	26.60	26.90	Ideal condition
9 2-Boom Jumbo*	D	14.00				106.80	93.70	13.10	13.10	Working condition

(Same ear muff:
((1st case) - operator does not move his neck or head, ideal conditions.
((2nd case) - operator under normal working conditions.

the same worker, and on the same machine (Table 6, No. 9). Under ideal conditions, as in the laboratory, the ear muff provided ideal results (26.9 dBA), while under working conditions, attenuation was only about half of that (12.6 dBA).

Assuming that ear muffs are excellent attenuators (which they are not), and that a miner is working in noise levels of 115 dBA (Jumbo-Three Drills), then he would have to wear his muffs 95 percent of the drilling time to lower his exposure to within the 85 or 90 dBA limit. Taking his muffs off for 12 minutes in a four hour drilling period would over-expose the miner to noise. Most hearing loss occurs in the first five years of exposure to noise[26]. A man who has worked in noisy environments for 25 years gains little practical benefit from even the most powerful muffs[27]. Of course, safety organizations in mines must be capable of performing the task of controlling attenuation of ear muffs[28].

CONCLUSIONS

The main problems encountered in ear muffs are caused by the ear cushion seal against the head and their functional design. In comfort tests it was demonstrated that ear muffs with large cushion areas were favoured (Tables 1 and 2). Laboratory tests showed that a difference exists in attenuation between muffs, and a difference also exists in attenuation characteristics between factory (ANSI Z 24.22-1957) and laboratory tests. Methods using short measurements for the determination of a noise exposure index, and modes of control for good muff wearing, were developed in the Elliot Lake Laboratory. Tests in mines showed that only three ear muffs of all those examined have good attenuations:

- No. 5, model E: (23.3 dBA)
- No. 6, model F: (19 dBA)
- No. 10, model J: (22.1 dBA).

All three ear muffs are worn with the compression band passing behind the head. The No. 10 muff has a support strap which improves comfort and maintains a good fit during wear. Causes of poor attenuation are numerous: bad mounting of ear muffs on helmets, improper fitting, interference by hair and eye glasses, improper wearing by miners, unsatisfactory enforcement by supervisory personnel, incomplete training of miners, etc. There was poor agreement in attenuations between laboratory tests and field tests.

Results of this research have indicated that none of the currently manufactured ear muffs tested in this study contain all of the characteristics desirable in an ideal unit.

RECOMMENDATIONS
1. The results suggest that tests, such as those developed in the Elliot Lake Laboratory for ear muff attenuation, should be obligatory.
2. Because of unsatisfactory ear muff attenuation in working conditions, it should be a mandatory requirement that workers wear both ear muffs and ear plugs if the noise level is higher than 105 dBA (various references in the literature recommend 110 dBA).
3. It is recommended that miners use support straps to maintain effective attenuation and positioning of ear muffs which are worn behind the head.
4. Foremen must be capable, through experience and training, of helping and controlling miners to wear their ear muffs properly.
5. The program should be introduced to new miners on hiring.
6. When purchasing ear muffs, practical attenuation results should be taken into account, because the greatest noise reduction is not always given by ear muffs which have the best attenuation characteristics in the laboratory. A new standard is necessary for tests to be uniform under working conditions. This standard would be the impetus to manufacturers to improve their products, and to consumers to develop better judgement in selecting equipment.

ACKNOWLEDGEMENTS
The author wishes to thank all of the mines that have supported the Elliot

Lake Laboratory, and the many colleagues in the mines and the Elliot Lake Laboratory involved.

Thanks are also extended to Dr. P.W. Alberti, Professor of Otolaryngology and Occupational and Environmental Medicine, University of Toronto for granting the opportunity to prepare this paper, and R. Tervo, Manager, Elliot Lake Laboratory, CANMET, Energy, Mines and Resources Canada for helpful suggestions.

REFERENCES
1. Working environment: atmospheric pollution, noise and vibration; Report IV (1); International Labour Conference, 63rd Session 1977.

2. Gales, R.S. Auditory presentation of information; in Human Engineering Guide to Equipment Design; McGraw-Hill Book Co. Inc; 1963.

3. Zwislocki, J.J., Design and testing of earmuffs. J. Acoust. Soc. Amer., 27, 11-55, 1955.

4. Shaw, E.A.G., Thiessen G.J., Improved cushion for ear defenders; J. Acoust. Soc. Amer., 30, 24-36, 1958

5. Neely, K.K. Noise and hearing conservation. Defence Research Medical Laboratories; Review Paper No. 671; Toronto.

6. Shaw, W.A. et al, OSRD Report 5122. U.S. Dept of Commerce, Washington, D.C.; PD 22849, 1945.

7. Zwislocki, J.J., Factors determining the sound attenuation of produced by earphone sockets. J. Acoust. Soc. Amer., 27, 146-155, 1955.

8. Santi, R. Women in mining: the progress and the problems. Mineral Bulletin MR 152, E.M.R. Canada; 1976.

9. Kennedy, J.B., Neville, A.D., Basic statistical methods. 2nd edition; A. Dun-Donnelly, New York, 1976.

10. Savich, M., Practical problems of hearing protector use in Canadian Mines. CANMET, Minerals Res. Prog., Mining Res. Lab Div Report MRP/MRL 80-(OP). Energy Mines and Resources Canada, 1980.

11. Hughes, J.G., Lomaev, O., An anthropometric survey of Australian male facial sizes. Am. Ind. Hyg. Assoc., 33, 77-78, 1972.

12. Hertzberg, H.T.E., Daniels, G.S., Chruchill, E., Anthropometry of flying personnel - 1950. W.A.D.C. Technical Report 52-321.

13. Hertzberg, H.T.E., Anthropometric survey of Turkey, Greece and

Italy. Pergamon Press, 1963.

14. Herman, H., Dumetriscu, H., Investigations into anatomophysiological conditions of gas masks. Report of Research into the Protection of Workers, Institute of Scientific Research for Labour Protection, 2, Bucharest; 1967.

15. Russell, M.F., May, S.P., Objective test for ear muffs. J. Sound and Vibration; 44, 545-562, 1976.

16. American National Standards Institute, Method for the measurement of the real-ear attenuation of ear protectors at threshold. ANSI Z 24.22-1957.

17. American National Standards Institute, Method for the measurement of real-ear protection of hearing protectors and physical attenuation of ear muffs. ANSI S 3.19-1974.

18. Nixon, C.W., Knoblack, W.C., Hearing protection of ear muffs worn over eye-glasses. Aerospace Medical Research Laboratory, Wright-Patterson Air Force Base, Ohio; AMRL-TR-74-61, 1974.

19. Shaw, E.A.G., Private communication, 1977.

20. Industrial noise manual, Second Edition; Amer. Indust. Hyg. Assoc., 1975.

21. Savich, M., Wylie, J., Noise attenuation in rock drills, Can Min J: 96, 39-44, 1975.

22. Kroes, P., Roy, F., Lempert, B., List of personal hearing protectors, Publication No. (NIOSH) 76-120, 1976.

23. Barton, C.K., A single number rating for effective noise reduction, Sound and Vibration; 7, No. 2, 23-25, 1973.

24. EPA to label hearing protectors, National Safety News; 86; July 1977.

25. MSA. Mine Safety Appliances Company; data from 1977 sales literature.

26. Damongeot, A., Efficacite et comfort des protecteurs indivuels contre le bruit. Travail et Securite; Sept. 1973.

27. McGinty, L., Noise - a standard error. New Scientist; 73, 1040, 452-454, 1977.

28. Savich, M.U., Attenuation of ear muffs in Canadian mines; Can Min and Met Bull; 812, 58-65, 1979.

26 NEW DESIGN CONCEPTS IN PERSONAL HEARING PROTECTORS

A. G. Gorman

The author's Company has been deeply involved in hearing protection and noise reducing headsets for nearly thirty years. Many of the markets served have very severe noise problems and so there has been a continual need to design and produce the best possible noise reducing devices. Some products are for use in continuous noise levels as high as 145 dB(A) and others are used to protect against impulse noise up to 190 dB peak. Another requirement for maximum noise reduction is in communications headsets. Noise levels are still tending to increase and so is the need for greater intelligibility of communications. Thus the demand for the most effective possible hearing protection and noise reduction continues to increase.

Some twenty years ago the Company started to manufacture, under licence, the liquid filled cushion patented by Shaw & Thiessen. This component undeniably improved hearing protector performance by a large amount but due to factors such as cost, weight, possibility of leakage and so on the liquid seal has not become universally applicable and in Europe today its acceptability is, if anything, unfortunately declining. It has therefore become necessary to produce hearing protectors of at least equal performance by other means.

Consideration of this problem led to the sobering conclusion that following the invaluable work of Shaw and Thiessen, Zwislocki, Bekesy and others in the late 1940's and the 1950's no further real progress had been made. Many variations on the theme had appeared but nothing basically new or better had been produced. The need to do better, forced a careful examination of hearing protector theory so that designs could be optimised and it seemed that the earlier work with circumaural protectors had left some doubt in various areas such as:

1)   The exact formula for low frequency attenuation and indeed for attenuation at any frequency.

2)   The limits to achievable attenuation.
3)   The reason why using earplugs in addition to a circumaural protector, added only a little more attenuation.

Shaw[1] for instance wondered at one time whether the inside or the outside area of the earcushion should be used in connection with attenuation calculations and he used an average of the two areas. Zwislocki[2] who developed an expression for low frequency attenuation basically similar to that which will be presented in this paper, considered that earshell depth was important.

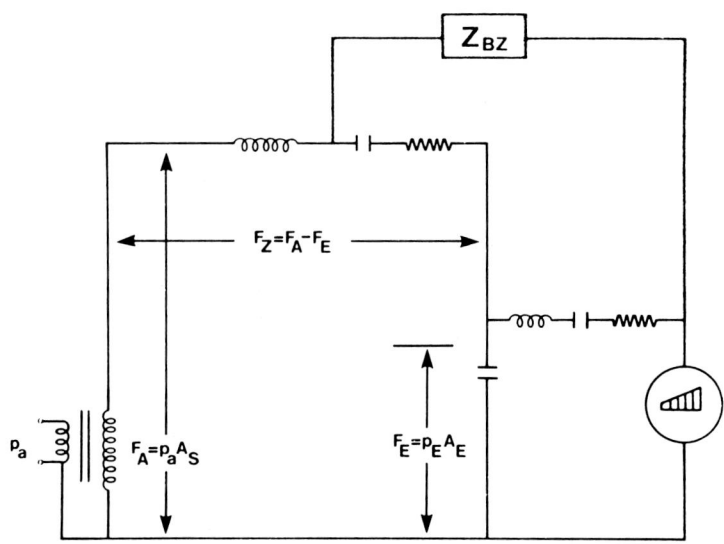

Figure 1.   Circumaural Hearing Protector. Simplified Equivalent Circuit. The inductance, capacitance and resistance near the top of the diagram are referred to in the text as M_m the earshell mass, C_m the resultant series compliance of earcushion platform and skin and R_m the resultant series resistance. The shunt capacitance is the earshell volume V_s. Z_{B2} is described in the text. The remaining components represent the ear drum and middle ear.

The ultimate limit to attenuation at middle and higher frequencies has long been recognized as due to bone conduction (for instance by Zwislocki[3] and Nixon[4]) but the levels found did not equate to the remarkably consistent levels of attenuation provided above about 1kHz by a wide variety of protectors. The very moderate increase of attenuation obtained by the wearing of earplugs as well as muffs has never been adequately explained. These various doubts needed, if possible, to be resolved. This paper will present an improved formula for attenuation and will describe an important bone conduction path which has not been previously isolated. The resultant improvement in knowledge of hearing protector design and of objective test method limitations will be detailed. Two new protector concepts which have arisen from the research, will also be presented.

ATTENUATION FORMULA

The attenuating system undoubtedly has the form of a half section low pass filter but lacks the classical source and terminating resistances and has a high insertion loss at low frequencies due to the splitting of the shunt capacitance into two series elements with the output taken from across one of these elements. This is shown in Figure 1 ignoring for the moment the uppermost path containing the element Z_{B2}. A careful consideration of the acoustic input and output conditions, leads to the following general formula for the sound attenuation of a circumaural hearing protector.

$$\text{Attenuation AdB} = -20\log_{10} \frac{A_e + A_c}{\frac{\omega V_s}{A_e \rho c^2} \sqrt{R_m^2 + \left[\omega M_m - \frac{1}{\omega}\left(\frac{A_e \rho c^2}{V_s} + \frac{A_c}{C_m}\right)\right]^2}}$$

A_c	= Contact area between earcushion and head	m^2
A_e	= Area of earcushion opening	m^2
M_m	= Mass of earshell assembly	kg
C_m	= Specific Compliance of earcushion and skin	m^3/N
R_m	= Resistance (mechanical) of earcushion	N s/m
V_s	= Volume of earshell cavity	ml
ρ	= Density of air	1.2 kg/m^3
c	= Velocity of sound in air	344 m/sec
ω	= $2\pi f$	

The main simplifying assumption made, is that the wavelength is large compared with the dimensions of the earshell. This obviously limits the usefulness of the expression to the lower frequencies. It is also assumed that the earshell parameters can be taken as lumped and that the movement of the earshell is piston-like on a line through the ears. All possible shunt paths are ignored in this basic expression and will be dealt with subsequently.

Considering frequencies sufficiently below the system resonance the situation simplifies to that shown in Figure 2 again ignoring the path Z_{B2}. The expression for low frequency attenuation then, in turn, simplifies to:-

$$AdB = -20\log_{10} \frac{A_e + A_c}{A_e + \frac{V_s A_c}{A_e C_m \rho c^2}}$$

A_e = Area of earcushion opening
A_c = Contact area between earcushion and head
V_s = Volume of earshell cavity
C_m = Specific Compliance of earcushion and skin
ρ = Density of air
c = Velocity of sound in air

All units are the same as in the general expression.

All symbols have the same meanings and units as for the complete expression. This is not the place to go through the proof of the expressions; this will be done elsewhere. Consideration however of the simplified expression for low frequencies shows it to be similar to Zwislocki's[2] if the following points are borne in mind:

1) Zwislocki's term Z_m is replaced by $C_m/A_c = 1/Z_m$

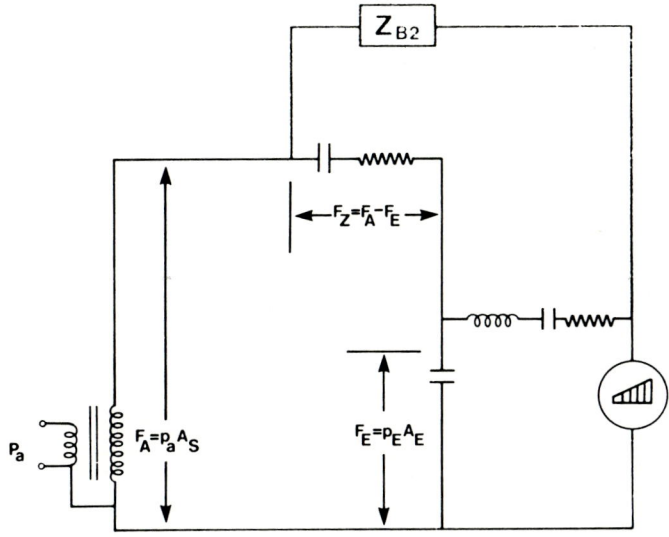

Figure 2. Circumaural Hearing Protector. Low Frequency Equivalent Circuit. This diagram omits the earshell mass M_m and applies to frequencies well below the mass-stiffness resonance. Remaining elements have the same references as Figure 1.

2) The earshell contained volume is retained as a volumetric term.

3) The area of the earshell volume is not limited to the inside (or the outside) area of the earcushion.

The term C_m/A_c is the <u>referred</u> value of the earcushion, skin and platform compliances all in parallel and expressed in this way, allows investigation of variation in the area terms, automatically adjusting for the consequent variation in referred effective series compliance.

The second and third points are important and reveal that there is complete freedom to decide the form of the earshell volume. This includes allowing the diameter of the earshell volume to be greater than the earcushion outer periphery. Earshell depth is not of itself an important dimension.

For given values of, say, V_s and C_m the area terms can be optimised to produce the most efficient device and using this technique it has been possible to design protectors having the same low frequency attenuation as with the liquid seals, with similar earshell volumes. If the optimisation of the area terms is taken to its logical extreme then a very interesting device results and this will be referred to later.

Going on now to another requirement, one of the important properties of the liquid seal was that it introduced considerable mechanical resistance into the system. (Much of this resistance was due to the properties of the underlying skin tissue, the skin being the significant series impedance at low frequencies when a liquid seal is used.) The result was that the hearing protectors with liquid seals were resistance controlled between about 100 and 500 Hz. This resistance together with the earshell volume was the main contributor to the attenuation around 250 Hz and so the property had to be duplicated with the non-liquid earcushions. Figure 3 shows the theoretical effect of varying resistance on a protector of the type considered by Shaw & Thiessen. The non-idealised curve is of an actual protector measured on a real head. The 12 dB (mass controlled) and 6 dB (resistance controlled) slopes can be seen and the dependence of this protector on the mechanical resistance is evident.

The realisation of the appropriate compliance and resistance in an earcushion is by no means a simple matter and each manufacturer must arrive at his own favourite techniques.

BONE CONDUCTION
Turning now to the effect of bone conduction, Figure 3 shows the attenuation theoretically continuing to increase at 12 dB per octave. This does not happen in practice. The horizontal solid line beyond 1 kHz is an approximate average of the attenuation achieved in this region by high quality protectors. The reason will be explained after some factors which are _not_ the fundamental cause of the limited attenuation, have been disposed of. It is instructive to consider Figure 4 which shows the complete equivalent circuit of a hearing protector. The element M_m is

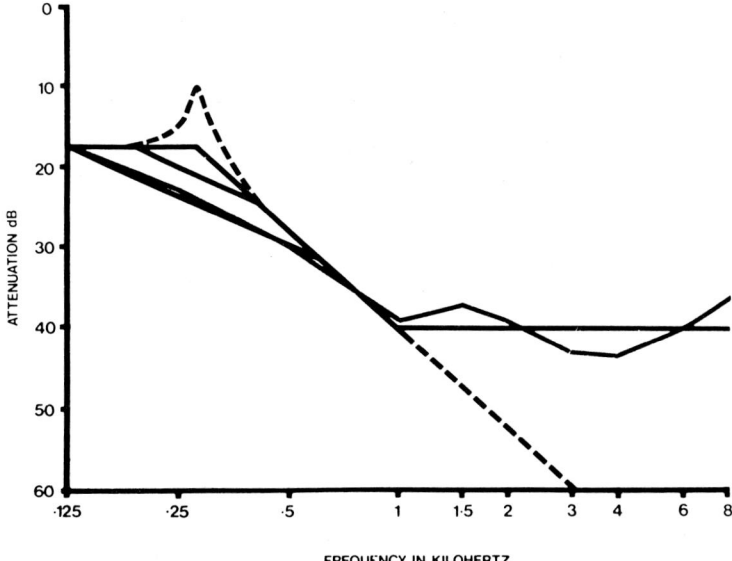

Figure 3. Circumaural Hearing Protector. Theoretical Performance. The effect of increasing mechanical resistance is shown. The lower dashed line shows the theoretical performance above 1kH$_z$. The horizontal solid line above 1 kH$_z$ shows an average of the actually achieved. A curve of a high performance protector with liquid seals, is superimposed.

the earshell mass and the three paths $C_f R_f$, $C_p R_p$ and $C_c R_c$ are the impedances respectively of the flesh under the earcushion, the earshell platform on which the cushion sits and the earcushion itself. V_s is the earshell volume. In addition there are various elements which are not designed in and which might conceivably reduce attenuation. The properties of the headband, being in series with the main transmission path, are more likely to increase than to decrease the performance. In practice most headband designs have only small effects. The element Z_L representing leakage under the earcushion is a serious problem. Long or thick hair, spectacles sidearms, or badly designed or damaged earcushions, can cause sufficient leakage to significantly reduce attenuation at the lower frequencies. The leak is normally fairly resistive and so its impedance does not rise noticeably with frequency. The leak can thus have an effect extending across the entire frequency range and so can

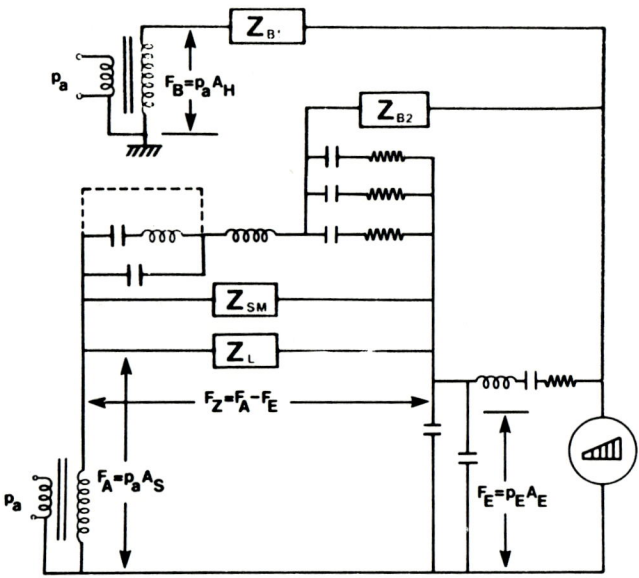

Figure 4. Circumaural Hearing Protector. Equivalent Circuit. All elements from Figures 1 and 2 retain their references. Elements to the left of the earshell mass, represent headband parameters. Z_{B1} is free-field bone conduction. Z_{B2} is the muff induced signal path. Z_{sm} is earshell break-up. Z_L is leakage under the earcushion.

alone be the cause of reduced attenuation above 1 kHz. Even if this leak is completely eliminated however, the attenuation limitation remains. Element Z_{sm} represents transmission via break up of the earshell material. Unless an earshell is very badly designed or made in some very unsuitable material, earshell break-up is not in fact the cause of the limited attenuation as demonstrated by objective measurements. Standing waves within the earshell might also reduce attenuation but these are easy to eliminate sufficiently to demonstrate that they are not responsible for the problem.

Element Z_{B1} represents bone/body conduction. Such conduction has been extensively investigated by von Gierke, Bekesy, Zwislocki, Nixon and others but their results have never quite explained the actual maximum attenuations produced by high quality protectors. An assumption was however made that the bone conduction transmission was unaffected by

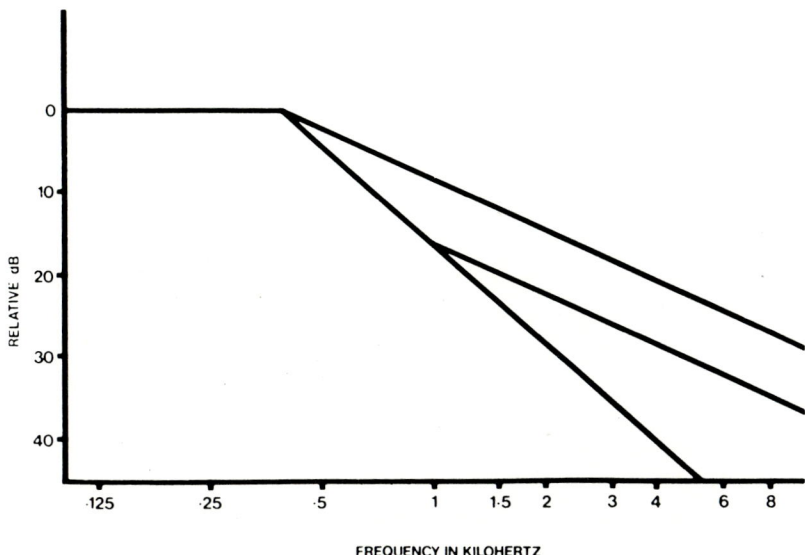

Figure 5. Circumaural Hearing Protector. Bone Conduction. The bone conduction is constant up to the resonance frequency (here 0.4 kHz). It then falls at 6 dB or 12 dB/octave dependent on the value of R_m the series mechanical resistance.

the wearing of the earmuff. It has now been found that this is not so. The element Z_{B2} in Figures 1, 2 and 4 represents a bone/body conduction path caused by the very wearing of the protector. Reverting to the simplified circuit of Figure 1 consider the force F_z across the series elements of the protector. The possible effects of this force are normally completely ignored as the preoccupation is with the force F_E which, after division by the relevant area term, yields the sound pressure P_e at the ear. For a good protector giving, say, 40 dB attenuation above 1 kHz, F_z is about 100 times F_E and for practical purposes equals the input force F_A. What effect does this force have physically? It is bearing on the head around the pinna as a mechanical force and so applies a bone conduction signal to the skull.

Several factors operate to increase the bone conduction transmission compared with the free-field values. First the area of contact between the earcushion and the head is less than the projected area of the earshell by a factor of about 2:1. Further a part of the earcushion sits below the

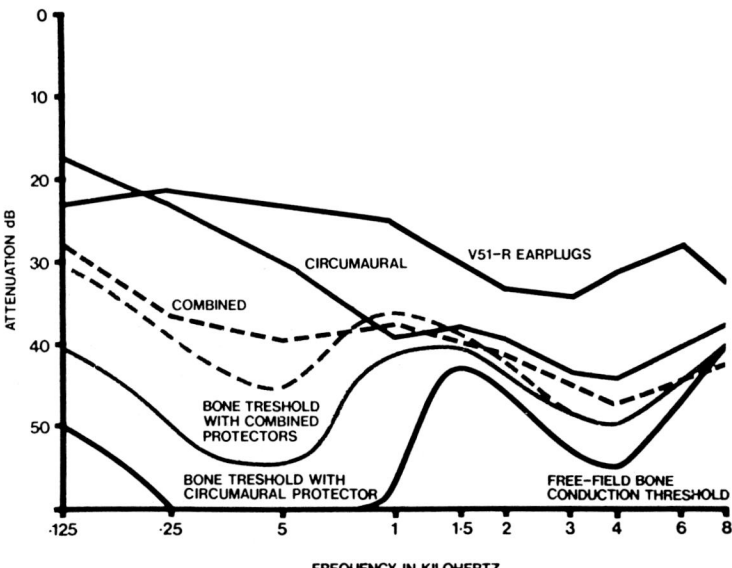

Figure 6. Circumaural Hearing Protector. Performance Limits. The curves clearly show the protector enhanced bone conduction and its effect on the attenuation of the muffs above 1 kHz and on muffs combined with plugs at all frequencies.

base of the skull so the force is concentrated within an area less than the total area of the earcushion. Due to the bony profile of the side of the head further force localization effects occur. All these points together cause the mechanical force at the lowest frequencies at three points around the ear to be some 3-4 times greater than might be expected. At higher frequencies, above the system resonance, the force decreases. The decrease is initially at 12 dB/octave but at even higher frequencies the resistance Rm predominates and reduces the slope to 6 dB/octave. For a protector with a high value of Rm the force will never fall at more than 6 dB/octave above the turnover frequency. These characteristics are summarized in Figure 5.

The three areas around the ear on which the mechanical forces largely concentrate are the mastoid process behind the ear and the prominences just above and infront of the ear. This latter area has a bone conduction sensitivity some 10 dB greater than the mastoid process or the area above the ear and this is a further important factor in the enhanced bone

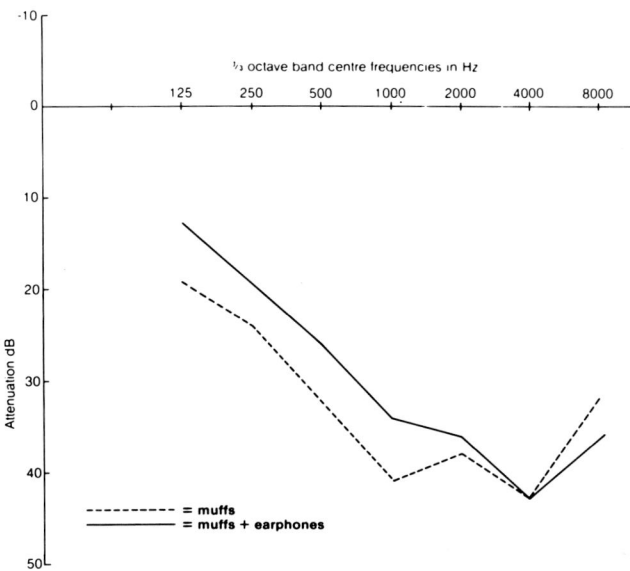

Figure 7. BS 5108 Test Results Amplivox sonogard Earmuffs With/Without Earphones. (After J.A. Chillery, 1978). An extreme instance where blocking the meatus decreased the attenuation compared with muffs alone.

conduction transmission. The effect of the enhanced bone conduction is shown in Figure 6. The lowest curve is Zwislocki's measurement of the free-field bone conduction threshold. The next curve up is the enhanced bone conduction threshold resulting from the effects noted above. The shape and position of this curve above 1 kHz relative to the curve labelled Circumaural, should be noted. The limiting effect of the increased bone conduction is clearly seen. The double humped shape of the attenuation curve with reduced attenuation around 1.5 or 2 kHz is typical of a great variety of hearing protectors and demonstrates the universal occurrence of the bone conduction path. It will be evident from Figure 5 that a moderate performance protector with light weight earshells and thus a higher frequency system resonance will have a higher level of bone transmission in the 1-8 kHz range and so even though the protector may achieve only about 35 dB average attenuation in this range, bone conduction still sets the limit and imposes the characteristic shape on the response curve.

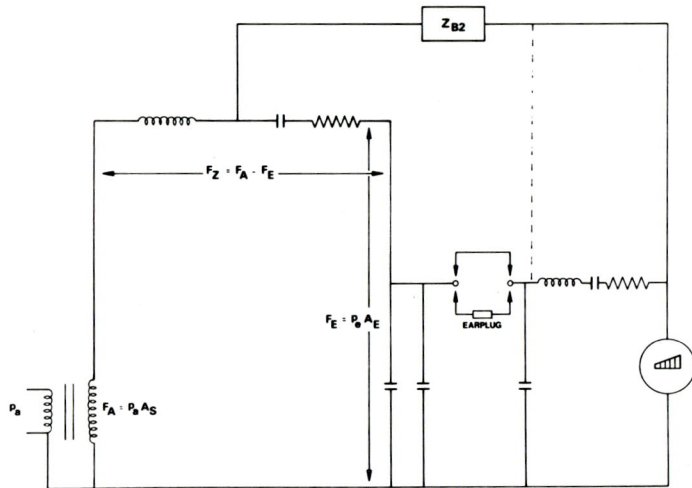

Figure 8. Circumaural Hearing Protector. Significant Bone Conduction Path. The transmission along the muff induced signal path is greatly increased when the ear canal is not open.

Below about 1 kHz or so, bone conduction is not a limitation at the levels of attenuation we normally achieve. The most interesting effect of all however, occurs when an earplug is worn together with a circumaural protector. The enhanced bone conduction caused by the circumaural protector seems to produce a sound pressure at the eardrum by vibration of the anterior wall of the meatus. This sound pressure is therefore very sensitive to blocking of the meatus and when an earplug is also worn the bone transmission is further increased by very approximately 10 dB at the lowest frequencies. Thus instead of the attenuations of the muff and plug adding arithmetically, the further increased bone conduction produces an absolute barrier and limits the otherwise achievable attenuation by, as much as 10-30 dB. The two dashed curves of Figure 6 show the subjectively measured performance of muff plus plug compared with the calculated bone conduction level. Chillery[5] noticed an extreme case of the effect discussed here when he measured the combined attenuation of a liquid seal type muff and a personal earmould fitted with an earphone. The attenuation of the combination was actually less at most frequencies than for the muff alone. His results are shown in Figure 7. It is

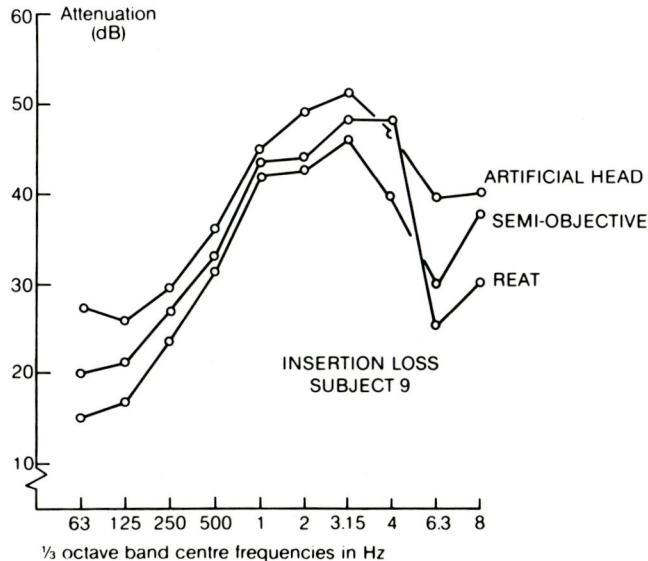

Figure 9. A Comparison of Mean Values for a Single Subject With Mean Measurements on the Artificial Head. (After G.M. Rood, 1978). The meatal microphone of the semi-objective method measures the meatal sound pressure produced by the muff induced signal path.

conceivable here that the size and rigidity of the earmould caused increased mechanical transmission from the tissue under the earcushion, direct to the meatus. The path of the enhanced bone conduction transmission is shown in Figure 8. It is quite clear how the resultant meatal sound pressure will vary depending on whether the meatus is open or blocked. Rood[6] has measured the attenuation of a hearing protector by three methods i.e., subjective threshold shift, semi-objective using a real head in a passive role and objective with an artificial head. An example of his comparative results is shown in Figure 9. The semi-objective results mirror the limited attenuation measured subjectively at 1, 2 and 3 kHz. The objective results are higher in the same frequency range, as would be expected from the absence of the bone conduction in the artificial head. Rood's semi-objective test employed a miniature microphone in the bowl of the ear. It gives further support to the notion that the enhanced bone conduction produces a sound pressure in the meatus, this being accurately measured in the semi-objective test.

Attenuation of hearing protectors in the 1-8 kHz range is normally sufficient in all but the most exceptional circumstances. The greater understanding of the bone conduction limitation of attenuation does not therefore, immediately lead to better hearing protection. It does however provide or confirm variously the following information.

CONCLUSIONS

1) Bone conduction is not the limit to performance of current muff designs below about 1 kHz.
2) Above about 1 kHz bone conduction is the limitation to muff performance with existing designs of muffs.
3) Muffs and plugs combined cannot provide much more attenuation than muffs alone.
4) Objective measurements (with any well designed artificial head) must be optimistic above about 1 kHz.
5) Semi-objective measurements are likely to be as meaningful as subjective threshold shift at least in the 1-3 kHz region.
6) As the enhanced bone conduction is largely confined to a small area forward of the ear it is intriguing to consider that it might be possible to construct an artificial head with a vibration pick up at this point to simulate the subjective situation.

Points 4, 5 and 6 above deserve further comment because the ability to meaningfully measure protector performance is an essential part of the design process. Subjective threshold shift measurements of protector attenuation are time consuming, difficult and expensive. There has therefore been much consideration of alternative objective measurement methods. At the very least these must correctly rank-order protectors of different subjective performance at all frequencies and must be reliable and repeatable. At best they would permit absolute measurements and perhaps eventually replace the subjective method. Arising from the various investigations carried out in the author's Company, it is felt possible to make the following comments with some confidence.

a) The subjective threshold shift method is accurate at all frequencies except the lowest where physiological noise causes an over estimate of attenuation by very approximately 5 dB. Otherwise, except for intentionally non-linear devices, the attenuation determination is valid at high noise levels.

b) Attempts to produce an absolute objective method have been plagued by lack of understanding of the basic mechanisms determining attenuation at various frequencies. There has thus been much discussion of objective/subjective correlation and some workers have considered their equipment and results to be correct when objective measurements have agreed with subjective results. With sufficient knowledge of the mechanisms operating, one can see that objective-subjective agreement is an almost certain guarantee that the objective results are incorrect. First, the objective low frequency attenuation should be some 5 dB lower. Then other errors, up to 30 dB at 125 Hz, will occur depending on how closely the compliance and resistance of the artificial head surface, duplicate an average real head. Above 1 kHz objectively measured attenuation will be high unless the earshells suffer break-up or the artificial head has unwanted mechanical transmission. There are other difficulties with absolute objective measurement but those noted are the major ones. It was with the various fundamental difficulties in mind that a proposal was made to ISO WG17 (Measurement of attenuation of Hearing Protectors) to proceed with a _comparative_ objective measuring system using a very simple and repeatable test fixture. The author does not believe any artificial head has yet been developed which permits accurate absolute measurements. Accuracy at low frequencies will require a reliable, repeatable simulation of flesh impedance. A new polyurethane based material holds out some promise in this respect. Accuracy at and above 1 kHz will demand the inclusion of a simulated enhanced bone conduction path. This may be easier than previously thought possible.

c) The semi-objective method is, in the author's view, accurate at all frequencies except for one significant effect. As the measuring microphone is at the outer rather than the inner end of the

EXPERIMENTAL HEARING PROTECTOR PERFORMANCE

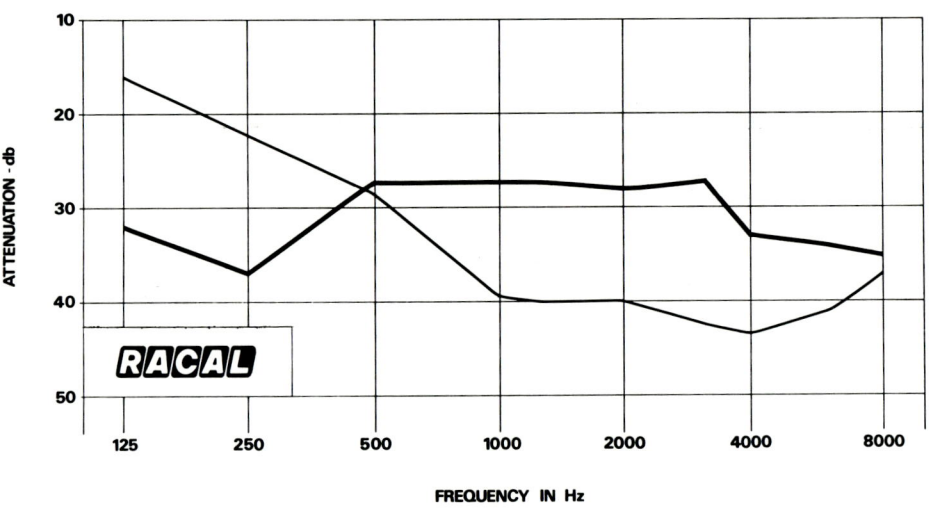

Figure 10.   Performance Curve of the 30 dB(A) Protector.

meatus, errors may be introduced at frequencies where longitudinal resonances are likely. Rood's differences between semi-objective and subjective results at 4 and 8 kHz may be due to this cause. The similarity between semi-objective and subjective results at 1-3 kHz has already been noted. At low frequencies the semi-objective figures are some 5 dB below the subjective, very much as should be expected.

NEW DESIGNS

The various investigations into protector theory have also enabled routine designs of conventional hearing protectors to become more definitive and it is now normal to predict accurately the average of subjective threshold shift measurements to within $\pm$ 1.5 dB at low frequencies. This has increased the confidence in releasing tooling drawings for protectors intended to be perhaps only a few dB different from some other model. There are also two completely new protectors to date and the first arose

EXPERIMENTAL HEARING PROTECTOR PERFORMANCE

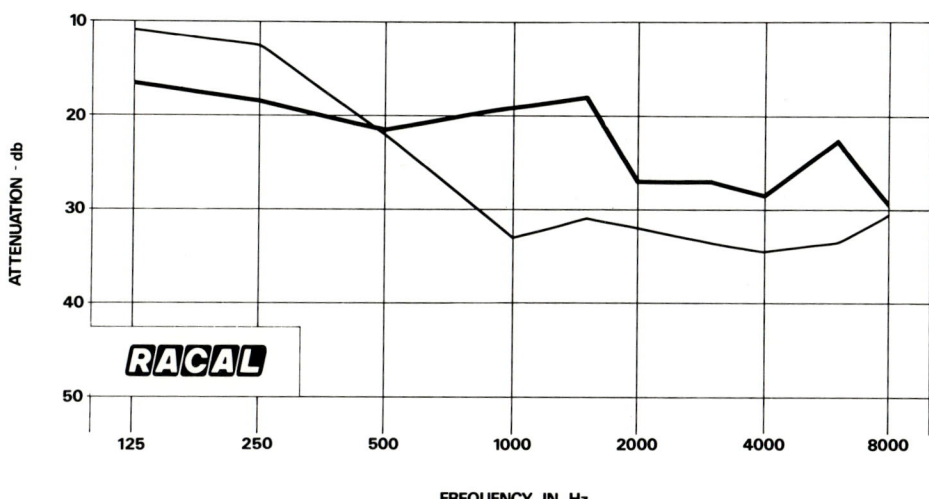

Figure 11.   Performance Curve of the 18 dB(A) Protector.

from taking the formula for low frequency attenuation to its logical limit. This yielded a device with earshell volume of about 20 cm^3, a weight of about 75 gm (2.6 oz) and a subjective attenuation of about 30 dB average across the range. Figure 10 shows the response curve. The aim was to achieve a low frequency attenuation of 30 dB with a small device and the relatively flat response was not intentional. Its presence led to an unexpected effect. Subjects wearing the device for fit and comfort tests reported that the protector was not attenuating although test results showed the performance to be as illustrated. The reason for the remarks turned out to be a result of the fairly flat response. Because the whole spectrum had been more or less equally attenuated the normal characteristically muffled sound quality had disappeared. Speech could be heard with remarkable clarity and hence the subjects' comments. The level response had removed the upward masking effect which occurs in hearing protectors of usual response. The point having been appreciated various practical means of intentionally producing a flat response have now been developed and are the subject of patent applications. One example of a muff with about 18 dB(A) attenuation to wide band noise, has its response curve shown in Figure 11.

Quite apart from the bonus of remarkable ability to hear clearly when wearing these level response devices, there is the additional and perhaps very important feature that a single figure attenuation value can be quoted which is quite independent of the noise spectrum. It should be pointed out that the two new devices shown are both experimental at this time. The 30 dB(A) model has problems of fit and sealing but these will be further studied. The 18 dB(A) device is definitely practicable and has applications in noise reducing communications headsets as well as in simple hearing protectors. Another interesting point is that the level response protector has no requirement for earshell mass and so the lightest possible materials can be used provided that various other requirements are met by good design.

In conclusion the author would state that his Company, being a manufacturing concern, conducts research only to the point where the fuller understanding achieved permits the product range to be usefully improved. It is not therefore suggested that all matters mentioned in this paper e.g. the protector enhanced bone conduction, are researched to the point where nothing useful remains to be found. Work has stopped at the point where the effect has been demonstrated to exist and when it has been sufficiently quantified for its influence on product performance and design to be determined. More research oriented establishments may be interested to consider whether more knowledge of it would further assist the understanding of hearing protector performance or the design of objective test methods. What is encouraging is to have found already, that hearing protector design possibilities have in no way reached their limit. On the contrary it is obvious that a variety of improved designs, suited to particular requirements, can be achieved.

REFERENCES
1.   Shaw, E.A.G., Thiessen, G.J., Improved Cushion for Ear Defender, J. Acoust. Soc. Amer., $\underline{30}$ 1-58, 1958.

2. Zwislocki, J., Design and Testing of Earmuffs, J. Acoust. Soc. Amer., 27, 11-55, 1955.

3. Zwislocki, J., Factors Determining the Sound Attenuation Produced by Earphone Sockets, J. Acoust. Soc. Amer., 27, 146-155, 1955.

4. Nixon, C.W., von Gierke, H.E., Experiments on the Bone-Conduction Threshold in a Free Sound Field, J. Acoust. Soc. Amer., 31, 8-59, 1959.

5. Chillery, J.A., Hearing Protector Attenuation Measurement Using a Standard Loudness Balance Technique, ISVR Memorandum 575 1-78, 1978.

6. Rood, G.M., A Comparison of Methods of Measuring the Acoustic Attenuation of Hearing Protectors, RAE Tech. Memo FS160 2-78, 1978

27
PERSONAL HEARING PROTECTION: PROBLEMS ASSOCIATED WITH THE HEARING PROTECTION PHASE OF THE HEARING CONSERVATION PROGRAM

Larry H. Royster and Susan Reece Holder

INTRODUCTION

A significant volume of information presently exists in the general scientific literature concerning the effectiveness of hearing protection devices (HPDs), especially with regard to controlled laboratory or in-the-field studies. They have extended the basic knowledge of how well HPDs attenuate sound in controlled environments and how much HPDs may affect speech communication in noise. However, there exist in the literature only a limited number of studies concerning HPDs that have considered in any significant detail the real-world interaction between the HPD and the individual employee who is required to wear HPDs daily. The evaluation of this interaction can be very difficult since practically, the typical industrial production schedule or environment cannot be significantly altered. Therefore, the researcher is limited as to the type and magnitude of information that may be obtained. However, because the shop floor is where the problems occur which limit the actual effectiveness of HPDs, it is the real-world environment that must be dealt with if the protection limits of HPDs are to be established.

In defining the problems that limit the effectiveness of HPDs at least four sources of information are potentially available: (1) the individual who must, or should, wear the HPDs provided; (2) the nurse or individual(s) responsible for the fitting and/or issuing and reissuing of HPDs; (3) the individual in management who has the responsibility for implementing and maintaining an effective HCP; and (4) the audiometric data base. These four sources of information are usually adequate when attempting to define and solve an existing problem related to the HP phase of a hearing conservation program (HCP).

The effectiveness of the HPD provided in preventing an on-the-job noise induced hearing loss can only be established by properly evaluating the existing audiometric data base. The laboratory produced real-ear PHD attenuation data is only an indication of the ultimate protection available. Regardless of the magnitude of the noise reduction rating (NRR) or real-ear attenuation values specified at different octave band frequencies, the HPD being worn by the employee is not satisfactory if hearing loss still occurs from occupational noise.

In evaluating the effectiveness of the HCP in preventing an on-the-job noise induced hearing loss it is essential that an appropriate reference population matched at least by race, sex, and age characteristics be utilized[1,2] for comparison with the audiometric data base. As an example, if one of the existing presbycusis data bases[3-6] were used as the reference population, an effective program would probably be judged ineffective if the population consisted of only white males, or it might be classified as an excellent program if the population consisted of only black females.[7] This is discussed in greater detail elsewhere[8].

This paper presents several observations made by the authors as a result of evaluating the hearing protection (HP) phases of industrial and non-industrial HCPs, observations made by OSHA inspectors as part of their routine noise inspections and during special educational training sessions, and comments made by nurses and management personnel responsible for the implementation of the HP phase. In addition specific problems observed concerning the design of HPDs, problems encountered by the employee and the employer as a result of having to wear HPDs, and problems encountered by the employer as a result of having to implement the HP phase of the HCP are discussed.

GENERAL OBSERVATIONS
Characteristics of Effective HCPs (HP phase)

The key features of an effective HP phase are, in order:

1. The requirement by management that the HPD provided be worn properly by the employees. As part of this requirement, failure of the employee to wear regularly the HPD provided must result in his/her termination of employment with the company, which should occur only after the employee has been given a notice in writing of the company's intent to terminate his/her employment for failure to use appropriately the HPD provided.

To date over 40 industrial and nonindustrial HCPs have been evaluated for effectiveness in preventing an on-the-job noise induced hearing loss by analysis of their audiometric data bases. The HCPs that were found to be acceptable had in common the characteristic mentioned above: company policy, enforced by management, required employees, management, and visitors to wear the HPDs provided when in an identified noise-hazard area. No correlation was observed between the amount of funds spent, number of educational programs (EP) developed and implemented, etc., and the effectiveness of the HCP in protecting the employee's hearing. However, the EP does play a very significant part in educating the employees about the HCP and in answering the many typical questions generated by an HCP.

2. The existence of a key individual. This person may be the safety director, an engineer, a company nurse of any individual who is given the responsibility for conducting the audiometric examinations and for issuing and fitting the HPDs. The existence of a key individual is a common characteristic of all known successful HCPs.

3. An active communication line between all management and nonmanagement segments of the company. It is very important that the first line employees know that it is their responsibility to ask _anyone_ to leave an identified noise-hazard area if that person is not properly wearing the required HP. Failure of management to wear HPs when in a noise-hazard area, regardless of the time spent in the area, is one proven way to downgrade the employee's respect for the HCP as well as for management.

4. The availability of HPDs that are "potentially effective" for preventing hearing loss in the existing noise environment. For a HPD to be "potentially effective" the device must be practical for employees to use so that they will be worn properly, and they must provide the appropriate attenuation of environment noise level.

The above four characteristics -- an enforced requirement that HPDs be worn properly by all individuals in an identified noise-hazard area, the existence of a key individual, an active communication line between the various levels of management and between management and the employees, and the availability of HPDs that are "potentially effective" -- have been observed to be common elements of effective HCPs.

Observations Made by OSHA Inspectors and Private Company Personnel
As part of OSHA-NC noise inspection reports, the inspector is required to complete an HCP evaluation survey. Included as part of the survey is an overall assessment of the various phases of the HCP; that is, the existence of acceptable sound surveys, educational programs, engineering and/or administrative controls, the issuing and fitting of HPDs, and the audiometric testing of the noise exposed population. With respect to the HP phase, the inspector indicates if HPDs were available to the employee, what type of HPDs were available, and if the proper fitting procedures were followed when necessary. Ninety-four noise inspections covering the period of June 1977 to June 1979 were analyzed to assess the quality of HCPs across North Carolina.[9]

The percentages of the companies, divided according to company size, that have made available at least one type of HPD are shown in Figure 1, while Figure 2 demonstrates the percentages of these companies that had properly fitted the HPDs issued, such as the V-51R and Comfit. The data in Figure 2 show a trend for proper HPD fitting procedures to be more common among larger companies. This trend was also found for other HCP phases: companies employing 100 or fewer workers were found to have satisfactorily implemented all HCP phases in 30% or less of the inspection reports available. For North Carolina industrial workers who

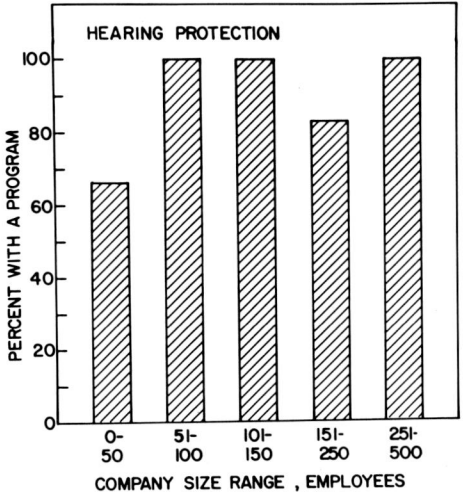

Figure 1. The percent of the companies that had made available at least one brand of HPD, classified by company size.

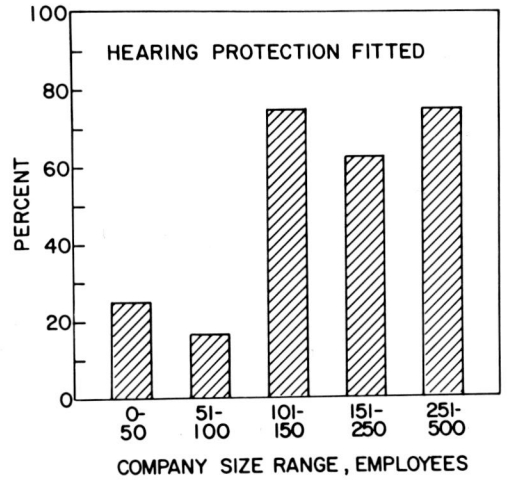

Figure 2. The percent of the companies that followed acceptable HPD fitting procedures classified by company size.

are exposed to significant noise levels, those workers employed by companies with 100 or fewer employees are less likely to be protected by an effective HCP.

A group of 30 OSHA inspectors were requested to identify the phase of

Table I. The Most Significant Problem Areas of the HCP Including a Support of Management Category as Identified by 30 OSHA Inspectors

HCP Area	Percent
Education	14
Noise Surveys	0
Engineering and/or Administrative Controls	4
Hearing Protection	35
Audiometric Testing	10
Support of Management	37
Total	100

the HCP considered by them to present the greatest difficulty to management in achieving compliance with the OSHA noise regulations. Many inspectors identified management-related problems, rather than a particular HCP phase, as the major weakness in the implementation of HCPs. Therefore, support of management was added as the sixth area as shown in Table I which shows the general distribution of the OSHA inspectors' responses.

They identified problems related to the support of management in 37% of the responses. The second most often identified area was the HP phase of the HCP.

In order to obtain a slightly different point of view from within a company's administrative structure, 25 area supervisors and audiometric technicians from one company were also presented with the same questions asked of the OSHA inspectors during two consecutive yearly educational refresher seminars. Their responses are presented in Table 2.

Whereas the OSHA inspectors identified the support of management and the HP phase as being approximately equal problem areas, the supervisors and technicians identified the HP phase as the dominant problem area.

Table 2. The Most Significant Problem Areas of the Company's HCP as Identified by 25 Area Supervisors and Audiometric Technicians of One Company During Two Consecutive Yearly Refresher HCP Training Seminars.

HCP Area	Percent '79	Percent '80
Education	22	18
Noise Surveys	0	2
Engineering and/or Administrative Controls	5	7
Hearing Protection	35	35
Audiometric Testing	14	19
Support of Management	24	19
Totals	100	100

The company supervisors and technicians identified the audiometric testing phase as a problem area more often in '80 than '79 mainly because production management was becoming less willing to send the employees on a regular basis to obtain their annual hearing tests. However, the support of management was identified as a problem in a lower percentage of the responses listed in '80 even though management was responsible for the decreasing support for the audiometric testing phase of the HCP.

It is important to note that both of the groups surveyed, in spite of their different perspectives, identified the HP phase as a major problem area to the company in attempting to establish an effective HCP.

The same group of OSHA inspectors was requested to identify problem areas encountered by employees in wearing HPDs. As part of the normal noise inspection procedures, three employees are identified and their daily noise doses established. A private conference is held with each employee for the purpose of identifying health and safety problems including those associated with the wearing of HPDs. The problems identified by the OSHA inspectors have been classified into five broad combined problem areas as indicated in Table 3. Again to obtain similar information from a different point of view, 20 on-site

Table 3. Distribution of Observed Employee-Related Problems While Wearing HPDs as Documented by a Group of 30 OSHA Inspectors While Conducting Routine OSHA Noise Inspections

	Problem Areas Identified	Percent
1.	General Discomfort, Sore Ear Canals, etc.	45
2.	Ear Canal Irritations, Infections, Headaches, etc.	11
3.	Speech Interference, Inability to Hear Warning Signals, Change in Machine's Noise Characteristics, etc.	13
4.	Improper Fitting of HPDs	18
5.	General Negative Type of Responses, Nuisance, Keeping Up With HPDs, Structural Failure of the HPDs, etc.	13
	TOTAL	100

Table 4. Distribution of Employee-Related Problems as Identified During 20 of the In-the-Field HPD Utilization Surveys

	Problem Areas Identified	Percent
1.	General Discomfort, Sore Ear Canals, etc.	32
2.	Ear Canal Irritations, Infections, Headaches, etc.	25
3.	Speech Interference, Inability to Hear Warning Signals, Change in Machine's Noise Characteristics, etc.	6
4.	Improper Fitting of HPDs	4
5.	General Negative Type of Responses, Nuisance, Keeping Up With HPDs, Structural Failure of the HPDs, etc.	33
	TOTAL	100

interviews were conducted with nurses and others involved in the HP phase concerning the utilization of HPDs in industry. These interview results were analyzed and separated into the same five problem areas, as presented in Table 4.

As would be anticipated, the individuals in industry who were responsible for the fitting of HPDs identified more problems related to the structural failure of HPDs, keeping up with the HPDs and irritations of the ear canal linings, than the OSHA inspectors. These individuals would also be less likely to criticize themselves for the improper fitting of the HPD provided.

One significant question is whether regular wearing of HPDs creates significant medical or nonmedical problems for the wearer? In attempting to answer this question, several different approaches are being utilized to collect the necessary data. These approaches include an analysis of OSHA noise inspection files, the on-site surveying of individuals in North Carolina responsible for the issuing and fitting of HPDs, and a nationwide phone and on-site survey of individuals respon sible for the fitting and issuing of HPDs.

Based on the survey information gathered to date in North Carolina, the V-5IR style of HPD is the most widely used HPD. The Comfit brand is the second, and the E-A-R plug is the third most frequently provided device. The materials used in the manufacture of the Comfit brand of HPD have proven to be very stable when exposed to the typical industrial environment.

An initial evaluation of the data suggests that the need to wear HPDs in industry does not create any significant medical problems. However, the study has identified several problems associated with the wearing of HPDs that must be dealt with effectively in order to achieve a successful implementation of the HP phase of the HCP. They will now be discussed.

Problems Associated with The HPD
1. The most common problem observed is for the V-5IR HPD to

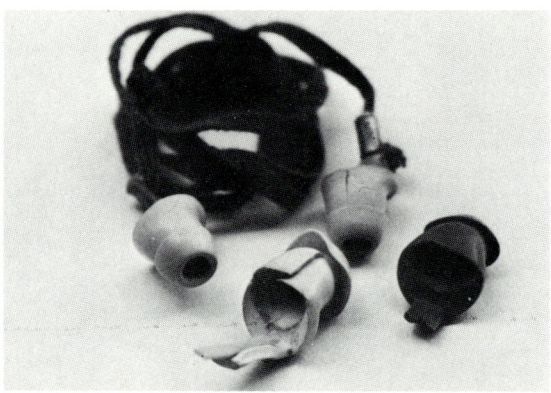

Figure 3. The most common type of problem encountered was the tendency of the V-5IR style of HPD to become hard and crack. Shown are samples of the HPD's collected.

become hard. It may then slightly irritate the ear canal lining, and it may separate along the mold line as shown in Figure 3. This problem is not new;[10] and can be minimized if an active, on-going "free" HPD replacement program is implemented. However, 18% of the industries surveyed only provided the employees with the initial pair of HPDs free. As a result, many employees were observed to wear their HPDs until a complete failure occurred, until the HPDs were lost, or until an active nurse, supervisor, or program technician observed the inadequate HPD and insisted on its replacement. The safe use period for the V-5IR design is estimated to be about three months.

2. HPDs with attached strings are becoming popular with management because string visability provides a way to identify employees who are wearing the HPDs. Employees also like them because of ease of handling. The second most common HPD failure identified is the separation of the string from the Comfit brand of HPDs as shown in Figure 4. In order to minimize the temporary threshold shift (TTS) or permanent threshold shift (PTS) that may result from too rapid a removal of a HPD, the connecting string provided is not permanently attached. However, the existing design often fails, resulting in the loss of one or both of the ear plugs. As a result, the employee is prematurely required to purchase a new pair of HPDs. Unfortunately, several nurses had

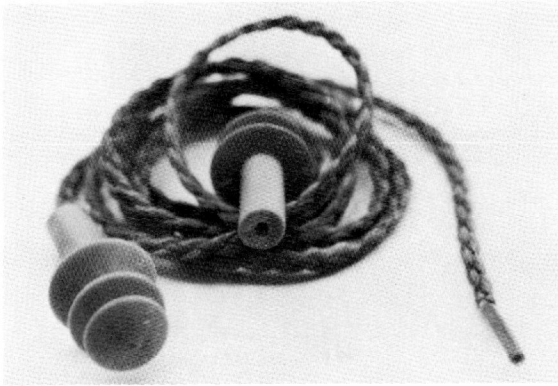

Figure 4. The attached string frequently separated from the comfit brand of HPD.

developed a solution for this problem: they permanently glued the string to the ear plugs.

Problems Encountered by the Employee

As would be expected, the number one complaint by the employee concerns the general discomfort experienced when attempting to wear HPDs. The discomfort is usually temporary for a majority of the employees who complain; however, for some employees the discomfort may last for several months or longer. An investigation is presently underway to attempt to identify some possible underlying causes of this discomfort in terms of the general distributions of the employees' ear canal sizes, the availability of different brands and sizes of HPDs, environmental conditions, and the race, sex, and age characteristics of the populations studied.

The tendency for different race and sex subpopulations to exhibit different ear canal sizes has long been known by individuals responsible for fitting HPDs in industry. In order to define better this distribution, the HPD fitting information from the recordkeeping files for one large corporation was collected and analyzed in terms of HPD sizes -- extra small (ES), small (S), medium (M), large (L), and extra large (EL). The general distributions of the HPD sizes fitted to different sex and race subgroups of the population are shown in Figures 5 and 6. The population

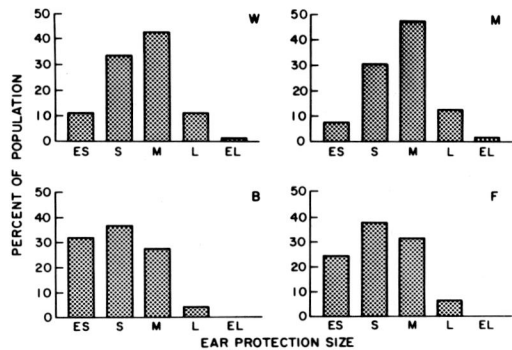

Figure 5. The distribution of HPD sizes as worn by one industrial population that utilized the V-51R style of HPD for different race and sex groupings.

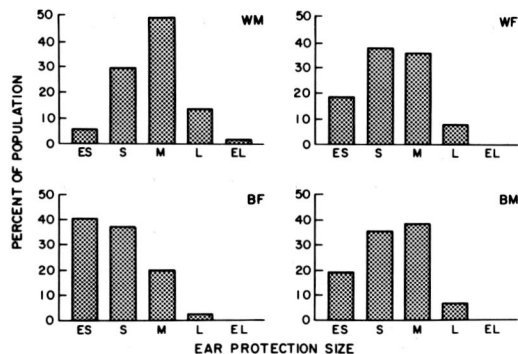

Figure 6. The distribution of HPD sizes as worn by one industrial population that utilized the V-51R style of HPD for different race and sex groupings.

consisted of 693 white males (WMs), 591 white females (WFs), 207 black females (BFs), and 135 black males (BMs). The HPD used was the V-51R design.

As shown in Figure 6, the WM population was determined to exhibit the largest relative ear canal diameter; the BM and WF populations exhibit similar distributions and relative ear canal diameters; and the BF population exhibited the smallest relative ear canal diameter. The data presented in Figure 6 becomes important in light of a second general observation: several companies whose HPD purchasing records were analyzed had not purchased any ES or EL sizes of HPDs. Obviously, for the populations where a significant number of the employees are not WMs, a number of complaints of discomfort would be anticipated by the employees who had to wear HPDs a size too large. It is also obvious that employees requiring an EL HPD would not be adequately protected by the smaller HPDs provided.

The data presented in Figure 6 also reveal a second very important fact: the relative mean ear canal diameter indicated for each subpopulation is slightly smaller than would be anticipated if an "outsider" had conducted the fitting of the HPDs utilized by the company. However, it should be noted that the data shown are for an industrial population where the HCP has been judged to be the most effective program studied to date.[13]

The above observations seem to lead one to the following conclusions:
1) the most effective HPD is the one that can be and will be worn in a given environment;
2) HPDs are not worn in the real world in the same manner that is required when conducting laboratory or controlled field studies;
and
3) as a result of real-world limitations, HPD attenuation data obtained in the field will show significantly less attenuation than the published real-ear attenuation data obtained in labs.

In addition to discomfort, a second problem often encountered by the employee is an irritation of the ear canal lining that is associated with the wearing of HPDs. A strong association has been observed between the number of complaints concerning ear canal lining irritation and the utilization of the V-51R style of HPD. As noted earlier, the V-51R design tends to become hard and separate along the mold line. This tendency seems to be employee-dependent and may become noticeable to some employees very soon (within one or two weeks) after they start wearing this style of HPD. This condition has often been linked with the type of materials used in the manufacture of the V-51R HPD. However, the problem can be significantly minimized by replacing this type of HPD every three months or when they begin to harden.

A third common problem concerns the difficulty encountered by many employees when attempting to communicate in noise while wearing HPDs. It is commonly reported in the literature that employees working in high noise levels will hear warning signals and communicate better in the noise when wearing HPDs. However, individuals responsible for fitting and reissuing HPDs very often report the opposite; that is, many employees encounter significant difficulty when attempting to communicate in noise while wearing HPDs. A study of this type of complaint has identified two conditions in which the problem seems to be very real. The first is for an individual who already exhibits a significant hearing loss, usually of the typical high frequency type, who, when wearing an effective HPD, encounters a significant problem in attempting to communicate in noise. The second problem situation occurs, even for individuals with only a mild high frequency hearing loss, when male and female employees attempt to communicate with each other in noise while wearing HPDs. The male employees often complain of an inability to communicate effectively with the female employees.

This situation has most likely also produced other detrimental side effects. For example, in many of the industrial environments investigated the percentage of the first line workers that are female has been steadily increasing. On the other hand, first line supervision still consists mainly of male employees, many of whom exhibit a significant high frequency hearing loss. As a result, many of the supervisors would be expected to have greater difficulty communicating with the general female employees than with the male employees. Therefore, part of the bias against female employees that is often observed in industrial environments may be related to a basic communication problem between the sexes in noise; this difficulty is most likely amplified by the wearing of HPDs.

A problem that is mainly limited to the employees who require an ES HPD is the difficulty encountered when attempting to insert the user-moldable HPDs. Because of the smaller relative ear canal diameter among BFs, this population more often than any other has been observed to complain about having to use the Norton and E-A-R moldable type of HPDs.

Earmuffs are utilized only by approximately one percent of the industrial employees in North Carolina who are required to wear HPDs. However, a limited number of complaints were received concerning the tendency for the ear canal to become uncomfortably hot and to perspire, especially during the summer months, when earmuffs were being worn. Still, it has also been noted that some employees who are required to work outdoors in the wintertime or in cold storage areas prefer earmuffs because of their ability to provide warmth. Wearers also complained of the discomfort from headband pressure. An analysis of the survey data base indicates that the three most important requirements of HPDs indicated by employees are comfort, ease of keeping up with the HPD, and minimum day-to-day cost. These requirements in fact limit the practical utilization of the earmuff type of HPD in general industry.

A limited number of reports have been documented concerning temporary or permanent injury to the ear resulting from too rapid a removal of an ear plug style of HPD. In two cases, too rapid a removal of a single ear plug resulted in a significant TTS in comparison to the employee's baseline hearing test. The remaining three cases involved ear plugs with attached strings that were removed too rapidly by a pull on the strings. In one instance, the string was caught in the equipment; in one the employee wearing the HPD was responsible for removing his HPD too rapidly; and in the remaining case a fellow employee grabbed the string, resulting in too rapid a removal of the HPDs.

A large majority of the problems complained about by the employees are real; however, a significant number of the problems result from a lack of knowledge concerning the effects of wearing HPDs. These problems may or may not ever be revealed by the employees. To give an example, during the presensation of an educational session for employees at a furniture manufacturing company, one employee in the back of the room asked, "Will the wearing of ear protectors affect my sex life?" Of course, as one would anticipate, the room was immediately filled with laughter and the speaker moved onto the next topic. However, after the session was over the individual was drawn aside and asked to further explain his question concerning the wearing of his HPDs. It seems that the way he was turned on was for his wife to blow softly into his ear canal; therefore, he was afraid that the wearing of HPDs would affect the sensititivy of his ear canals. This type of concern expressed by one employee at one facility is most likely representative of other odd types of real personal problems that are in the minds of employees. It is important that an attempt to made to deal with the real and imaginary problems that employees face through the presentation of regular educational programs concerned with the utilization of HPDs and the resulting benefits.

Another major consideration of the employee who is required to wear HPDs is the resulting cosmetic effects. Often this concern is in conflict with management's desire to provide HPDs that can be readily seen at a distance, easily identified if dropped into the product, etc. However, most individuals are concerned about their external appearance. Often this part of the employee's general attitude toward HPDs is overlooked. Therefore, when possible, the employer should provide a selection of HPDs for the employee to choose from.

How Effective are HPDs?
A very significant question concerns the use of HPDs in industry: if worn properly, will the HPD provide adequate protection for the employee in preventing an on-the-job noise induced hearing loss? Here, "worn properly" refers to the practical utilization limits of HPDs as used by employees in the real world. The HPD sizes and ear plug insertion procedures commonly used in laboratories to obtain published real-ear attenuation data are often not practical for use in industrial environments. If individuals who are responsible for measuring HP attenuation data and specifying fitting procedures were required to wear the evaluated HPDs eight hours a day, five days a week, in the same manner as was required in the laboratory, the present trend for HP real-ear attenuation data to improve would quickly be reversed. Unfortunately, individuals

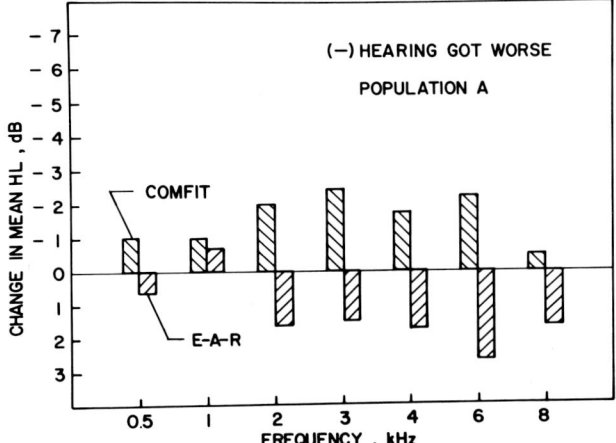

Figure 7. The shifts in the measured mean hearing levels between the first and second hearing test by HPD and audiometric test frequency.

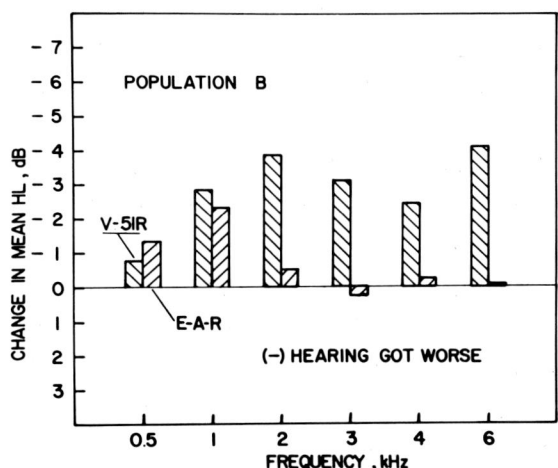

Figure 8. The shifts in the measured mean hearing levels between the first and second hearing test by HPD and audiometric test frequency for a group test 8 minutes after leaving the noise environment.

who are responsible for the fitting and issuing of HPDs seldom wear them for any significant length of time.

To obtain a better estimate of the real-world attenuatin capabilities of different HPDs, a series of in-the-field HPD evaluations is presently underway. Two studies have been completed[11,12] and the general findings are presented as Figures 7 and 8. In Figure 5, the changes in mean hearing level (HL) at different audiometric test frequencies between the initial and final audiometric tests are presented for employees in one industrial population (Population A) when wearing two different brands of HPDs. The two HPDs evaluated were the Comfit and E-A-R brands. Figure 8 displays a similar data set obtained for a different industrial population (Population B). In Figure 8 the two HPDs evaluated were the Hear Guard (V-51R) and the E-A-R brands. The measured daily equivalent A-weighted sound pressure levels were approximately 95 dB for both industrial environments.

For both sound exposures, the utilization of the published real-ear attenuation data, including a reduction of two standard deviations, would have resulted in a prediction that no significant TTS would have resulted. However, a significant TTS was indicated by the employees who wore the Comfit and Hear Guard HPDs and a significant difference in the measured TTS values was established between the employees who wore the Comfit, Hear Guard (V-51R), and the E-A-R HPDs. The employees who were wearing the E-A-R HPDs exhibited significantly less TTS in the frequency range where the majority of the acoustic energy was concentrated. These findings do correlate with the observed changes in the population's HLs over a period of several years. The data seem to support the notion that HPDs, as used in the real world by employees who are sincerely trying to protect their hearing, provide significantly less attenuation than would be indicated by the published real-ear attenuation data or by the NRR.

Problems Encountered by Management

It is not unusual to hear of the many types of problems encountered by the employee when attempting to wear HPDs; however the employer frequently faces problems, real and imaginary, as a result of having to develop and implement the HP phase of a HCP.

The most significant initial concerns occurring, especially in smaller business establishements, is difficulty in obtaining information necessary to make good decisions with respect to the procedures to be followed in implementing the HCP. The employer often turns to the local industrial association or the company's legal staff. Unfortunately, these two groups are limited in their knowledge of the areas and requirements of a HCP; however, they have been observed to be more than willing to supply advice. As a result, several industry vs. government legal confrontations have occurred in which the cost of complying with the noise regulations would have been significantly less or no greater than the legal fees eventually paid by the company.

A potential problem that management seems to fear the most is that the employees, if required to wear the HPDs provided, may unionize the plant if not already unionized. Unionization as the result of a mandatory program requiring the wearing of HPDs has not been observed when the requirement of wearing the HPDs provided was an integral part of the HCP when it was initially implemented. However, significant problems have been encountered by management when an incomplete HCP was implemented initially and at a later date a change in policy was implemented requiring the wearing of HPDs.

Many employess have been observed to resist the proper wearing of the HPDs provided in any way possible. Although some employees may have justifiable reasons for resisting the utilization of HPDs, many do not. It is simply that some employees would just as soon suffer a hearing loss as be bothered with the wearing of a HPD. Of course, these individuals are often the ones who also resisted the wearing of safety glasses, safety shoes, and other types of safety equipment. This type of blatant resistance to the wearing of HPDs cannot be tolerated if an effective HCP is to be implemented and maintained.

A further concern for management is the selection of appropriate HPDs for the employee to choose from. Even after the HPDs to be used have been selected, management must be on the lookout for potentially harmful employee-environment-HPD combinations. One hazardous combination has been observed to occur when insert types of HPDs are used in environments where toxic chemicals are in use. Care should also be exercised in selecting the styles and colors of HPDs to be made available to employees working in the vicinity of uncovered food products.

Another potential problem that management must face is the possibility of creating a safety hazard when an employee who is required to work in a high noise level area and who exhibits a significant high frequency hearing loss is required to wear HPDs. If this employee fails to hear a warning signal as a result of having to wear a HPD and in injured, then management may be forced to assume the responsibility for the accident. A solution to this type of problem is to review the HLs of all employees who are required to wear HPDs and transfer the potentially affected employees to an area without a noise hazard.

It is anticipated that new legal problems will develop as the legal profession becomes better educated about the general effects of noise and about the requirements of the different phases of the company's HCP. As an example, an employee at one production facility in North Carolina tripped and fell down the stairs leading from a noise hazard area. The employee's supervisor, who was in the vicinity, did not immediately respond to the fallen employee's call for help. The employee that was injured sued for compensation as a result of the injury received and claimed that the injury was aggravated because the supervisor did not immediately respond to his calls for help. The lawyer, while cross-examining the supervisor, pointed out several times that the supervisor was wearing a HPD and, as a result, could not hear the employee's call for help as well as he normally could have. The company lost the initial court trial, but the case has been appealed. If the lawyer had requested that the supervisor be given an audiometric exam, and if the supervisor had exhibited the typical industrial noise exposed WM HL characteristics, she possibly could have established an even more damaging case against the company.

Management is also sometimes caught in the middle of an employee vs. physician conflict with respect to the employee's ability to wear HPDs. Unfortunately a significant number of the smaller industries often turn to the local physician for advice when the employee complains of problems associated with the use of HPDs. Experience in dealing with and assisting physicians in providing this type of service over several years clearly points out the almost total lack of basic knowledge on the part of these individuals in the HCP areas. One should not assume that all physicians possess the knowledge necessary to administer a HCP. However, upon request physicians often accept responsibility for giving audiometric exams, determining the adequacy of a HPD, deciding if the HPD used was the cause of an employee complaint, or determining if the employee's work environment caused a complaint. It has also been observed that the physician's diagnosis is often made without ever visiting the employee's work environment.

It is not uncommon for management to start receiving statements from a local physician that certain employees at a given facility cannot wear the HPDs issued due to the type of environment where the employee works. However, once management realizes what is happening they should notify the affected employees that if they desire to continue working at their present work station, they will be required to wear the HPDs provided. The notices being received from the physician will subsequently stop.

As a further example that a physician may be uninformed about HPD use, consider the case of a female employee who complained to her family physician that the wearing of HPDs caused her to cough. The physician then notified company management that the tendency of an individual to cough when required to wear HPDs was a well-known medical fact. In order to avoid eventually encountering problems between company management and the local physician who assists the company with the HCP, it is essential that the physician be educated regarding the essential phases of an effective HCP and the realities of HPD use.

A very significant decision that must be made by management is the selection of the HPD replacement policy to be followed. A characteristic of all successful HCPs evaluated to date is the availability of free replacements if HPDs become worn out or in any way become defective.

The company must take the initiative in replacing ineffective HPDs. As an example, management at one company sets up a HPD replacement station at the factory exit gates once each quarter and freely replaces all worn out HPDs.

Management committed to an effective HP phase of the HCP will often have problems maintaining proper HPD fitting procedures. There is a strong tendency for the mean earplug size to become smaller. Some employees will ask a fellow employee, who wears a smaller size HPD, to purchase a smaller HPD for them. A limited number of Japanese-made HPDs, obviously significantly smaller than the typical HPD worn by the WM population in American industry, have been purchased by employees. These types of problems can best be handled by maintaining accurate HPD fitting records and by on-the-spot checking of the employee's HPD size as well as the condition of the HPDs being worn. Once the employee knows that the nurse, technician, or individual responsible for the proper fitting of the HPDs will leave his/her normal work station and conduct on-the-spot checks of the HPDs being worn, the tendency of the employees to wear a smaller HPD size will be significantly reduced.

While conducting on-the-spot surveys concerning problems associated with the use of HPDs, the individuals responsible for fitting and issuing of the HPDs have identified several significant HCP-related problems that were not known to the next higher level of management. Not only were the problems identified significant, but in many instances solutions to the problems were very simple to implement. The fact that management failed to discover these problems was a result of inadequate communication between the parties involved. If management is to minimize the real cost of not having an effective HCP, especially the HP phase, then a sincere effort is necessary to insure that adequate communication lines are maintained.

CONCLUSIONS

If a company is to minimize the number of problems encountered when establishing and trying to maintain the HP phase of a HCP, then the program must exhibit four charactertistics: (1) an enforced requirement that HPDs be worn properly by all individuals in identified noise-hazard areas; (2) the existence of a key individual; (3) an active communication line between the various levels of management and between management and the employees; and (4) the availability of HPDs that are "potentially effective."

The cost of maintaining a very effective HP phase of a HCP is minimal on a per employee basis. However, the real cost of not having an effective HP program is potentially very significant.

REFERENCES
1. Royster, L.H., Thomas, W.G., Age Effect Hearing Levels for a White Nonindustrial Noise Exposed Population, (NINEP) and Their Use in Evaluating Industrial Hearing Conservation Programs, Am. Ind. Hyg. Assoc. J., 40, 504-511, 1979.

2. Royster, L.H., Driscoll, D.P., Thomas, W.G., J.D., Royster, Age Effect Hearing Levels for a Black Nonindustrial Noise Exposed Population, (NINEP), Am. Ind. Hyg. Assoc. J., 41, 113-119, 1980.

3. Robinson, D.W., Sutton, G.J., A Comparative Analysis of Data on the Relation of Pure-Tone Audiometric Thresholds to Age, NPL Acoustics Report AC 84, 1978.

4. Corso, J.F., Age and Sex Differences in Pure-Tone Thresholds, Arch. Otolaryngol., 77, 385-405, 1963.

5. Hinchcliffe, R., The Threshold of Hearing as a Function of Age, Acoustics, 9, 303-308, 1959.

6. Spoor, A., Presbycusis Values in Relation to Noise Induced Hearing Loss, Int. Audiol., 6, 48-57, 1967.

7. Royster, L.H., Royster, J.D., Thomas, W.G., Representative Hearing Levels by Race and Sex in North Carolina Industry, J. Acoust. Soc. Amer. 68, 551-566, 1980.

8. Royster, L.H., Royster, J.D., Methods of Evaluating Hearing Conservation Program Audiometric Data Bases, in Personal Hearing Protection in Industry, ed. P.W. Alberti, Raven Press, New York, 1981.

9. Holder, S.R., Royster, L.H., An Analysis of OSHA-NC Noise Surveys, (June 1977 to June 1979). Proc. of the Special Session in the Evaluation and Utilization of Hearing Protection Devices, (HPDs) in Industry, L.H. Royster Ed., Spring 1980 Meeting of the N.C. Regional Chapter of the ASA. D.H. Hill Library, N.C. State University, Raleigh,

N.C.

10. Scott, C.E., Thomas, W.G., Royster, L.H., Determination of In-Use Attenuation Values for Selected Ear Plugs, Proceedings of the Eighty-Fifth Meeting of the Acoust. Soc. Amer., P.83, 1973.

11. Royster, L.H., Lilley, D.T., Thomas, W.G., Recommended Criteria for Evaluating the Effectiveness of Hearing Conservation Programs, Am. Ind. Hyg. Assoc. J., 41, 40-48, 1980.

12. Royster, L.H., Effectiveness of Three Different Types of Hearing Protection Devices in Preventing a Temporary Threshold Shift, J. Acoust. Soc. Amer., 66, Supp 1, S62, 1979.

13. Royster, L.H., Evaluation of the Effectiveness of Two Different Insert Types of Ear Protection in Preventing TTS in an Industrial Environment, Am. Ind. Hyg. Assoc. J. 41, 161-169, 1980.

28 Hearing Protector Programme Establishment

Denis Else

INTRODUCTION

It has always been obvious that hearing protectors cannot protect unless they are being worn and it has long been recognised that getting people to wear hearing protectors is not easily accomplished. Conversely, when hearing protectors are made available to people with noisy jobs, some choose to wear them even when little effort is expended on the hearing protection scheme; there are, for example, records of people wearing earplugs in the last century. The amount of effort and the mix of elements that is necessary to achieve a high usage of hearing protectors depends upon the particular circumstances associated with the noise problem.

Circumstances in which a high usage of hearing protectors can more easily be accomplished are:

> exposure to very high noise levels; short periods of exposure; a young workforce; a workforce new to the company; a workforce new to the trade; stationary job site (i.e., little need to move from area to area whilst performing job); absence of need to communicate; lack of other danger in the area; a workforce without previous history of noise exposure.

Circumstances which make it more difficult to achieve a high usage of hearing protectors are:

> exposure to noise levels which only slightly exceed recommended limits; exposure for long periods each day without opportunity for breaks from the noise; older workforce; highly skilled jobs in which some information is received via the ears; a need to communicate; jobs in which people need to move from area to area; other recognisable dangers in the area; a workforce with many years unprotected exposure to noise; the need to wear other protective equipment on the head; hot environments.

SELECTING HEARING PROTECTORS

Hearing protectors should be chosen to reduce the noise level at the wearer's ears to below the recommended limit for unprotected exposure to noise. They cannot be chosen from simple measurements of the A-weighted level of the noise, because the reduction in sound level depends upon the particular frequency spectrum of the noise. This could be very important: for example, an earmuff might reduce the noise level from a mostly high frequency noise by as much as 35 dB(A) but the same earmuff worn in the low frequency noise from a compressor house might only provide about 10 dB(A) reduction in sound level.[1]

Although many companies perform the correct measurements and calculations there are many earmuffs purchased without any prior calculation of whether they adequately reduce the noise level. It is also common to find small areas for which the correct measurements and calculations are not made even in companies which attempt to follow the correct procedures - this is usually as a result of areas being missed during the initial survey, e.g., the compressor house.

Possible interactions between hearing protectors and other forms of personal protection equipment should be considered during the initial selection of hearing protectors. For example, the wearing of spectacles can significantly reduce the protection provided by earmuffs because the spectacle arms create leakages around the earmuff seals as quantified by Nixon et al (1974).[2] Where possible, alternative forms of hearing protectors should be available, e.g., earmuffs as alternative to earplugs for people who suffer permanently or temporarily from outer ear infection, irritation or skin sensitivity.

CORRECT FITTING OF HEARING PROTECTORS

There are two stages at which hearing protectors can be incorrectly fitted: initially when the hearing protectors are selected and fitted to the individual worker; and at each time the hearing protector is fitted prior to entry into the noisy area.

Re-usable Earplugs - Because of the large variation in ear canal sizes, earplugs must either be designed for universal fitting or supplied in a range of sizes. Supervision is necessary during the initial fitting; if the earplugs are supplied in a range of sizes (often five sizes) the correct size must be chosen (some manufacturers provide a tool for guaging ear canal diameters, others expect the correct size to be found by trial and error from the range available). It should be noted that different sizes may be required for left and right ears of the same individual. Clearly, the user must be given adequate instruction to ensure he or she can routinely fit the earplugs correctly.

Disposable Earplugs - supervision is necessary during the initial fitting of most types of disposable earplugs. If made from loose glass fibre material the user must be given adequate instruction for both forming the earplug and inserting it in the ear canal. If it is a pre-formed plastic coated glass fibre earplug, or polyurethane foam, adequate instruction must be given on inserting the earplug in the ear canal and adjusting the fit. Note - it is not uncommon to find people dividing pre-formed glass fibre earplugs into two pieces, one for each ear.

Earmuffs - it is highly desirable that users be given an opportunity to select from a range of earmuffs all of which are capable of reducing the level of noise to below recommended limits. The earmuff which is most suitable for the majority of users doesn't necessarily provide an adequate comfortable fit on the minority users. Some earmuffs are larger than others, some have more adjustment in their headbands -relying on just one type of earmuff will reduce the likelihood that all users will achieve adequate, comfortable fit.

Earmuff users need to be instructed to wear earmuffs with their pinna inside the earmuff shells rather than pinned under the seal. They also have to be supervised to make sure they achieve adequate fit in practice and do not for instance wear the earmuffs resting on part of a cloth beret or other head covering.

THE USAGE OF HEARING PROTECTORS IN PRACTICE

Robinson (1968)[3] showed that the risk of hearing loss from exposure to continuous noise can be predicted from a knowledge of the cumulative A-weighted sound energy received by the ears and it therefore follows that the effectiveness of a hearing protector is actually governed by the protector's ability to reduce A-weighted noise dose rather than its ability to reduce A-weighted sound <u>level</u>.

It has been shown (Else, 1973[4]) that the removal of hearing protectors for very short periods during noise exposure seriously reduces the <u>protection</u> (protection is defined as the reduction in equivalent-continuous sound level afforded by the wearing of the hearing protectors) afforded by the protectors. The relation between the protection and the percentage of the exposure duration for which the hearing protector is worn is shown in Figure 1; the hearing protector is assumed to provide infinite attenuation, i.e., in this simplified case it is assumed that no noise reaches the ears whilst the hearing protectors are worn.

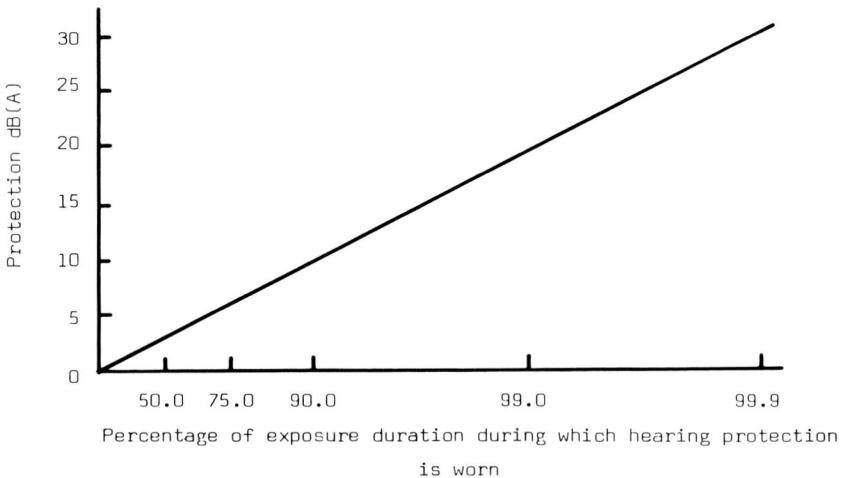

<u>Figure 1.</u> The effect of removing a hearing protector for short periods of time. The theoretical case of a hearing protector which provides infinite attenuation. (3dB rule)

It can be seen from Figure 1 that no hearing protector can provide more

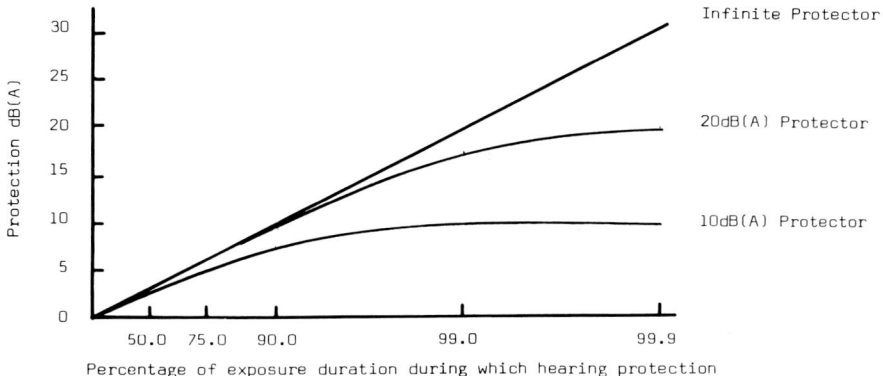

Figure 2. The effects of removing hearing protectors for short periods of time. Comparisons of the protection afforded by hearing protectors which reduce the instanteous sound level by 10 decibels and 20 decibels respectively. (3dB rule)

than six decibels of protection if it is worn for less than 75 percent of the exposure duration. Similarly if it is necessary to protect a person exposed continuously for eight hours per day to a sound level of 120 dB(A) even an infinite attenuation hearing protector would have to be worn 99.9 percent of the exposure duration, i.e., removing the protectors for one minute will result in the person receiving twice the recommended daily maximum noise dose. (A recommended maximum daily noise dose equivalent to 90 dB(A) for eight hours per day has been assumed for this example.)

In practice hearing protectors do not provide infinite attenuation and therefore some noise energy is immitted whilst the protectors are worn. The relation between the protection provided and the percentage of the exposure duration for which the protector is worn is shown in Figure 2 for hearing protectors which reduce the instantaneous sound level by 10 dB(A) and 20 dB(A) respectively (Else, 1976).[1] The equivalent curves assuming a 5 dB trading relationship between noise level and duration of exposure are shown in Figure 3. Clearly if a high-attenuation hearing protector is removed for part of the noise exposure then the same degree of protection, or greater, could be achieved with a hearing protector which provides less instantaneous reduction in sound level, provided that it would be worn for a sufficiently high percentage of the exposure duration.

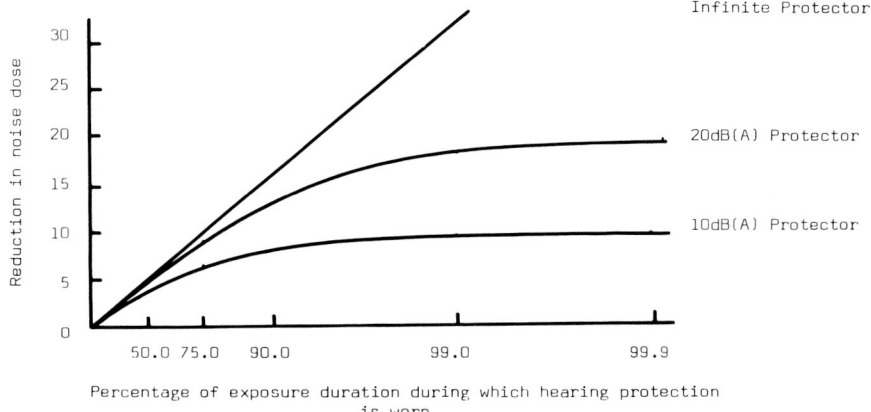

Figure 3. The effects of removing hearing protectors for short periods of time. Comparisons of the reduction in noise dose afforded by hearing protectors which reduce the instanteous sound level by 10 decibels and 20 decibels respectively. (5dB rule)

How comfortable a hearing protector is and whether it can be worn for the full duration of exposure in the particular environment by people who may also have to wear other forms of personal protective equipment are vital factors that should be considered during the initial selection. User trials are usually the only way of discovering how acceptable, comfortable or compatible a particular type of hearing protector will be for a particular application. Unfortunately, it is quite common to find that people exposed to noise levels only slightly in excess of recommended noise levels have been issued with high-attenuation earmuffs - the high attenuation is often obtained at the expense of comfort and as a result of high usage of earmuffs is not achieved.

MAINTENANCE AND CLEANING OF HEARING PROTECTORS

Most hearing protection schemes need to have incorporated within them provisions for cleaning, maintenance and the issue of replacements.

All non-disposable types of hearing protectors require cleaning -the frequency of the cleaning depends on the type of protector and the

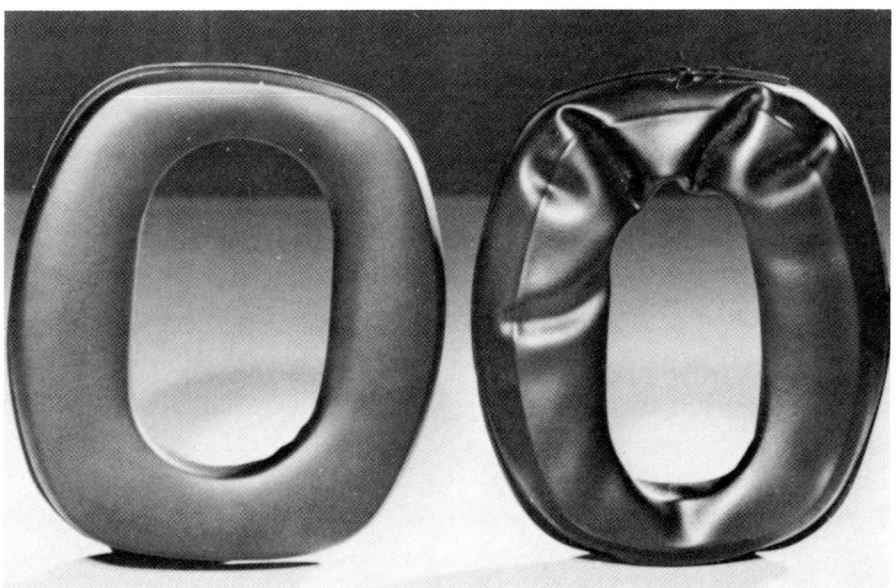

Figure 4. Comparison of new and used earmuff cushions.

environment in which it is used. The cleaning is necessary for two reasons: to reduce the risk of irritation of the skin of the outer extremities of the ear canal or the skin surrounding the ears; and because people are unlikely to want to wear hearing protectors if they are dirty.

Earmuff seals are likely to need replacement frequently because most seals become less compliant as a result of contact with natural hair oils, perspiration and hair dressings. Figure 4 shows a comparison of a new seal with one that had been used for three months in a foundry environment. Many manufacturers now make available spare seals or replacement parts which include seals and the inner foam inserts for earmuff cups. The complete earmuff or parts of an earmuff are likely to have to be replaced as a result of: wear in the adjustment mechanisms; damage resulting from the earmuff being dropped; distortion resulting from exposure to intense heat; or as a result of normal wear and tear.

Earplugs, because they are simpler devices tend to require less maintenance. However, many of the earplug materials become less pliable as a result of cleaning, exposure to natural oils and perspiration. Replacements are also necessary when earplugs are lost. Even with disposable earplugs there may be a need for maintenance -not of the earplugs themselves but possibly of the machines used for dispensing them. Damage to dispeners or failure to replenish them can easily result in earplugs not being available at the time when operators need to use them.

Users are unlikely to notice the deteriorating condition of their hearing protectors because the changes are insidious. Someone has to compare new and used hearing protectors side by side before decisions can be made about the replacement of all or part of the hearing protector.

PROVISIONS FOR EDUCATION AND TRAINING

Education and training are important. Set out below are the most commonly involved individuals and groups and indications of the information they would probably need to have presented to them.

Selector of Hearing Protectors (also assumed to be the individual responsible for the hearing protection scheme): noise exposure limits; methods of selecting hearing protectors; how to calculate A-weighted sound level beneath hearing protectors from octave band analysis; effects of removal of hearing protectors for short periods of time; possible effects of wearing hearing protectors on other dangers; methods of selecting hearing protectors to obtain adequate fit; <u>plus</u> all information listed for other classes of people involved with the scheme.

Users of Hearing Protectors: how the ear works; how ear is damaged by noise; what it is like to suffer occupational deafness (tape recordings if possible); magnitude of the risk; responsibilities in law; how to fit the hearing protectors; when and where (for most circumstances it will be necessary to mark the noisy areas) the protectors should be worn, including need for very high usage; faults to look for in hearing protectors; what to do with damaged hearing protectors; action that should be taken if piece of earplug lodges in ear canal or if skin irritation develops subsequent to wearing hearing protectors; need to maintain voice level; probable loss in directional hearing; probable need to relearn auditory cues.

Storeman: Dangers of issuing wrong type of hearing protector; need for correct assessment of protection afforded against particular type of noise exposure.

Maintenance and Cleaning Staff: How to clean and maintain the equipment; how to assess damage, wear and need for replacements.

Supervision and Management: How ear works; how ear is damaged by noise; what it is like to suffer from occupational deafness; magnitude of risks; responsibilities of supervision and management in the hearing protection scheme; need to achieve very high usage; company procedures for noise control, hearing protector maintenance, cleaning and issuing; effects of hearing protectors on directional hearing, voice level and auditory cues; need to set example even though noise exposure may be relatively low because exposure infrequent and not prolonged.

The provisions for education and training of all of the individuals and groups listed above should cater for the three stages listed below:

1. Initial Training on introduction of the scheme: broadly as itemized above.
2. Refresher Training: it is not adequate to rely on a "once and for all" burst of interest in education and training -there is a need to refresh people's interest by the use of films, tapes, tape-slides or lectures.
3. Education and Training for New Employees or New Entrants into Noisy Areas or the Management and Supervision of Noisy Areas: A system must exist to ensure that new starters into any of the above classifications receive the same degree of training as that given initially to the members of that classification. This can be difficult to arrange but it is, of course, vital to the long term success of the scheme. Note that it is vital that users of hearing

protectors receive this training <u>before</u> they go into noisy areas and whenever possible hearing protectors should be used during training, e.g., during training in works' training school if company has its own training school.

Supervision and Monitoring of the Hearing Protection Scheme

Hearing protection schemes are unlikely to work unless someone is given overall responsibility for the scheme. The responsible person is likely to have a largely co-ordinating and monitoring role although often the person will be also responsible specifically for the selection of hearing protectors.

Monitoring is required to ascertain:

a) <u>Whether people (including supervisors and management) are wearing the hearing protectors</u> - the person responsible should know what percentage wear the hearing protectors (probably by head count) and what action is being taken for those who are not wearing them.

b) <u>Whether hearing protectors are adequately maintained and cleaned</u> - the responsible person needs to monitor procedures for maintenance and cleaning to make sure the hearing protectors are likely to provide the calculated degree of protection.

c) <u>Whether training provisions are being carried out rather than falling into disuse.</u>

The responsible person needs to act upon the information gathered by monitoring the hearing protection scheme and where necessary gather together resources to supplement standard procedures, e.g., if usage of hearing protectors is declining because of hot weather or waning interest it may be necessary to increase awareness and interest by the use of poster campaigns, displaying articles on noticeboards, or by injecting interest via safety committees or safety representatives.

The person responsible for the scheme must also have action planned for consistent non-usage. There should be a system for considering alternative types of hearing protectors for the wearer who finds the issued types unacceptable. Some people have great dislike of putting earplugs into their ears - they may need to be given the chance to use light-weight earmuffs even though the noise level does not warrant such high attenuation. It is probable that some people will develop some sort of skin irritation whilst they are wearing the earplugs or earmuffs - it will be necessary to ascertain the probable cause of the irritation (e.g., is cleaning adequate, is the individual sensitive to the materials of the hearing protectors, or cleaning agents or other materials in the work environment).

There must be a procedure for taking action for people who refuse to wear hearing protectors because they do not believe that noise could damage them - more training may be necessary although it is more likely that some form of personal counselling will be necessary and perhaps agreed disciplinary procedures. The responsible person will also have to cope with: changes in earmuffs design which make those that were initially selected no longer available, and changes in the noise environment which necessitate checking the adequacy of the hearing protectors against the new noise spectra.

COMMITMENT OF MANAGEMENT

A major determinant of whether a high usage of hearing protectors will be achieved is the degree to which management are committed to health and safety generally (as evidenced perhaps by the degree of effort put into other problems - e.g., it is unlikely that a very high usage of hearing protectors will be achieved if the eye protectors which have been issued are not being worn), and noise exposure control in particular.

Commitment of management to noise exposure control may be evidenced by their responses to some of the following questions:

1) Do management wear hearing protectors when walking through noisy areas?
2) To what extent are supervisors encouraged to wear hearing protectors and are sanctions applied if they do not wear them?
3) Has the company procedures for ensuring new machines are vetted to make sure noise levels are the lowest practicable?
4) To what lengths have the company gone in testing feasibility of control measures aimed at controlling noise at source?
5) What level in the management hierarchy is given to the person responsible for the hearing protectors scheme?
6) Is the hearing protection scheme underpinned by written procedures?

DANGERS ASSOCIATED WITH THE USE OF HEARING PROTECTORS

Many potential wearers of hearing protectors express concern that the protectors will put them at greater danger, e.g., Sugden[5], reported that some foundrymen who had worn hearing protectors gave this as their reason for ceasing to use protectors. Other authors have expressed concern that hearing protectors could, in some circumstances, present a further hazard to the wearer, e.g., Coles and Rice[6], Dunn[7], Burns[8], Else[1]. Atherley and Noble[9], Atherley and Else[10] and Else[1] found evidence, from their laboratory studies of directional hearing, to support claims made by foundrymen that earmuffs reduced their ability to determine the direction of sounds. In my experience earmuffs noticeably decrease directional hearing in many circumstances in industry - although often earmuff users make up for this by making greater use of visual cues.

It is often very difficult to establish in individual cases whether the wearing of hearing protectors could put the wearer or others in greater danger. However, whenever people are issued with hearing protectors some thought should be given to possible adverse effects brought about by hearing protector usage. In some cases it may be adequate to just urge the new wearers of hearing protectors to exercise caution but in other cases it may be necessry to change the method of working to eliminate obvious dangers which might be increased by the use of hearing protectors.

Establishing a successful hearing protection programme is not just a question of selecting the best hearing protectors. Many of the decisions which have to be taken whilst the programme is being established require competent informed interpretation of available data against the background of the local circumstances. A hearing protection programme should not be considered established until: all the people who should be wearing hearing protectors habitually wear them at all times during exposure; the systems for selecting and maintaining the protectors can be relied upon to ensure they are capable of providing adequate protection; the systems for training can be relied upon to ensure all people will wear the protectors correctly; and the whole scheme is underpinned by written procedures to ensure that people continue to be adequately protected whilst at the same time pressure is maintained to move towards control of noise at source.

REFERENCES
1.   Else, D., Hearing Protectors, unpublished PhD thesis University of Aston in Birmingham 1967.

2.   Nixon, C.W., Hearing Protection of earmuffs worn over eye glasses. Aerospace Medicine Research Laboratories, Wright-Patterson Air Force Base, Ohio 1974.

3.   Robinson, D.W., The relationship between hearing loss and noise exposure Aero Report Ac32 National Physical Laboratory England 1968.

4.   Else, D., A note on the protection afforded by hearing protectors Implications of the energy principle. Ann. Occup. Hyg., 16, 81-83, 1973.

5.   Sugden, D.B., Some notes on the provision of personal hearing protection for fettlers at an iron foundry. Ann. Occup. Hyg. 10, 263-268, 1967.

6.   Coles, R.R.A., Rice, C.G., Earplugs and impaired hearing. J. Sound and Vibr. 3, 521-523, 1965.

7.   Dunn, J.G., Skills analysis used for the investigation of accident risk in power-saw operation: AP Note 21 Applied Psychology Department University of Aston in Birmingham, 1970.

8. Burns, W., Noise and Man: Second edition London, John Murray, 1973.

9. Atherley, G.R.C., Noble, W.G., Effect of ear defenders (ear muffs) on the localisation of sound. Brit. J. Indust. Med. $\underline{27}$, 260-265, 1970.

10. Atherley, G.R.C., Else, D., Effect of ear muffs on the localisaton of sound under reverberant conditions. Proc. Roy. Soc. Med. $\underline{64}$, 203-205, 1971.

29 How to Motivate People in the Use of Their Hearing Protectors

Hans Lofgreen, Mats Holm, and Ronald Tengling

It is easier to provide hearing protectors than to persuade the workforce to use them. They are frequently uncomfortable and it takes time to become accustomed to them. Unlike hard hats or protective gloves or safety goggles, the danger of <u>not</u> using hearing protectors is by no means apparent.

There are two traditional methods of motivation: to force or to reward. Provided that there is enough incentive, these methods will work, but the incentive must be great. Experience has shown that attempting to enforce the use of hearing protectors without incentive or explanation, doesn't work; the majority of people resist attempts to force them to do something unpopular or incomprehensible, even if supposedly to their own benefit.

Reward is potentially a better stimulus in an industrial setting than force. The greatest reward for using hearing protectors is, of course, the long-term one: retaining hearing. However this is a difficult concept to grasp, particularly for young workers. A more immediate reward is needed. There <u>is</u> a shorter-term reward which results from the regular use of hearing protectors. After about two weeks of use, during which workers adapt to the initial discomfort, many feel less fatigued and irritable and have an increased sense of well being. This is the result of cutting out the extra-auditory effects of noise which may include general stress reactions, physical disorders, mental and emotional difficulties, performance loss - problems that may extend into leisuretime activities.

The first major hurdle is to persuade a work force to try hearing protectors and to help them persevere with them in the initial weeks of use.

Case Example:
At the Austrian engineering firm of Bunzl & Biach, a combination of rewards and intensive information was tried. Of their 1700 employees, 300 in three different departments were exposed to noise levels in excess of 85 dB(A).

Previous attempts to enforce the use of hearing protectors by means of signs that warned workers that it was their DUTY to use hearing protectors had failed to have any effect. A motivation package was therefore carefully prepared by the company, an educational psychologist, the Austrian Health Insurance Authority and the local Bilsom representative.

The psychologist, Dr. P. Weingarten from Vienna stated the theoretical strategy as follows:

1. As the rewards of wearing protectors only become evident to the wearer after a period of regular use, some more immediate reward is needed to persuade the employee to overcome any initial difficulties.
2. The immediate reward should be in a form not normally associated with hearing conservation.
3. Once the wearer has crossed the resistance threshold, the fact that he feels better for using the protectors will be sufficient reward in itself and the external reward can be withdrawn.
4. The resistance threshold should be as low as possible. In other words, the hearing protectors supplied should be the most comfortable ones available.
5. If the majority of the workers use protectors, the group-dynamic effect will influence the rest to follow suit.

It was decided that the immediate reward for using hearing protectors should be the chance of winning a prize by being awarded tickets in an internal lottery. The whole noise exposed workforce was fully informed about the conditions and rules of the lottery and prizes were prominently displayed. The prize included a bicycle, records, glassware and kitchen utensils.

All the noise-exposed workers were issued with Bilsom earplugs and the supervisor made random checks to see if they were being correctly used. If so, the worker was given a lottery ticket. The checks, though randomized in time, were planned so that every worker was checked the same number of times. the supervisor also made "fake" rounds so that there was no means of knowing beforehand when a check would be made. A single worker could be awarded up to five lottery tickets.

The campaign, including the information phase, lasted 3 months. At the end, the lucky winners were given their prizes and the first check on the number of regular users was made.

Table I shows the results of the campaign which were impressive - the number of users had risen from 7% to 61% of the exposed workforce. But what happened after the rewards had been removed? What was the long term affect of the programme? Three months after its end the percentage of regular users had dropped to 58%, and one year later it was 62%. The lastest check, four years later showed that the number of regular users was maintained at around 60%. This lasting effect of the campaign demonstrates that once the initial resistance to the use of hearing protectors is overcome, it is probable that their use will become habitual.

This campaign was costly, not because of the actual prizes, but in terms of organization, manpower and effort. Not many firms are in position to launch a campaign of this type, but principle should be applicable in a more modest sense. If it is accepted that the rewards of wearing hearing protectors become self-evident after a short period of training, it should be possible to replace the glittering prizes with other means of

Table I Campaign Results

	Noise Area			TOTAL
	1	2	3	
No. of noise-exposed workers	200	70	30	300
Quota of Hearing Protector Users:	%	%	%	%
- before campaign	9	6	0	7
- at end of campaign	68	51	36	61
- 3 months later				58
- 1 year later				62
- 4 years later				61

persuasion.

At Bilsom we have devised an intensive action motivation campaign, which is intended to parallel the ongoing general hearing conservation measures. It should be used to increase the pace and heighten awareness over a short period of time; its sole aim is to persuade people to persevere with hearing protectors for two weeks or so. The theme is: "take it gradually". As theme or symbol for the campaign we are using a hearing cell spokesman. Hearing conservation is a serious subject, but we feel that a lighter approach has a better chance of getting our message across.

Initially the appropriate supervisors are briefed by the Safety Department or similar organization in the company. They must be fully aware of the need for, and the applicability to their own plant, of a hearing conservation programme. A campaign kit has been designed to help them persuade the work force. It is intended for issue to first line supervisor (fig. 1). When an intensive motivation campaign of this type is carried out, it is of the utmost importance that maximum interest is generated around it. It should receive as much publicity within the company as possible. A genuine show of interest on the part of top management is essential.

The campaign is designed to be conducted in the following stages:

The supervisor calls in the noise-exposed workers in his department and tells them about the campaign. This completed, he issues each of them

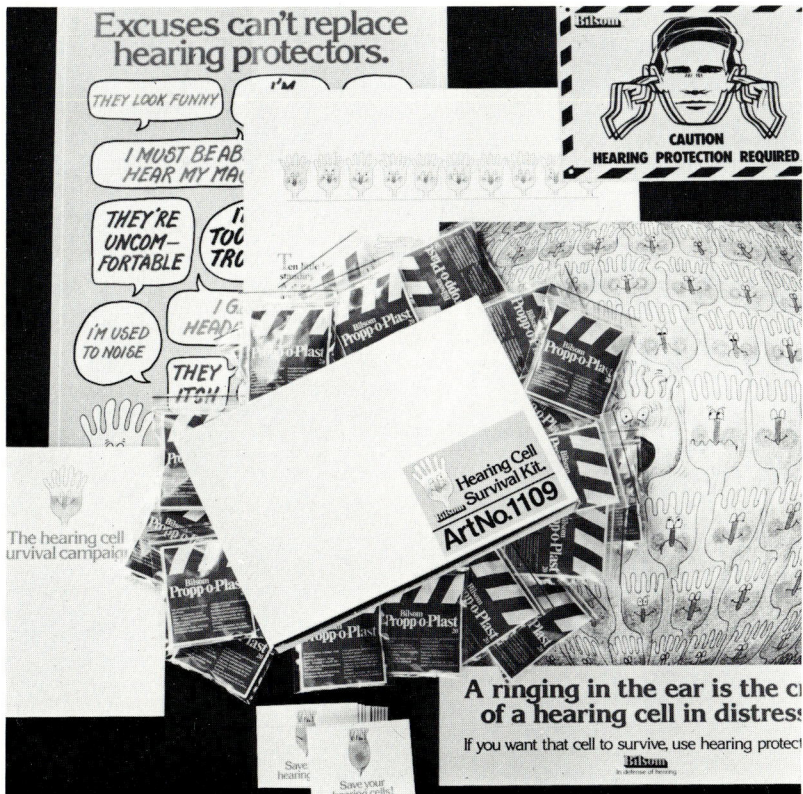

Figure 1. Components of the Bilson Motivation campaign kit.

with a pocket pouch of earplugs together with a pocket-size booklet. The booklet explains in simple terms how the hearing cells are gradually destroyed by noise. It also contains information on hearing tests and how easy it is to use hearing protectors. Most importantly, it gives the schedule for the two-week self-administered program for getting used to protectors. The employee is encouraged to increase wearing time a little each day. His objections are anticipated and answered. The pouches contain 10 pairs of Propp-o-Plast disposable earplugs. These pre-shaped plugs of soft fiber generally have high acceptance.

The supervisor puts up the posters and warning signs where they can best be seen. He makes regular checks to see that the plugs are being used. The ammunition to meet the most usual objections is given in his manual.

Visitors to the department, even if only passing through, are firmly requested to use protectors. At the end of the first week the supervisor checks on progress and issues a fresh supply of protectors.

At the end of the two-week period the supervisor reports back to the safety department on the results of the campaign.

The campaign outlined above has already been used in a number of companies with considerable short term success. However its long-term effects have yet to be evaluated.

30 Employee Attitudes Towards Hearing Protection as Affected by Serial Audiometry

S. J. Karmy and A. M. Martin

INTRODUCTION

The debate as to the value of industrial audiometry has proceeded in the United Kingdom for at least the last decade. The arguments discussed by the various protagonists have ranged from the resolution required of audiometric measurement if serial audiometry is to act as a reliable biological monitoring tool, through various medico-legal considerations, to the suggestion that a possible additional benefit to be derived from industrial audiometry could be an increase in hearing protector usage by employees participating in an audiometric programme. Investigation of the hypothesis linking hearing protector usage to the performance of industrial audiometry forms the basis of this paper.

Examination of the literature shows the diversity of opinion on the benefits to be obtained from a programme of monitoring audiometry[1-18]. However, even the author who, perhaps, has written most persistently against the use of industrial audiometry, concludes in one of his papers that "research has so far concentrated upon the technical aspects of audiometry. The wider aspects of audiometry have not been the subject of adequate research despite the many recommendations for its use"[1]. It is the contention of the authors of the present paper that the effect of monitoring audiometry on the usage of hearing protection within a plant in which no other means of noise control can be effected, constitutes one of the wider aspects referenced in the quotation given above, and that any increase in ear protector usage observed in response to a programme of monitoring audiometry, would represent a substantial additional benefit to both the employee and the employer. Hence, any cost benefit analysis performed upon the merits of industrial audiometry would be more likely to result in the conclusion that monitoring audiometry is a worthwhile exercise.

Pelmear[12] states that usage of ear protection rises in factories in which audiometry is regularly performed. However, Pelmear concedes that this statement was based upon casual observation,[14] and not a controlled study.

This paper presents the results of a study which was designed to investigate those parameters which most affect the success of a hearing conservation programme in industry, and as such evaluated the effect of monitoring audiometry upon ear protector usage by employees working in excessive industrial noise. Comparison was also made of the relative merits of audiometry and the presentation of educational material designed to raise the awareness of noise as a hazard to the hearing, in terms of the increased usage of hearing protection achieved.

METHOD
The experimental design
The site chosen for the study was large, and was owned by a single company. The industrial complex consisted of a large number of closely grouped plants on several thousand acres of land. The general diversity in nature of the plants with a noise problem was thought to increase the overall applicability of the results obtained from the research programme. The site also possessed a well-equipped medical centre, with audiometric facilities, which acted as a locus for coordination of the study.

Eight plants were selected for participation in the experiments, and were sub-divided into four groups. The selection and allocation of plants to each of the groups was made after consideration of six factors. These were: the measured noise levels, the distribution of noise sources and employees within the plants, the type of industrial process undertaken on the plants, the approximate size of the workforce, the levels of ear protector usage pre-dating the beginning of this study, and finally, the criterion that no plant participating in the research programme should have been exposed to educational material describing the hazard to the hearing represented by excessive industrial noise later than 18 months prior to commencement of the study. Care was also taken to ensure that employees from each of the plants did not come into contact with employees from other plants participating in the study.

The noise levels within the various plants were measured using both sound level meters, and personal noise dosemeters. It was stressed to those employees who carried a personal noise dosemeter for a working shift, that the results of the noise measurements would be used for research purposes only, and would not be shown to either management or trade union bodies. It would appear from comparison of the results of the noise dosemeter survey, and the sound level meter survey, that under the conditions pertaining to this study the noise dosemeter readings returned by employees were accurate representations of their exposure to industrial noise. The results of the dosemeter measurements for each plant are shown in Figure 1.

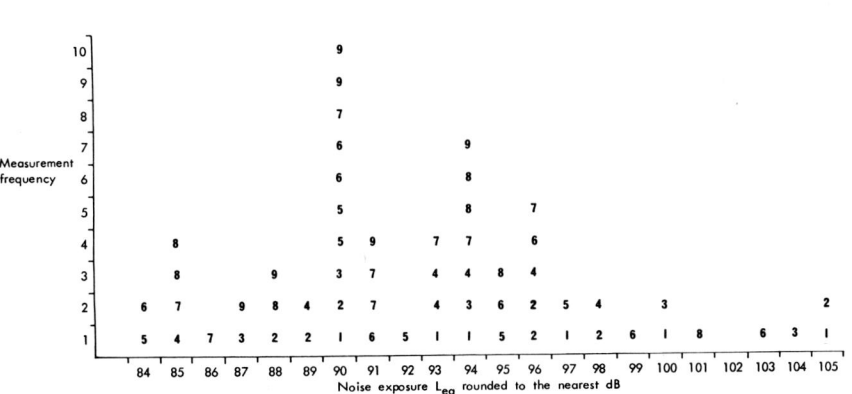

Figure 1. The distribution of L_{eq} noise exposure measurements made in the eight plants.

The optimum grouping of the plants in respect of the six factors described above is shown in Figure 2. A different treatment was assigned to each group. Serial monitoring audiometry was performed on employees working in plants belonging to Group 1. Employees on plants within the second

Audiometry	Education	Audiometry and Education	Control
Plant 1 N = 198	Plant 3 N = 311	Plant 5 N = 224	Plant 7 N = 143
Plant 2 N = 175	Plant 4 N = 180	Plant 6 N = 247	Plant 8 N = 238

Figure 2. The experimental plan and the treatments.

group were exposed to educational material describing the hazard to the hearing represented by excessive industrial noise. Employees from plants of the third group were subjected to both serial audiometry and an educational programme, whilst the fourth group of plants acted as a control.

The Treatments
1. Education

A video tape was produced using site and university facilities, for use in the research programme. This video tape was seen by all employees on any plants within a group in which education was a treatment, except in the case of Plant 3. On this plant only shifts W and Z saw the video tape, in order that a precise estimate of the effectiveness of the film could be made by comparing hearing protector usage by employees on these two shifts with that observed on shifts X and Y.

The centre portion of the video tape consisted of a commercially produced film "It's Nice to Hear" which described the necessity to use ear protection in excessive noise, and industrial noise as a hazard to the hearing. The film was recorded with the permission of the company to whom the film belonged, Bilsom International Ltd. The initial and final sections were recorded both at the university and on the industrial site. These sections were designed to achieve the general aims of the hearing conservation programme, to promote the usage of hearing protection, and to increase employee cooperation with specific research programme activities, such as the completion of certain questionnaires on noise, and attendance at the site Medical Centre for an audiometric test, where appropriate. The video tape was 20 minutes in length, and was watched by groups of a convenient size at times which did not disrupt plant production.

A poster campaign was the second educational method used in the research programme. Quantities of six designs of poster advocating the use of hearing protection were obtained, and regular poster changes were effected on the relevant plants during the research period.

2.   Audiometry

The audiometric tests performed as a part of the research programme were required to fulfil two functions. Firstly, encouragement of employees to use hearing protection, both by implication and by direct encouragement from the medical staff performing the test. Secondly, to provide a measure of the hearing acuity of employees working in the relevant plants.

Each individual required for an audiometric test was requested to attend the site Medical Centre on two occasions separated in time by approximately 9 to 18 months. Second appointments were made for those individuals who failed to attend the clinic on the appropriate day. A further appointment was made for those individuals who failed to respond to these requests. After making allowance for those employees who left their plants during the study, approximately 80% of the appointments for an initial audiometric test were kept. Figure 3 shows this attendance percentage analysed by plant, reaching in the best case 95% and in the worst 60%.

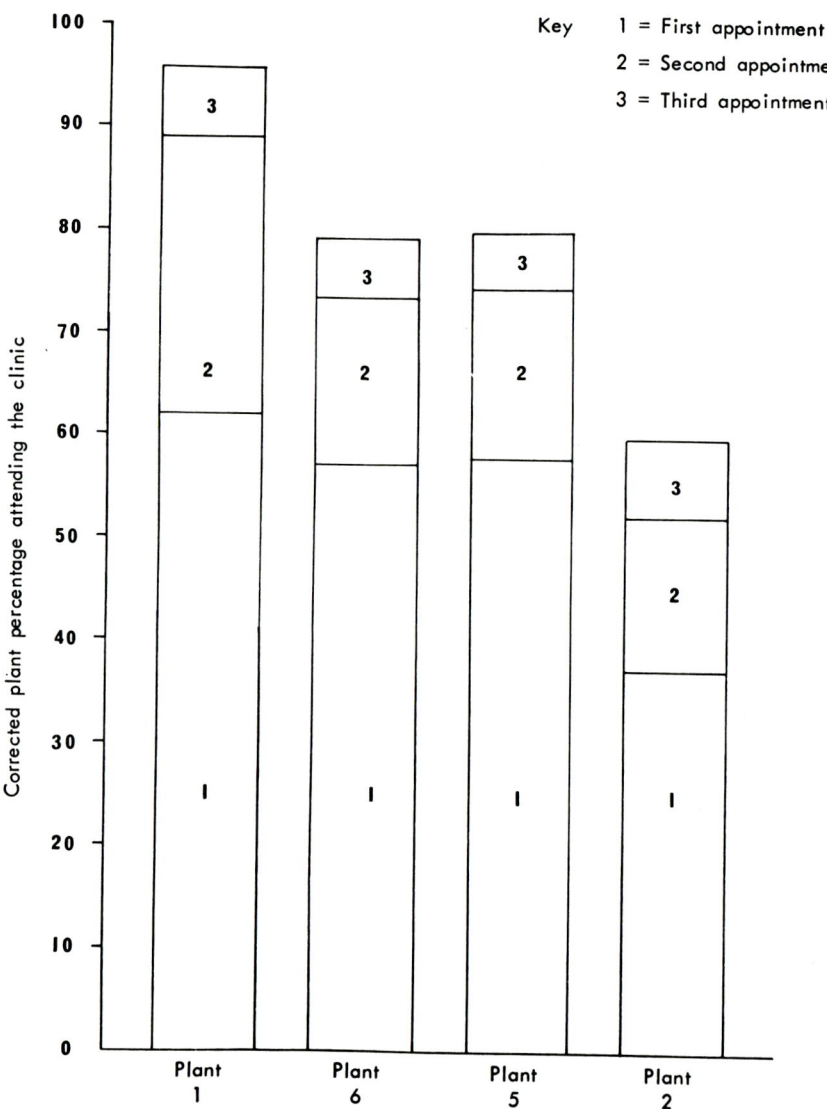

Figure 3. The percentage of the plant population attending the Medical Centre for a first audiometric test.

Agreement had been reached prior to commencement of the research programme, with trade union and management bodies, to the effect that all information pertaining to individual employees obtained during the study, would be confidential and seen only by members of the University research group. Accordingly employees were not officially informed of the results of their audiometric test, and it is felt probable that this policy resulted in only 56% of the employees who attended the clinic for an initial audiogram returning for their second 9 to 18 months later. The attendance for a second audiometric test was distributed between plants in a similar manner to that shown in Figure 3.

It was decided to call only a few men from each plant for audiometric test each day, rather than to test intensively for a period of several weeks, in order that employees might appreciate that the programme of audiometry was an on-going exercise. In this manner employees on these plants would receive a constant stimulus towards increasing their use of hearing protection in a noisy environment.

Methods of Measuring the Success of the Treatment on the Plants

1.   Attitude Questionnaires

Questionnaires designed to measure the attitudes held by employees towards components of a hearing conservation programme were specially developed during the study. The questionnaires were dispatched prior to commencement of the plant treatments and at their termination, thus monitoring any attitude change over the experimental period. Care was taken to ensure that a sufficiently long period was allowed to elapse between dispatch of the first round of attitude questionnaires and the commencement of the plant treatments, in order to prevent any possible interaction. Full results from the questionnaires will be reported in a later paper. Initial results have been described in an earlier paper[19].

2.   The Usage of Hearing Protection

The attitude questionnaires were of value in assessing the change in employee opinions resulting from the plant treatments. However, attitude change is not always mirrored by a behavioural change. Accordingly 160 visits were made to plants participating in the main study, to measure the percentage of employees using hearing protection whilst working in an area containing a noise hazard. An increase in this percentage was used as an index of the success of the relevant plant

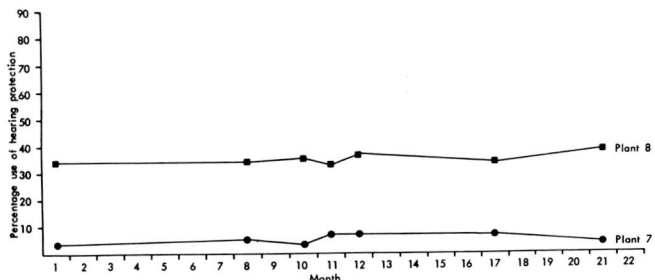

Figure 4. The percentage usage of hearing protection in the control plants over the experimental period.

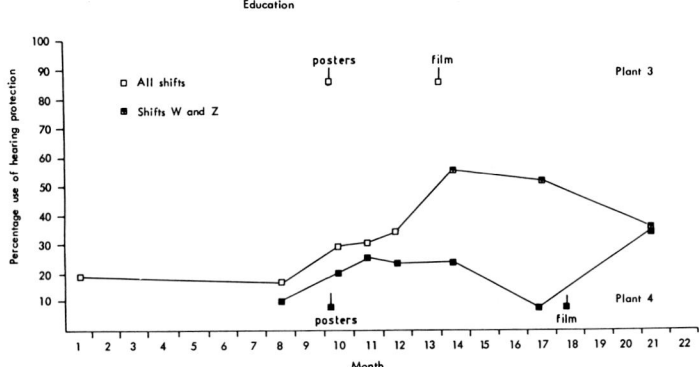

Figure 5. The percentage usage of hearing protection in the plants receiving education as a treatment over the experimental period.

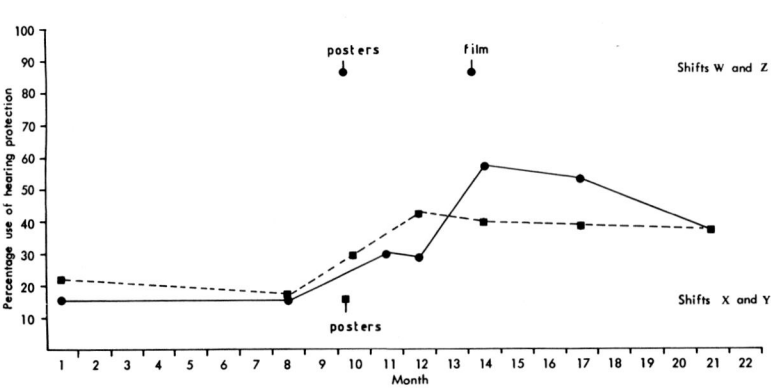

Figure 6. The percentage usage of hearing protection in plant 3, by shifts.

EMPLOYEE ATTITUDES

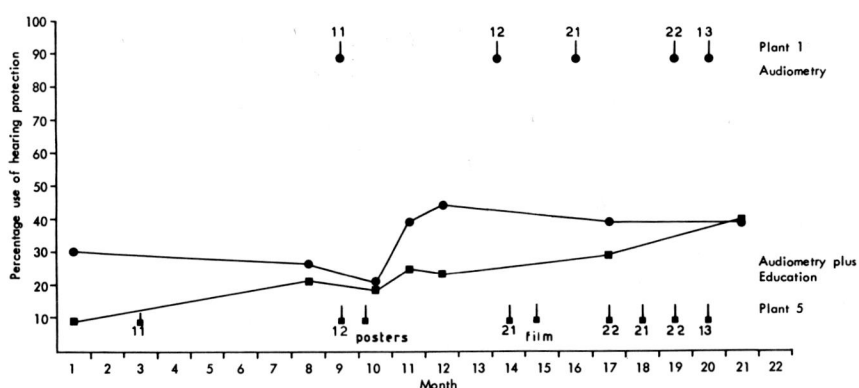

Figure 7. A comparison of the percentage usage of hearing protection in plants 1 and 5 over the experimental period.

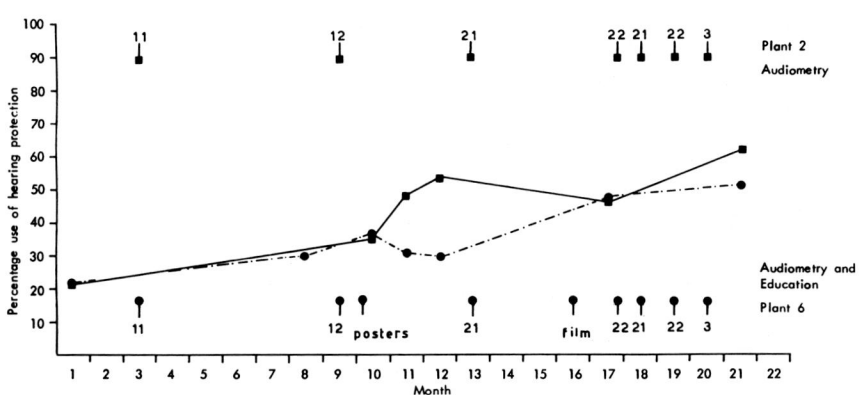

Figure 8. A comparison of the percentage usage of hearing protection in plants 2 and 6 over the experimental period.

Key to figures 7, 8 11 and 12
The two digit numbers used in the above figures represent the starting date of different stages of the audiometric survey.

11   First audiometric test, first appointment
12   First audiometric test, second appointment
21   Second audiometric test, first appointment
22   Second audiometric test, second appointment
13   First audiometric test, third appointment

treatment.

The visits were made to the plants at random times of the day, with the provision that no visit was made to a plant at a time when it was known that a substantial proportion of the workforce would either be taking a meal or work break. Observation of hearing protector usage was made without prior warning to the employees, and passage around each plant was rapid, following a pre-set path which had been chosen to permit examination, as far as was possible, of all individuals present in an area containing a noise hazard. Any employee who was not wearing earmuffs and had a hair style such that his ear canals could not be observed was deemed to be not wearing ear protection. These individuals comprised a very small proportion of the workforce.

RESULTS AND DISCUSSION

The results of the assessment of hearing protector usage during the experimental period in each of the eight plants are given in Figures 4, 5, 6, 7 and 8. On average each data point plotted represents the percentage of employees wearing hearing protection on three of the four shifts operated by the company, except in the case of plant 4 which employed only day workers. Plant 4 was therefore visited twice at different times on a single day to obtain the estimate of plant hearing protector usage.

The time at which each of the various treatments was initiated is also shown on the figures. The two-digit numbers shown above the curves relating to those plants whose employees attended the Medical Centre for audiometric tests, represent the commencement of various phases of the audiometric survey on these plants. The key to these digits is given prior to Figure 7.

The results will be examined in four sections. Firstly, the change in hearing protector usage observed in the control plants. Secondly, the effect of education upon the usage of hearing protection; thirdly, the effect of serial audiometry upon the use of ear protectors; and finally, the relative effectiveness of audiometry and education in increasing the

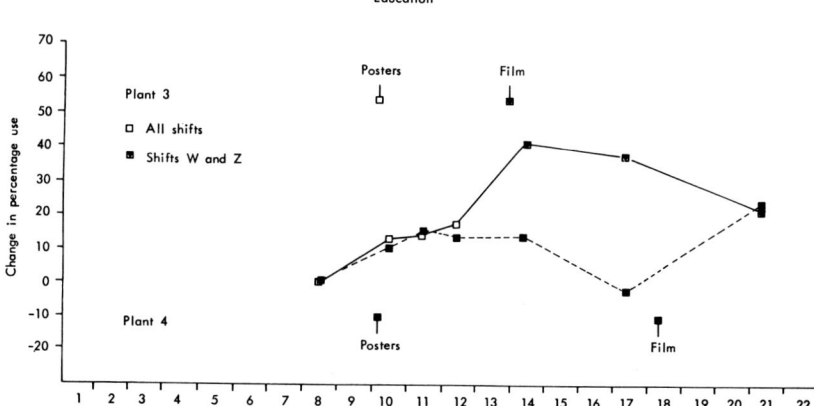

Figure 9. The change in hearing protector use in the plants receiving education as a treatment over the experimental period.

wearing of hearing protection on an industrial site.

1. The Control Plants

Figures 4 and 13 show the hearing protector usage on the control plants during the experimental period. As can be seen, no significant change in the usage of ear protection in these plants was measured. Therefore any change in hearing protector usage observed in the non-control plants can be ascribed to the experimental treatments.

2. The Effect of Education Upon Hearing Protector Usage

Figure 9 shows the change in hearing protector usage occurring as a consequence of the poster campaign used in the plants receiving education alone. It can be seen that in both plants, the poster campaign has resulted in an increase in the number of employees using hearing protection, of approximately 15% between months 8 and 12. The observations made in month 12 represent the last measurements of hearing protector usage obtained prior to showing the film on plant 3.

Two steps were taken to ascertain if the use of hearing protection would have continued to increase on plant 3 without the additional educational

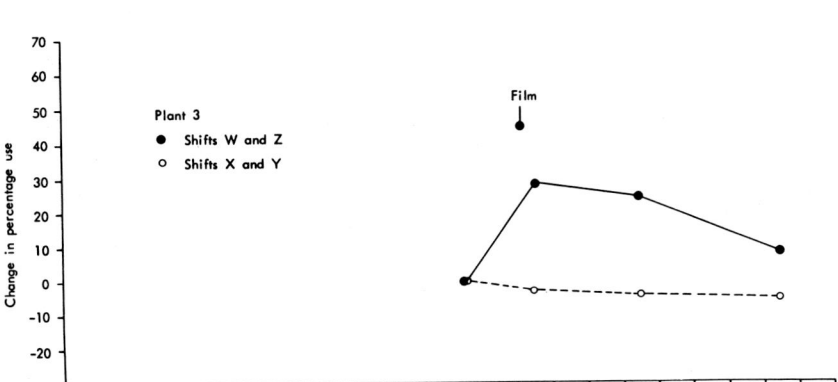

Figure 10. The change in hearing protector use in plant 3, by shifts, over the experimental period.

effect of the film. Firstly, as described in the section on Education, the film was shown to only two of the four working shifts on plant 3. Secondly, the showing of the video tape on plant 4 was delayed for approximately 5 months.

Lacking the additional benefit of the film, the hearing protector usage on plant 4 remained approximately constant between months 12 and 14, and then decreased, until the video tape was shown in month 18. A showing of the video tape on plant 3 appears to have prevented this decrease from occurring, and increased the usage of hearing protection on the plant by approximately a further 25%. A similar increase in the percentage usage of ear protection by employees working in plant 4 was also observed when the film was shown in month 18. This finding would imply that the observed effects of the showing of the film, and of the poster campaign, are additive.

The data shown in Figure 10 reinforce the point made in the previous paragraph that hearing protector usage by shifts W and Z would not have risen to the level observed in month 14 on plant 3 had the film not been shown. From the data obtained from shifts X and Y, which did not see the

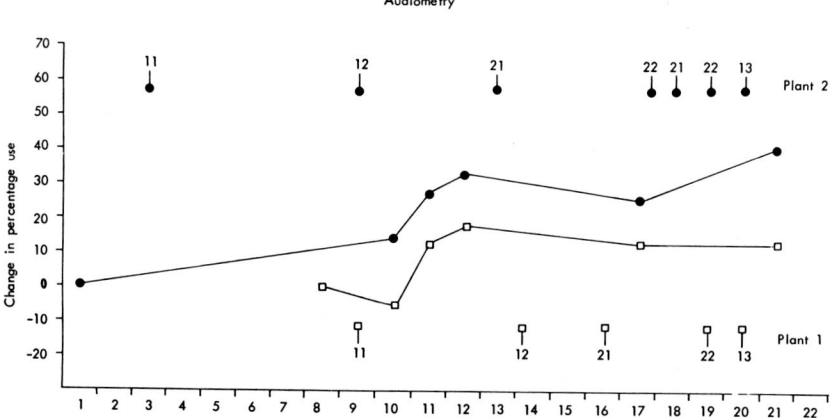

Figure 11. The change in hearing protector use in the plants receiving audiometry as a treatment, over the experimental period.

film, it would appear that the effects of the poster campaign alone lasted for at least 12 months. Figure 9, however, indicates that the poster campaign on plant 4 became ineffective after approximately 7 months.

Showing the video tape to only two shifts out of the four in plant 3 also enabled the length of time for which the educational film remained effective, to be assessed. Referring again to Figure 10, the curve for shifts W and Z shows that after an initial increase in the level of ear protector usage, which can be ascribed to the effects of the video tape, the number of employees wearing hearing protectors decreased regularly in the following months. Extrapolation of the hearing protector usage curves for shifts W and Z and shifts X and Y would indicate, given that a poster campaign and an educational film have additive effects upon the usage of hearing protection, that the overall effectiveness of the film had become negligible within 11 months of the original showing.

3. <u>The Effect of Serial Audiometry Upon Hearing Protector Usage</u>

Figure 11 shows the change in the use of ear protection by employees on those plants assigned audiometry as a treatment.

The maximum gain was made on plant 2, in which the wearing of hearing protectors increased by approximately 40% over the experimental period. The programme of audiometric tests did not produce such a large change in hearing protector usage in plant 1. The maximum increase observed was approximately 20%, decreasing to approximately 15% by the end of the experimental period. The overall gains observed in plants 1 and 2 do not correlate with the plant attendance figures for an audiometric test, as can be seen from Figure 3. Approximately 95% of employees working in plant 1 attended for an audiometric test, whilst the corresponding figure in plant 2 was 60%.

The difference between these two plants in terms of the increase in hearing protector usage observed during the experimental period is thought to be allied to the spacing of the audiometric tests in time.

The first round of audiometric tests was completed on employees from plant 1 in a period which was approximately 30% shorter than that used for employees in plant 2. Whilst this difference may have contributed to the greater number of individuals attending the clinic for an audiometric test from plant 1, it may have given the audiometric programme the ambience of a routine industrial health screening exercise, reducing the overall impact on the attitudes of the employees. Moreover, in testing employees from plant 2, the pattern of appointments for a second audiometric test in the monitoring series was altered, from that used for employees drawn from plant 1. This is thought to be responsible for the upturn in protector usage between months 17 and 21 observed on plant 2, as opposed to the unchanged percentage of employees using hearing protection measured over the same period in plant 1. It could be hypothesised that employees are responding to the stimulus represented by the onset of different phases of the audiometric programme rather than to the content of the stimulus itself.

Therefore, it is likely that if an additional stimulus is provided by ensuring that each employee is informed of the results of his audiometric test, it is possible that the benefit offered by industrial audiometry in terms of promoting the wearing of hearing protection on a plant, would be greatly increased.

The similarity in shape between the curves for plants 1 and 2 is of interest. The peaks in the numbers of employees wearing ear protectors occurring during months 10, 11 and 12, could have arisen as a consequence of the beginning of a major new phase in the audiometric programme. If it had been possible to make an assessment of protector usage in plant 2 soon after the inception of the audiometric programme on this plant, similar peaking might have been observed. An identical argument could be advanced for months 14 and 16 on both plants 1 and 2. Lack of such an observed peak in months 17 to 21 in the hearing protector usage curve for plant 1 could be ascribed to the previously stated argument; that is, the lack of variation in the pattern of the audiometric tests, allied to the shorter period of time used to complete the audiometric programme, could have reduced the impact.

4. The Effect of Both Education and Audiometry Upon Hearing Protector Usage

Figure 12 shows the increase in the percentage of employees wearing ear protectors on those plants in which the experimental treatment consisted of audiometry and an educational programme. Both plants 5 and 6 showed a similar response in that a progressive increase in hearing protector usage was observed, an increase which reached a maximum value at the end of the study period of approximately 30%. It would be unproductive to attempt to apportion this overall gain in terms of that to be ascribed to each of the three major components of the treatment; that is, the audiometric testing, the poster campaign, and the video tape. However, it is of note that the maximum change in hearing protector usage attained using both monitoring audiometry and educational material, was less than was achieved on plant 2 using audiometry alone. It is not to be suggested that any hearing conservation programme need contain only an audiometric component and no educational material, but rather that industrial monitoring audiometry could produce the desired effect in terms of increased usage of hearing protection, even if the educational component

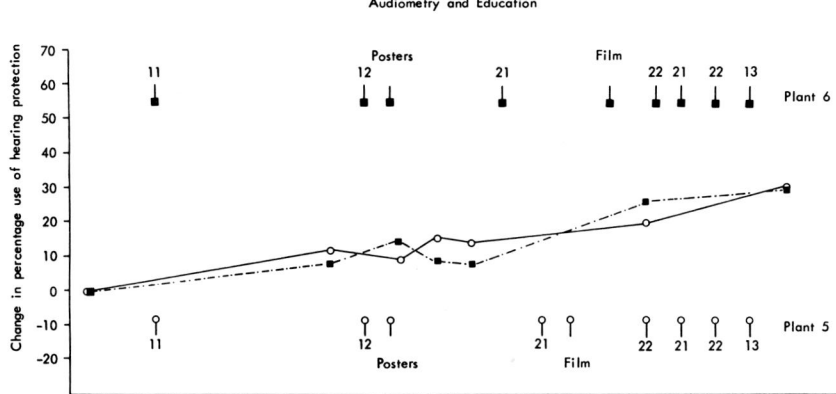

Figure 12. The change in hearing protector use in the plants receiving audiometry and education as a treatment over the experimental period.

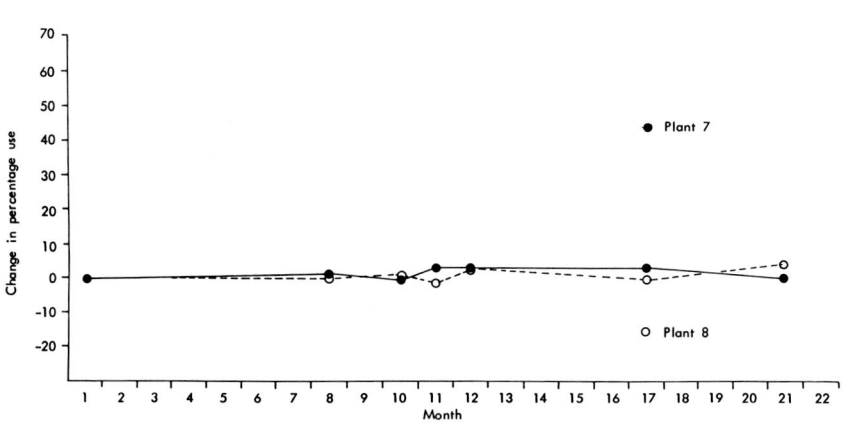

Figure 13. The change in hearing protector use in the control plants over the experimental period.

of the hearing conservation programme was to be kept in a low key, that is informative rather than of the nature of propaganda.

CONCLUSIONS

The results of the study showed that an educational programme designed to increase the awareness of a workforce that excessive levels of industrial noise represent a hazard to the hearing, was capable of improving the level of hearing protector usage on plants containing a noise hazard. The maximum effect of a film, in terms of achieving the desired increase in the number of employees making use of their hearing protectors, is greater than that of a poster campaign, but appears to decay within about 11 months. The results also indicated that it is best assumed that a poster campaign will become ineffective within 7 months.

The main finding of the study was that a programme of monitoring audiometry is capable of increasing the usage of ear protection on a plant. However, the overall success achieved is dependent upon maintaining the interest of the workforce in the audiometric programme, by not permitting it to fall into a routine pattern. It is also suggested that the plant employees respond to the stimulus afforded by the programme of monitoring audiometry, rather than to the content of the audiometry itself. This potential for industrial audiometry to act as a stimulus on the workforce to use ear protection would probably be increased if employees were informed of the results of their audiometric tests. It would also be beneficial if the minimum number of employees each day were called for an audiometric test, thus maximising the number of days each year for which members of the plant were attending the Medical Centre for a hearing acuity test.

It is also of note that the greatest increase in the numbers of employees using hearing protection on a plant participating in the study was observed in plant 2, in which audiometry was the only component of the treatment.

Whilst the plants receiving both industrial audiometry and education as a treatment showed a more regular increase in hearing protector usage over the experimental period than observed in response to either of the other two treatments, the overall result was not the summation of the effect of each of the two components of the treatment, audiometry and education. The same level of success, in terms of an increase in hearing protector usage was not observed in either of these two plants as was measured in response to audiometry alone undertaken in plant 2.

It is suggested that as audiometry can be used as a medium for employee education, traditional educational methods can be kept at a low intensity, that is, informative rather than attitude-changing exer cises. Thus the spacing in time between educational films could be increased on plants implementing programmes of industrial audiometry.

The major conclusion of the study is that industrial audiometry represents a very cost effective component of a hearing conservation programme, for in addition to its role as a monitor of physiological function, audiometry possesses a strong additional attribute in that it contributes significantly to employee education in the hazard represented by industrial noise, and is capable of changing behavioural patterns; in particular hearing protector usage.

ACKNOWLEDGEMENTS

The authors would like to acknowledge the invaluable assistance of Dr. S. Jenkin-Evans during the original research programme culminating in the work described in this paper. The authors would also like to thank Professor R.R.A. Coles for his much appreciated input into the research work, and the manufacturing company on whose site the study was conducted.

REFERENCES
1.   Atherley, G.R.C., Duncan, J.A., Williamson, K.S., The value of audiometry in industry. Journal Soc. Occup. Med. 23 19-21, 1973.

2.   Atherley, G.R.C., Problems of industrial audiometry. Ann. Occup. Hygiene. 7, 335-341, 1964.

3.   Atherley, G.R.C., Occupational deafness. Diagnosis, assessment and some pointers against audiometry. Update 7, 1565-1570, 1973.

4.   Burns, W., Robinson, D.W., Hearing and noise in industry. H.M.S.O., London, 1970.

5.   Burns, W., Robinson, D.W., Audiometry in Industry. J. Soc. Occup. Med. 23, 86-91, 1973.

6.   Harris, J.D., Letter to the editor. Sound and Vibration, June, 16, 1974.

7. Hartley, B.P.R., Howell, R.W., Sinclair, A., Slattery, D.A.P., Subject variability in short term audiometric recording. Brit. J. Indust. Med. 30, 271-275, 1973.

8. Howell, R.W., Hartley, B.P.R., Variability in audiometric recording. Brit. J. Indust. Med. 29, 432-435, 1972.

9. Karmy, S.J., Wright, A.P., Cooke, W.G., Industrial audiometry; the referral problem. Disorders of Auditory Function III, Ed. I.G. Taylor Academic Press. 197-209, 1979.

10. Martin, A.M., Industrial hearing conservation 2: audiometry. Noise Control Vibration and Insulation. March, 1976.

11. Noble, W.G., Monitoring audiometry: protection for whom?. 1978 Proc. of the 1978 Annual Conf. of the Australian Acous. Soc., Ed. Waugh, R.L., Macrae, J.H., National Acoustical Laboratories, Sydney, Australia. 164-177.

12. Pelmear, P.L., Hearing conservation. 1973. J. Soc. Occup. Med. 23, 22-26, 1973.

13. Pelmear, P.L., Hughes, B.J., Self-recording audiometry in industry. Brit. J. Indust. Med. 31, 304-309, 1974.

14. Pelmear, P.L., Personal Communication, 1975.

15. Somerville, E.T., Noise induced hearing loss and industrial audiometry. J. Royal Coll. Gen. Practitioners, 26, 770-780, 1976.

16. Taylor, W., The Weavers of Dundee. 1972, Trans. Soc. Occup. Med. 22, 37-43, 1972.

17. The editor. Letters to the editor. 1973. J. Soc. Occup. Med. 23, 22-26, 1973.

18. Wilmot, T.J., The meaning of modern audiological tests in relation to noise induced deafness. Brit. J. Indust. Med. 29, 125-133, 1972.

19. Karmy, S.J., Martin, A.M., Hearing conservation; attitudes in industry. Proc. of the 9th I.C.A. Madrid, 1977.

Personal Hearing Protection in Industry, edited by P. W. Alberti, Raven Press, New York ©

31 METHODS OF EVALUATING HEARING CONSERVATION PROGRAM AUDIOMETRIC DATA BASES

Larry H. Royster and Julia D. Royster

INTRODUCTION

There is a need for objective procedures for evaluating the effectiveness of a hearing conservation program (HCP) in preventing a noise induced hearing loss. The fact that a HCP is well thought out and well administered is no guarantee that the program is in reality effective. As a result of problems in the utilization of hearing protection devices (HPDs) and of limitations in the degree of protection afforded by HPDs in real-world environments, the only reliable estimate of the actual protection being provided comes from analyzing the audiometric data base.

The U. S. Departament of Labor has not had a consistent policy requiring employers to conduct audiometric exams and to evaluate the resulting data. Therefore, audiometric data are not available nationwide as an indicator of how well the hearing of noise exposed populations is being protected. Fortunately for North Carolina employees, general industry and the N. C. Department of Labor initially realized the potential benefits of including audiometric testing as part of an overall HCP. The recommendations developed for HCPs in North Carolina during the late sixties and early seventies included five phases as follows: education, sound surveys, engineering and administrative controls, hearing protection and audiometric testing. Equally important was a set of basic guidelines for conducting the audiometric exams, technician certification, audiometric calibration procedures, evaluating the audiometric data base, etc. In addition, the Occupational Safety & Health Administration (OSHA-NC) administrators considered the results of audiometric exams along with efforts on the part of the company in the other areas of the HCP in determining compliance or non-compliance with the noise standard.

As a result of the emphasis on audiometric testing, an extensive audiometric data base has been compiled for North Carolina employees working in industrial and nonindustrial high noise areas. Audiometric testing environments and procedures have been relatively consistent across the facilities that have implemented HCPs. Extensive initial educational programs developed in cooperation with OSHA-NC helped ensure consistent methods for companies which began their own testing programs. For companies which rely on private audiometric testing services, their procedures are monitored by reviewing the OSHA-NC health and safety reports. As part of the overall effort to assist industry in conducting and evaluating audiometric tests, and in conjunction with a grant awarded to N. C. State University by the Rockefeller Foundation, a program was initiated to define the characteristics of the industrial audiometric data base. The goals of this part of the grant objective were the development of general guidelines for evaluating industrial audiometric data bases, the development of a computer program for evaluating a company's audiometric data base that could be implemented in-house and the provision of a service to industry through the evaluation of the data.

To date over 40 industries in North Carolina and surrounding states have made their audiometric data sets available for analysis. The size of the data sets varies from 50 to 15,000 employees, and in some cases over 12 years of audiometric test results are included. For a significant number of the data sets, complete medical histories, audiometric and test room calibration results and general noise survey findings are available. Fortunately for both the employee and the employer, this very productive working relationship with industry has been maintained.

The analysis of the multiple data sets within the North Carolina data base has revealed several general characteristics which are consistent across data sources representing employees from different regions and socio-economic groups. The most important population parameters identified across data sets are the differences in hearing ability among race and sex subgroups and the "learning effect". Prior to the identification of these two parameters, attempts had failed to correlate changes in employees' mean hearing threshold levels ($\overline{HTL}$s) as indicated by the audiometric data with known employee noise exposures or with the proper use of HPDs. Only after the significant variance contribu-tions of the population race and sex composition and of the "learning effect" were accounted for during analysis did a consistent relationship become apparent between HTL data, noise exposures and the use of HPDs.

Several of the procedures developed to analyze audiometric data sets, discussed below, are used to assess HCP effectiveness. It is believed that the first order factors which influence the variability in industrial audiometric data sets have been isolated. However, as more data sets are analyzed, additional factors may be identified and simpler techniques may be developed for evaluating HCP audiometric data.

GENERAL CONSIDERATIONS

In attempting to evaluate the effectiveness of the audiometric testing phase of a HCP it is desirable to compare the $\overline{HTL}$s of the noise exposed employees with those of a reference population. There exist at least two possible but contrasting types of reference populations. One of the available presbycusis data bases could be used.[1] However, the developers of these data bases have attempted to exclude such contaminating effects as sociocusis, pathological problems, etc., in order to isolate the effects of advancing age on hearing. Since it can be assumed that the typical industrial population would exhibit the types of contamination that are minimized in presbycusis populations, a comparison made between the HTLs and the changes in HTLs over time - the HTL's - of an industrial population and those of a screened presbycusis population would unfairly penalize the credibility of the industrial HCP.

A more realistic type of reference population would consist of subjects who exhibit all of the pathological and non-occupational hearing hazards which affect the industrial population except, of course, industrial noise exposure. Such a population has been established and is referred to as a NINEP -- that is, a nonindustrial noise exposed population.[2]

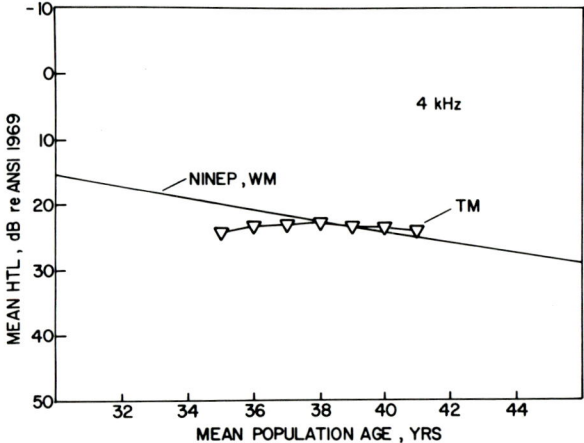

Figure 1. Variations in $\overline{HTL}$s at 4kHz over seven audiograms for a racially mixed total male (TM) INEP compared to the smoothed HTL curve for a WM NINEP at corresponding population ages.

Figure 1 shows the variations in the $\overline{HTL}$s at the 4 kHz audiometric test frequency over seven tests for a total male (TM) industrial noise exposed population (INEP). The population was restricted to only those employees who had each been given seven tests, and the mean age of this constant population at each test is indicated. Also shown plotted in Figure 1 are the smoothed HTLs with advancing age for the white male (WM) NINEP. One quickly realizes from these data, that whereas the HTLs for the WM NINEP are steadily worsening with age, the $\overline{HTL}$s for the INEP seem to improve with age as indicated by more sensitive $\overline{HTL}$s over several tests. This tendency for indicated improvement to occur in the $\overline{HTL}$s of an INEP at least partially protected from noise by a HCP known to be working has been termed the "learning curve" or "learning effect" for lack of a better description at this time.[3,4] If the NINEP had been given several audiometric tests over some time period, then a similar "learning effect" would be anticipated in their data.[3] However, the NINEP curve is obtained by smoothing the HTLs of subjects tested only once, so it is not influenced by the learning factor. Because this male INEP was known to have experienced a significant industrial noise exposure prior to the time of

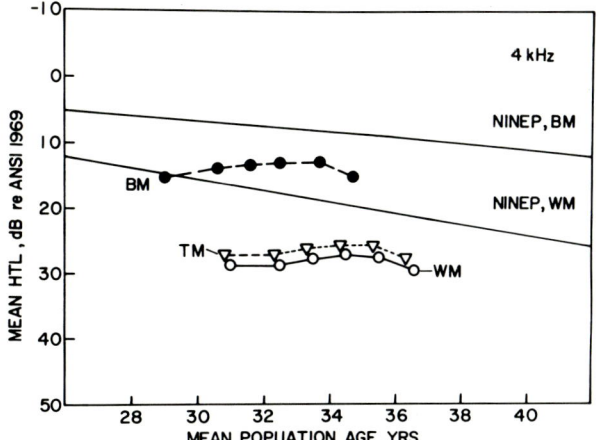

Figure 2. Variations in $\overline{\text{HTL}}$s at 4 kHz over seven audiograms for the WM, BM, and total male (TM) INEPs compared to the smoothed HTL curves for the WM and BM NINEPs at corresponding population ages.

their first audiometric test, the close approximation of the male INEP's initial $\overline{\text{HTL}}$ with the WM NINEP's HTL could not be justified. This lack of a substantial discrepancy between INEP $\overline{\text{HTL}}$s and NINEP HTLs has been noted in numerous data sets.[4]

Such conflicts can be eliminated by separating an INEP into subpopulations grouped by race and sex and then comparing these restricted INEP subgroups to NINEPs appropriately matched by race and sex classification. The resulting comparisons for another typical male INEP at the 4 kHz test frequency are shown in Figure 2. After separation by race the $\overline{\text{HTL}}$s for the BM and WM INEPs are observed to be appropriately poorer at the initial audiogram than the HTLs at the same age for their matching NINEPs. Due to the "learning effect" the INEP $\overline{\text{HTL}}$s for several successive tests approach their respective NINEP curves. When the "learning effect" diminishes, the curves may either become parallel, or they may diverge due to inadequately protected exposure to occupational noise.

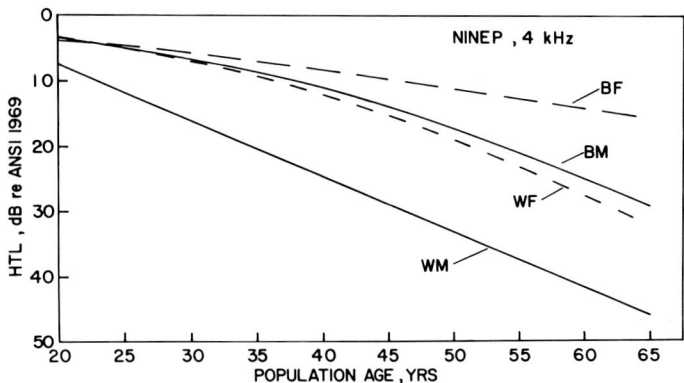

Figure 3. Smoothed HTL curves at 4 kHz for the BF, BM, WF, and WM NINEPs as a function of age.

Based on the relationship of the TM $\overline{\text{HTL}}$s to those of the WM and BM subgroups in Figure 2, one can easily visualize the variety of possible conclusions that could be reached regarding the effectiveness of the HCP associated with the data depending on the relative percentages of BMs and WMs in the INEP, and on which reference population was used for comparison. The BM NINEP exhibits significantly better hearing than the WM NINEP at every age. Equally importantly, the BM NINEP HTL curve also displays a smaller $(\overline{\text{HTL}})^1$ with advancing age over the age range shown. As will be elaborated upon later, one indication that a HCP is effective in preventing on-the-job noise induced hearing loss is approximately equal values for the $(\overline{\text{HTL}})$'s of an INEP and its matching NINEP.

Reference NINEPs for each race and sex group[3,5] have been established for use in evaluating the effectiveness of HCPs in protecting the hearing of INEPs. Presented as Figure 3 are the smoothed HTL curves for each NINEP at the 4 kHz test frequency. There are obvious significant differences in HTLs among the race and sex groups as a function of age. The BF, BM, and WF NINEP curves display increasing $(\overline{\text{HTL}})$'s with advancing age, similar to findings for presbycusis data bases, even though the NINEPs include some subjects with ear pathology, gunfire exposure,

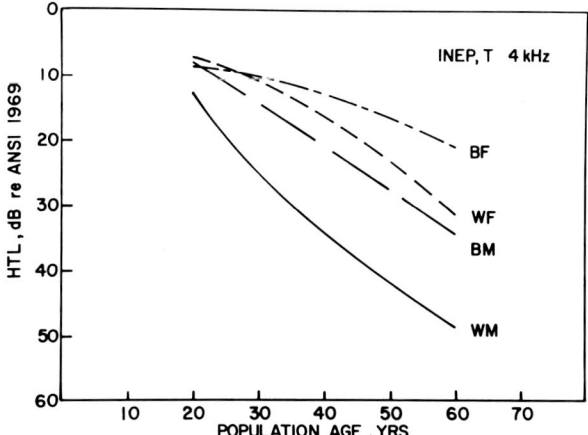

Figure 4. Smoothed HTL curves at 4 kHz for the BF, WF, BM, and WM INEPs as a function of age.

military service, etc. In fact, if the male presbycusis HTL data collected by Robinson and Sutton[6] were normalized to the median HTLs for our 18-year olds, the resulting presbycusis population curve would fall below (i.e., showing poorer hearing) the BM NINEP curve,[1] but with similar positive curvature. In contrast, note how the (HTL)[1] for the WM NINEP curve does not increase with advancing age, resulting in a near lack of curvature. This contrast is important because it may indicate that the WM NINEP's HTLs have been influenced significantly more by non-occupational noise exposure than those of the other NINEPs. The WF and WM NINEP data presented in Figure 3 are based on the addition of new subjects to the data which were previously published.[3]

Shown in Figure 4 are the smoothed HTLs at the 4 kHz test frequency for a large INEP plotted as a function of population age.[7] Comparison of Figures 3 and 4 reveals basic similarities between the NINEP and INEP data, but important differences are also evident. The effect of industrial noise exposure on HTLs is indicated by the contrast of the positive curvature for the BM NINEP curve with the near absence of curvature for the BM INEP curve. The comparable effect of industrial noise exposure on the WM HTL data results in an obvious negative curvature for the WM INEP curve.

The preceding examples illustrate the need to divide INEP audiometric data into race and sex classifications before attempting to assess the effectiveness of a HCP in protecting employees' hearing. These examples also demonstrate the need to compare the subgroup $\overline{\text{HTL}}$s with matched NINEP HTLs in order to determine the impact of industrial noise exposure while controlling for the pathological and non-occupational factors shared by INEP and NINEP subjects. In addition to nonindustrial noise exposure and industrial noise exposure, other factors which can potentially influence HTL measurements include the normal aging process or presbycusis, systematic variations in the mean temporary threshold shift for the population at the time of testing and the "learning effect".

If it is assumed that the employees who constitute an INEP had no experience with audiometric testing before their first industrial audiograms, then the magnitude of the mean industrial noise induced component of the population's hearing loss at the time of their first test could be estimated by comparing the initial audiogram $\overline{\text{HTL}}$ for the INEP with the HTL of the appropriate NINEP at the same population age. If the INEP had more prior experience in taking audiometric exams than the NINEP, this assumption would lead to an underestimation of the industrial noise induced component of the mean hearing loss indicated for the INEP by their initial audiograms. Assuming that the INEP and the NINEP subjects would experience similar changes in their HTLs over time if the effect of industrial noise exposure were eliminated, then the curves for the INEP and NINEP would become parallel with advancing age unless the INEP had already sustained severe hearing loss. Consequently, an estimate of the magnitude of the "learning effect" for the INEP under study can be obtained by identifying the point where the INEP and NINEP curves become parallel, then projecting a curve parallel to the NINEP curve backwards in time from that point to the time of the initial audiogram. The difference between the HTL value of this line and the $\overline{\text{HTL}}$ of the

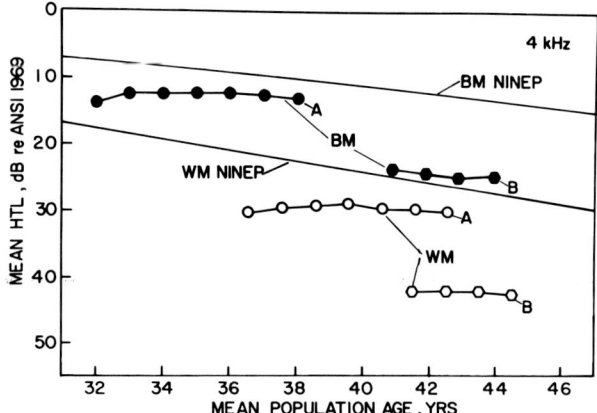

Figure 5. Variations in $\overline{\text{HTL}}$s at 4 kHz over seven audiograms for the BM and WM subgroups of two INEPs (A and B) compared to the smoothed HTL curves for the BM and WM NINEPs at corresponding population ages.

initial audiogram would be the amount of learning for that INEP assuming that no additional noise induced hearing loss were occurring.

As an illustration, consider the data in Figure 5, which represent the $\overline{\text{HTL}}$s measured at 4 kHz for two male INEPs which have been separated by race and restricted to constant groups of employees. For population A, whose hearing is protected by an effective HCP, the "learning effect" is estimated as 4-6 dB. Population B is not properly protected by an effective HCP; consequently, the potential "learning effect" is apparently cancelled out by progressive noise induced hearing loss for the BM subgroup, and the WM subgroup shows a limited "learning effect" since their $\overline{\text{HTL}}$s do not show the deterioration which would be expected due to unprotected noise exposure.

Support for the validity of the "learning effect" has been obtained by studying the changes in $\overline{\text{HTL}}$s for two industrial reference populations whose daily equivalent noise exposures based on a 3 dB doubling rate (L_{eq}s) were 85 dB(A) or less, for employees such as secretaries and warehouse personnel within industrial plants who are exposed to an L_{eq}

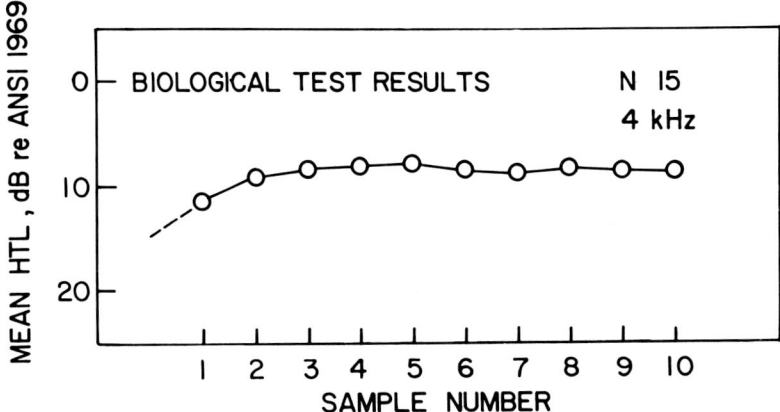

Figure 6. Variations in $\overline{\text{HTL}}$s at 4 kHz over ten audiograms for 15 biological test subjects.

less than 80 dB and for a group of 15 industrial nurses who provided biological checks of audiometric calibration. These nurses were first introduced to audiometric testing during a course to train them as industrial audiometric technicians. During training each individual received 3-4 hearing tests. Following training each nurse was required to take hearing exams approximately weekly for use as biological checks of the calibration and general operating condition of their audiometers. The resulting series of $\overline{\text{HTL}}$s at 4 kHz is presented as Figure 6. A "learning effect" of over 3 dB is indicated by these biological test series data. Since the individuals had received at least three complete audiometric exams prior to this series of measurements, the degree of learning would be estimated as greater if the $\overline{\text{HTL}}$s from the prior tests were available. One interesting similarity in the data presented in Figures 1, 5, and 6 is that the "learning effect" seems to reach an asymptote after 4-6 tests. When audiometric exams are given at intervals over either a short or long time period to a population whose hearing is not deteriorating due to unprotected exposure to excessive noise, measured $\overline{\text{HTL}}$s show apparent improvement in hearing over the first 4-6 tests.

The consistent pattern of significant differences found in the $\overline{\text{HTL}}$s of race and sex groups necessitates the subdivision of an INEP's audiometric

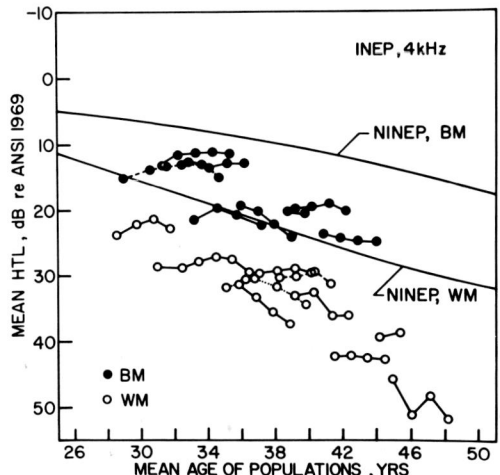

Figure 7. Variations in $\overline{HTL}$s at 4 kHz for BM and WM subgroups of ten INEPs compared to the smoothed HTL curves for the BM and WM NINEPs at corresponding population ages.

data by race and sex before attempting to evaluate the effectiveness of a HCP. Additional examples of the differences in $\overline{HTL}$s for BM and WM INEPs are shown in Figure 7, and similar differences have been reported between BF and WF $\overline{HTL}$s within INEPs.[7] Note in Figure 7 how the BM INEPs consistently fall below the BM NINEP curve and generally above the WM NINEP; likewise, the WM INEPs are grouped below the WM NINEP curve. The comparison of INEP group data to NINEP reference data enables the individual responsible for HCP evaluation to better isolate the noise induced hearing loss component of $\overline{HTL}$ changes. The magnitude of race and sex differences in $\overline{HTL}$s obviously requires that INEP subgroup data be compared to the HTLs of NINEPs matched by race and sex.

PROGRAM EVALUATION PROCEDURES
Individual and Population Evaluation Procedures
Evaluating the effectiveness of a HCP in preventing noise induced hearing loss requires at least two complementary procedures: the evaluation of the changes in each individual's hearing ability over time and the

evaluation of the total audiometric data set properly divided by race and sex into sub-populations and restricted to a constant group of employees.[8] It is very important that an individual's changes in hearing ability be properly documented and followed with appropriate response when significant shifts in HTLs are observed. However, a potentially superior procedure for evaluating the HCP's overall effectiveness is a detailed analysis of the population audiometric data. When a large data set is analyzed, small changes in the population's $\overline{HTL}$s of 2-3 dB or less become significant and meaningful because of the large number of subjects considered. Abnormal changes in the population's $\overline{HTL}$s, such as those indicated in Figure 2 between the 5th and 6th tests, have usually been traceable back to a change in the audiometric calibration procedure followed or the reference calibration utilized. In evaluating $\overline{HTL}$ data representing large restricted industrial populations, the evaluator should decrease his tolerance of threshold variability from the 5-10 dB range which is acceptable in lab or clinic testing of individual subjects to the much smaller tolerance range of 2-3 dB. Conversely, however, typical industrial audiometric test results for individual employees are characterized by much greater threshold variability than lab or clinic data because of the screening nature of industrial audiometry. It would be very unrealistic to assume that a shift of 10 dB from a previous industrial audiogram to a more recent test would represent a significant hearing deterioration, even for employees protected by an effective HCP.

If appropriately restricted subgroup data for an INEP are evaluated over time, significant small shifts in population $\overline{HTL}$s can be detected and the problems identified (poor calibration, improper HPD use, etc.) can be corrected before major shifts in individual employees' hearing ability begin to show up several years later.

Test-Retest Comparisons (TRCs)

One indicator of the changes occuring in population $\overline{HTL}$s is the percentage of employees who display shifts in their individual HTLs at various frequencies or frequency combinations. Shifts may be counted in several ways:

(1) by comparison of HTLs for a specific base hearing test to HTLs measured for later tests (first to second, first to third, etc.);

(2) by comparison of HTLs for an assumed baseline to HTLs measured for later tests (baseline to first, baseline to second, etc.);

(3) by sequential comparisons of HTLs for consecutive tests (first to second, second to third, third to fourth, etc.).

In making these comparisons it is important not only to look at the percentage of employees who indicated a worsening in their hearing based on the criterion selected, but it is equally important to consider the percentage of the population who indicated an improvement in their hearing.

Several criteria that have been used in evaluating the effectiveness of HCPs[4] are shown in Table I. Typical results obtained using categories 4, 5, and 10 are presented in Figures 8 and 9. The data shown were generated by first restricting the population by race and sex to a constant group of employees, then comparing thresholds between the first and second, first and third, etc., audiometric tests in both ears to see if shifts occurred which met the specified criterion. For category 4, as an example, the criterion for counting an employee is a HTL shift equal to or greater than 15 dB in either ear at any frequency indicated in Table I. If an employee's hearing improved by 15 dB or greater in either ear at .5, 1, 2, 3, 4, or 6 kHz, he was included in the "better" category. If his hearing got worse by the same amount, he was included in the "worse" category.

Based on our experience to date, the most important indicator generated using the TRC procedure is the ratio of the percent of the population that indicated better hearing at one or more frequencies to the percent of the population that indicated worse hearing at one or more frequencies (the %B/%W ratio). Shown in Table II are the observed $\%B_M/\%W_M$ ratios for several populations and the effectiveness of the corresponding HCPs as judged based on several different evaluation procedures. The $\%B_M/\%W_M$ ratio was obtained by identifying the maximum percent better

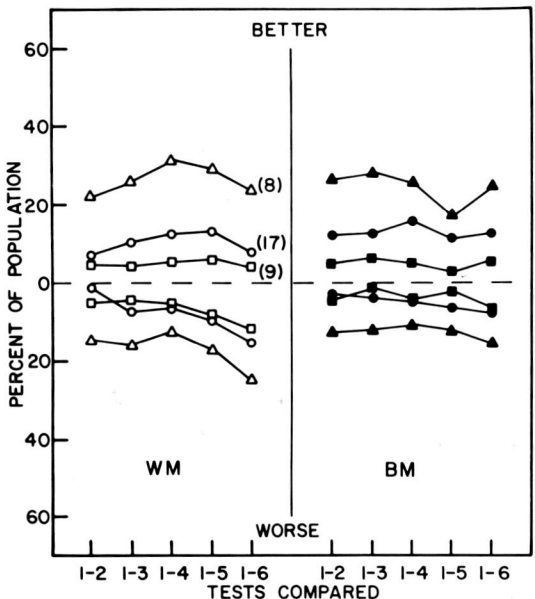

Figure 8. Percentages of WMs and BMs in one INEP whose shifts exceeded test-retest comparison criteria 4, 5 and 10.

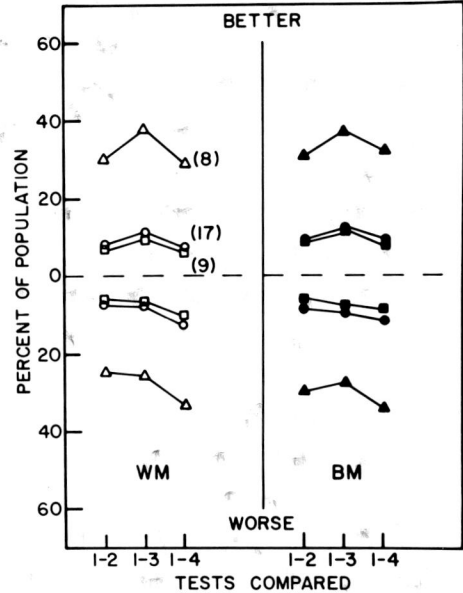

Figure 9. Percentages of WMs and BMs in another INEP whose shifts exceeded test-retest comparison criteria 4, 5 and 10.

Table I: Different Test-Retest Comparison (TRC) Categories Using Varying Shift Criteria and Frequencies. (Optionally 8 kHz could also be included where appropriate.)

Category	Criterion dB	Frequency Range kHz
1	> 10	.5,1,2,3,4,6
2	≥ 10	.5,1,2,3,4,6
3	> 15	.5,1,2,3,4,6
4	≥ 15	.5,1,2,3,4,6
5	> 10	2,3,4
6	> 10 > 15	.5,1,2,3 4,6
7	> 10 > 15	2,3,4 .5,1,2,3,4,6
8	> 10 > 15	.5,1,2 3,4,6
9	> 10 > 15 > 20	.5,1 2 3,4,6
10	≥ 8	4

($\%B_M$) value and the maximum percent worse ($\%W_M$) value out of those obtained by the TRCs for test 1 to test 2, test 1 to test 3, and test 1 to test 4, then forming a ratio of these maximum percentages. For industries where the HCPs are working and where employees' on-the-job noise exposures have been shown to be low, the $\%B_M/\%W_M$ ratios have been consistently greater than 1.25 over the first four years of audiometric testing.

Obviously the ratio of %B/%W would eventually go to zero if the base test procedure described above was applied indefinitely due to the population's normal aging process, nonindustrial noise exposures, etc. This procedure is useful in evaluating the effectiveness of the HCP over the first four years of audiometric testing for any constant subgroup involved in the program. The procedure can also be used in evaluating a HCP that has already been in effect for several years if a significant number of new employees were hired in a particular year; the audiogram from this year would become the TRC base test. One would simply restrict the population to the employees who were hired in that year and who had remained continuously with the company and had received four consecutive audiometric tests.

In addition to the base test comparison method, a second way of looking at the overall effectiveness of the HCP is to compare the hearing tests in a sequential manner; that is, by comparison of the HTLs for test 1 to test 2, test 2 to test 3, etc. (comparing HTLs for successive pairs of consecutive tests). Whereas the comparison of HTLs for each test to a fixed base reference test yields information that may be related directly to the overall trend in the population's HTLs, sequential comparisons of HTLs for pairs of consecutive hearing tests yield an indicator of the relative spread or variability in HTL shifts occurring from year to year. The data that were presented as Figures 8 and 9 came from two different INEPs. The HCP for the population represented by the data presented in Figure 8 has been judged acceptable in preventing an on-the-job noise induced hearing loss; however, the HCP represented by the data presented as Figure 9 has been classified as a marginally acceptable program. It is obvious that over the first 4-5 years of test results shown in Figure 8 for any TRC criterion, the percentage of the population showing better hearing exceeded the percentage showing worse hearing. However, for the population represented by Figure 9, the opposite trend developed over three years of test results. In addition, the spread of the data is greater for the population represented by Figure 9 than for the population represented by Figure 8.

The spread of the data can be estimated by determining the percentage of employees who exhibit either better or worse hearing in either ear at any frequency included in the desired criterion; the resulting "better or worse" percentage value is the %BW. For example, using the category 4 criterion defined in Table I, an employee would be included in the count for the %BW if he displayed a shift equal to or greater than 15 dB either better or worse in either ear at any included frequency. High values for the %BW indicate inadequate audiometric calibration or testing procedures, the

Table II   The Ratio of $\%B_M/\%W_M$ Using Category 4 Based on the First Four Audiometric Tests for Several WM INEPs and the Judged Effectiveness of Their Respective HCPs.

Population	N	$\bar{A}$*	$\bar{S}$*	$\%B_M/\%W_M$	Judged HCP Effectiveness
1	764	31	4	1.53	A*
2	89	36	5	1.46	A
3	4108	38	14	1.12	MA
4	177	39	16	.97	MA
5	513	35	2	.69	U
6	272	42	17	.49	U
7	91	36	1	.47	U
8	23	44	19	.46	U

*A - acceptable; MA - marginally acceptable; U -unacceptable.

$\bar{A}$ - population mean age, yrs.

$\bar{S}$ - population mean service, yrs. (Note! $\bar{S}$ does not reflect the total service because service to previous employers is not included.)

contamination of HTL measurements by significant temporary threshold shift (TTS) when employees not properly wearing HPDs are tested during their work shifts, etc. For each of the HCPs rated in Table II, three %BW values were calculated by comparing successive pairs of consecutive HTL measurements over the first four years of testing. The resulting three %BW values for each program were averaged to obtain the $\overline{\%BW}_{1-2.3-4}$ values which are presented in Table III.

The apparently inconsistent relationship between the $\overline{\%BW}_{1-2.3-4}$ values and the HCP effectiveness ratings becomes clear if the L_{eq}s, the audiometric testing procedures, and the employees' use of HPDs are considered. When the L_{eq}s for the populations represented in Table III are computed, population 2 shows the lowest L_{eq}, 85 dB or less. Except for populations 1 and 5, the other populations represented all are exposed to L_{eq}s in the 94-97 dB range. The highest L_{eq}s, in the 99-109 dB range,

Table III The $\overline{\%BW}_{1-2,3-4}$ Values Determined for Several WM INEP HCP's Using Category 4.

Population	$\overline{\%BW}_{1-2,3-4}$	Overall Judged HCP Effectiveness
1	29.5	A*
2	26.5	A
3	48.7	MA
4	62.3	MA
5	61.4	U
6	30.1	U
7	25.3	U
8	52.1	U

*A - acceptable; MA - marginally acceptable; U - unacceptable.

are found for populations 1 and 5, which represent employees working at two similar production facilities. The low values of $\overline{\%BW}_{1-2,3-4}$ for populations 1 and 2 may be attributed to their proper audiometric testing procedures and their minimal TTS contamination due to the high percentages of employees properly using HPDs, in spite of the contrasting L_{eq}s for these two populations. For populations 3, 4, and 5 the high values of $\overline{\%BW}_{1-2,3-4}$ reflect significant TTS contamination of HTLs since employees are tested during their work shifts, and since many employees fail to wear the HPDs furnished. However, the HCPs for populations 3 and 4 were still rated as marginally acceptable because the "learning effect" occurring among employees who were properly wearing their HPDs is partially offsetting the industrial noise induced hearing loss occurring for the unprotected employees. Populations 6 and 7 display low values of $\overline{\%BW}_{1-2,3-4}$ because they receive their audiometric exams only prior to work or when they have been properly protected by HPD use. These populations are required to wear the provided HPDs during only the first half of their daily work shift. Since their L_{eq}s are approximately 95 dB, their noise dose does not exceed the present OSHA criterion even though they are unprotected during the second half of their work day.

However, the significant hearing loss which occurs due to this unprotected noise exposure does result in unsatisfactory ratings of the HCPs for these populations.

Changes in the Population's $\overline{HTL}$s at 4 kHz

Since the "learning effect" seems to also be an indicator of the effectiveness of the HCP, then a significant correlation should exist between the changes in the population's $\overline{HTL}$s and the $\%B_M/\%W_M$ ratio described earlier. In evaluating the available data bases it was observed that very similar "learning curves" existed for the 3, 4 and 6 kHz audiometric test frequencies. Since the 4 kHz test frequency is often identified in the literature as the frequency where a noise induced hearing loss is most likely to become apparent first, 4 kHz was selected as the probable best estimator of the presence or absence of the "learning effect". In keeping with the procedure outlined earlier, the slope of the variations in $\overline{HTL}$s at 4 kHz ($\Delta \overline{HTL}_{4kHz}$) over the first four years of testing for a constant population may be approximated using a simple linear regression procedure. The data points presented as Figure 10 were obtained by plotting the $\Delta \overline{HTL}_{4kHz}$ for several WM populations against their respective $\%B_M/\%W_M$ ratios figured using the category 8 criterion. As expected, a strong correlation between the $\Delta \overline{HTL}_{4kHz}$ and the $\%B_M/\%W_M$ ratio was found across all the INEPs shown. Population E is exposed to an L_{eq} equal to or less than 85 dB. Population X is an industrial population whose data set and whose HCP have been studied extensively in-house and found to be exceptional from all standpoints. For each of the remaining populations shown it is known that the HPDs provided are not worn properly by substantial proportions of the employees.

The reliable relationship of the $\%B_M/\%W_M$ ratio to the $\Delta \overline{HTL}_{4kHz}$ among these WM populations provides an indicator of the degree of effectiveness of the corresponding HCPs in preventing industrial noise induced hearing loss. A recommended criterion for rating HCP effectiveness for WM INEPs based on this relationship of $\%B_M/\%W_M$ to $\Delta \overline{HTL}_{4kHz}$ during the first four years of testing[4] is presented as Figure 11. The protection of groups of WM employees in different production

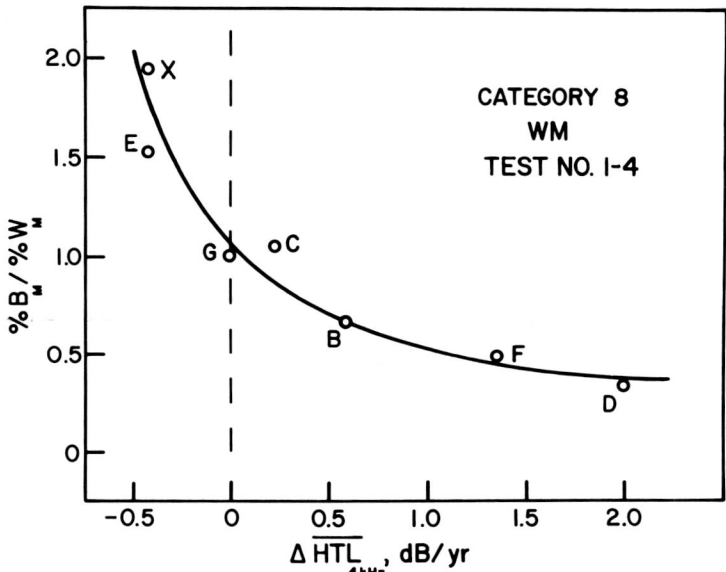

Figure 10. The %B_M/%W_M ratios for seven WM INEPs plotted as a function of the slope of changes in $\overline{HTL}$s at 4 kHz over the first four years of testing.

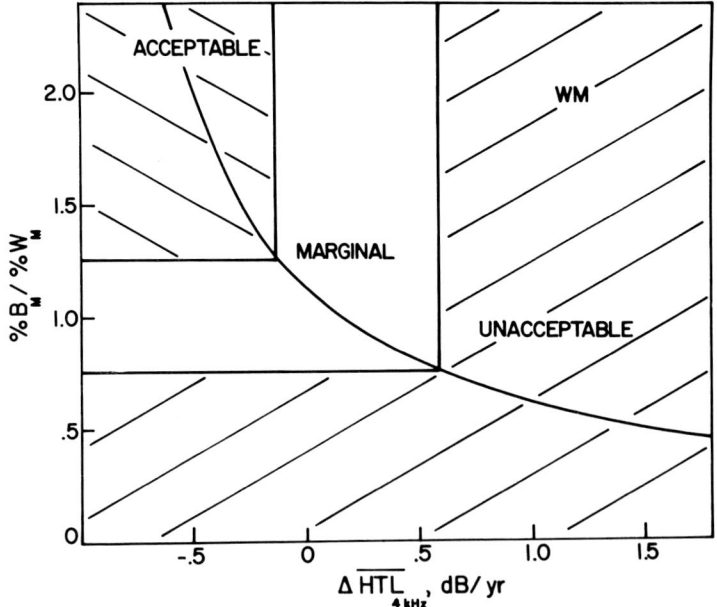

Figure 11. Value ranges of acceptable, marginally acceptable, and unacceptable HCPs for the %B_M/%W_M ratio and the slope of $\overline{HTL}$ changes at 4 kHz over the first four years of testing for WM INEPs.

areas within a facility may also be compared using this criterion. For older HCPs, the criterion may be used to assess program effectiveness in later years of testing by restricting analysis to a constant population of employees all hired in a selected year. For race and sex subgroups other than WMs, similar criteria for rating HCP effectiveness have been recommended[4] based on the relationship of $\Delta \overline{HTL}_{4kHz}$ to $\%B_M/\%W_M$ observed for INEP data sets. This relationship has been observed to vary somewhat among race and sex subgroups, especially for BFs; however, these variations may be due to the smaller numbers of data sets including these subgroups currently available in the INEP data base, as well as to their differing HTLs.

DIFFERENCES BETWEEN THE (HTL)'S FOR NINEPS AND INEPS

As previously mentioned, comparison of the rates of change for an INEP and its matched NINEP provides an additional indication of the effectiveness of a HCP. Once the "learning effect" has diminished, the curve representing $\overline{HTL}$ changes for an INEP should become parallel to the appropriate NINEP HTL curve if proper protection prevents further industrial noise induced hearing loss[3]. The (HTL)'s for the parallel curves would be equal and would be positive in value due to the hearing loss occurring from aging, non-industrial noise exposure, etc. On the other hand, if an INEP were not being properly protected, its $(HTL)^1$ would be a larger positive value than the $(HTL)^1$ of its matched NINEP due to the additional hearing loss resulting from industrial noise exposure.

A typical $\overline{HTL}$ curve for one INEP protected by an effective HCP is presented in Figure 12 along with the reference curve for the NINEP appropriately matched by race and sex. The circles on the smoothed HTL curve for the NINEP have been added to simplify comparisons with the INEP at the same age. The constant population represented by the INEP data points had received seven consecutive audiometric exams. Over the first four tests the $(HTL)^1$ for the INEP is negative due to the measured threshold improvement resulting from the "learning effect". After the fourth test, however, the $\overline{HTL}$ curve for the INEP shows a larger positive $(HTL)^1$ value than the NINEP HTL curve, indicating that some industrial

Table IV Smoothed Rate of Change in Hearing Threshold Levels for an All White NIINEP (HTL)^1 in dB/Yr.

Sex	Frequency (Hz)	Age, Yrs.									
		20	25	30	35	40	45	50	55	60	65
White Males	500	0.03	0.06	0.09	0.12	0.15	0.18	0.21	0.24	0.27	0.30
	1000	0.01	0.06	0.11	0.16	0.21	0.26	0.31	0.36	0.41	0.46
	2000	0.08	0.17	0.26	0.35	0.44	0.53	0.62	0.71	0.80	0.89
	3000	0.38	0.45	0.52	0.59	0.66	0.73	0.80	0.87	0.94	1.01
	4000	0.85	0.86	0.86	0.86	0.86	0.86	0.86	0.86	0.86	0.86
	6000	0.90	0.90	0.90	0.90	0.89	0.89	0.89	0.89	0.89	0.88
White Females	500	0.06	0.11	0.16	0.21	0.26	0.31	0.36	0.41	0.46	0.51
	1000	0.07	0.13	0.19	0.25	0.31	0.37	0.43	0.49	0.55	0.61
	2000	0.04	0.12	0.20	0.28	0.36	0.44	0.52	0.60	0.68	0.76
	3000	0.09	0.19	0.29	0.39	0.49	0.59	0.69	0.79	0.89	0.99
	4000	0.23	0.32	0.41	0.50	0.59	0.68	0.77	0.86	0.95	1.04
	6000	0.18	0.29	0.40	0.51	0.62	0.73	0.84	0.95	1.06	1.17

Table V   Smoothed Rate of change in Hearing Threshold Levels for an All Black NINEP

$(HTL)^1$ in dB/Yr.

Age, Yrs.

Sex	Frequency (Hz)	20	25	30	35	40	45	50	55	60	65
Black Males	500	-0.29	-0.23	-0.17	-0.11	-0.05	0.01	0.07	0.13	0.19	0.25
	1000	-0.07	-0.06	-0.04	-0.02	0.01	0.03	0.05	0.07	0.09	0.11
	2000	0.14	0.16	0.18	0.20	0.22	0.24	0.26	0.28	0.30	0.32
	3000	0.12	0.21	0.30	0.39	0.48	0.57	0.66	0.75	0.84	0.93
	4000	0.22	0.30	0.37	0.45	0.52	0.60	0.67	0.75	0.82	0.90
	6000	0.47	0.51	0.55	0.59	0.63	0.67	0.71	0.75	0.79	0.83
Black Females	500	0.05	0.05	0.05	0.04	0.04	0.04	0.03	0.03	0.03	0.03
	1000	0.16	0.14	0.12	0.10	0.08	0.06	0.04	0.02	0.00	-0.02
	2000	0.12	0.13	0.14	0.15	0.16	0.17	0.18	0.19	0.20	0.21
	3000	0.12	0.15	0.17	0.20	0.22	0.25	0.27	0.30	0.32	0.35
	4000	0.18	0.20	0.21	0.23	0.24	0.26	0.27	0.29	0.30	0.32
	6000	0.31	0.34	0.36	0.39	0.41	0.44	0.46	0.49	0.51	0.54

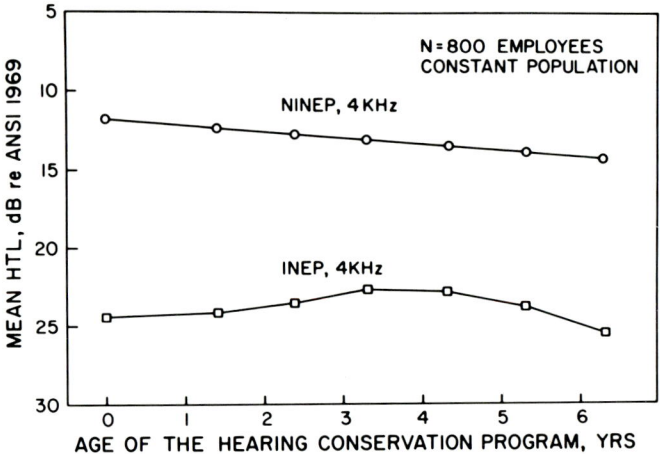

Figure 12. Variations in $\overrightarrow{HTL}$s at 4 kHz over seven audiograms for one INEP compared to the HTL curve for the matching NINEP at corresponding population ages.

noise induced hearing loss is occurring in addition to non-occupational hearing loss.

The (HTL)'s for NINEPs have been calculated[3,5] and are presented as Tables IV and V for each race and sex group as a function of age and test frequency. Note that the (HTL)[1] data presented in Table IV represent a recent update of the data base for which (HTL)[1] data had previously been published.[3] As an illustration of the variations in (HTL)'s for different race and sex NINEPs at the same age, the (HTL)'s at 4 kHz and age 35 years range from .23 dB/yr. for the BF NINEP to .86 dB/yr. for the WM NINEP.

CHANGES IN THE POPULATION'S POTENTIAL COMPENSATION COST

The implementation of an effective HCP has been consistently observed to result in a reduction in the potential compensation cost for noise induced hearing loss in the protected population. Translation of HCP benefits into a dollar figure representing the potential savings due to the HCP provides management with a simple summary figure to refer to when making decisions regarding the company's HCP. Potential compensation cost may be calculated using the recently revised AAO criterion[9] and/or the older AAOO criterion which is still used by most states. The potential compensation cost for an employee population has been shown to be highly dependent not only on the employees' noise exposure history, but also on the age, race and sex composition of the population.[10] The prevention of additional on-the-job noise induced hearing loss is not the only reason why implementation of an effective HCP reduces potential compensation cost. Since audiometric data from effective HCPs display "learning effect" improvements in measured $\overline{HTL}$s over the first 4-6 years of testing, the potential compensation cost also decreases over this time period. The resulting dollar value reduction can be quite dramatic. The magnitude of the "learning effect" appears directly related to the INEP $\overline{HTL}$ at the initial audiogram; for populations with larger $\overline{HTL}$s at 4 kHz (i.e., with poorer hearing) the magnitude of the "learning effect" is greater.

To illustrate reductions in potential employee compensation, Table VI shows the percentages of the race and sex subgroups of a constant INEP who were potentially compensable based on HTLs measured for their first audiogram and based on HTLs for their fourth audiogram. For the 7000 WM employees represented in Table VI the potential compensation cost per $1000 of compensation payable per employee dropped from $25.20 to $15.80. In a state where the maximum compensation payable is $25,000 for a total bilateral hearing loss due to occupational noise exposure, this represents a decrease in the total potential compensation cost from $4,410,000 to $2,765,000 --a potential savings of $1,645,000.

Table VI: Percentage of Employees in an INEP Divided by Race and Sex Who Were Potentially Compensable for Noise Induced Hearing Loss Based on Their First and Fourth Audiometric Tests.

Low Fence: $\overline{HTL}_{.5, 1, 2kHz}$ = 26 dB.

Audiometric Test No.	INEP Subgroup			
	WM	WF	BM	BF
1	20.3	15.0	8.2	4.3
4	12.4	10.0	2.7	0.0

In addition to the reductions in potential compensation cost due to proper wearing of HPDs and the "learning effect", changes in the composition of an INEP may also reduce potential cost. Over recent years the proportions of females and blacks in the work force have increased, and the growing percentage of these employees has reduced $\overline{HTL}$s for many INEPs. With the retirement of employees who had worked unprotected in noise during years prior to HCP implementation, $\overline{HTL}$s for currently protected INEPs will decline, also influencing the reduction in potential compensation costs for the INEP. When using potential compensation cost as an indicator of HCP effectiveness, it is necessary both to consider a constant population over time in order to see effects of population composition changes, and to consider the changing population in order to determine current potential compensation costs.

CONCLUSIONS

Several indicators of the effectiveness of HCPs in preventing occupational hearing loss have been developed based on analysis of population audiometric data. Although it is important to monitor individual employees' HTL shifts, analysis of audiometric data for a constant population permits superior assessment of overall HCP performance.

Significant differences in $\overline{HTL}$s among black and white males and females necessitate separating these subgroups of an INEP for analysis. In order to control for non-occupational hearing loss, NINEPs matched by race and sex to the INEP subgroups should be used as reference populations. When INEP $\overline{HTL}$s are compared to NINEP reference HTL curves, a "learning effect" resulting in better INEP $\overline{HTL}$s over the first 4-6 years of testing is apparent if the INEP has been properly protected.

One indicator of HCP effectiveness is the $\%B_M/\%W_M$ ratio. Based on the first four years of testing, a HCP is judged to be acceptable if the $\%B_M/\%W_M$ value is 1.25 or greater, or unacceptable if the value is less than .75. These values may be used in rating HCP effectiveness if the criterion selected for calculating TRCs is a shift ≥ 15 dB in either ear at any test frequency from .5 kHz to 6 kHz. This criterion has been found to be sensitive to HTL changes both across INEPs and also among subgroups within an INEP.

A second indicator, which estimates the reliability of audiometric calibration and testing procedures, the amount of TTS contamination in group data, etc., is the %BW. This statistic indicates the variability in HTLs between sequential pairs of consecutive audiograms. When the criterion used counts shifts ≥ 15 dB over the first four years of testing, the resulting %BW$_{1-2,3-4}$ statistic is $\leq 30\%$ for HCPs with acceptable audiometric testing procedures and minimal TTS contamination of HTLs. For HCPs which have completed additional years of testing, the %BW for the most recent years of testing should drop and should stabilize around a lower value once the "learning effect" has diminished.

The "learning effect", or measured improvement in $\overline{HTL}$s for protected INEPs over the first 4-6 years of testing, has been identified as a characteristic of at least the 4 kHz audiometric data for effective HCPs. Consequently, the presence of a "learning effect" can be used during the early years of a HCP's existence as an indicator of program acceptability. When the change in $\overline{HTL}$s over the first four years of testing is approximated by fitting a linear regression line to the $\overline{HTL}$ values at 4 kHz, the slope of the resulting $\Delta \overline{HTL}_{4kHz}$ line will be -.2 dB/yr. or a larger negative value for an acceptable HCP. Although the "learning effect" has been discussed only for the 4 kHz test frequency, the effect has also been observed to occur at 3 kHz and 6 kHz.

The correlation between %B$_M$/%W$_M$ and the slope of $\Delta \overline{HTL}_{4kHz}$ calculated using the results of the first four tests may also be used to rate HCPs as acceptable, marginally acceptable, or unacceptable by plotting these two statistics against the value ranges for WM INEPs shown in Figure 11. Value ranges of these statistics for other race and sex subgroups of INEPs are presently being refined.

Once the "learning effect" has ceased to influence $\overline{HTL}$s, the effectiveness of a HCP may be judged by comparing the rate of change - the

$(HTL)^1$ - of the curve representing the INEP's $\overline{HTL}$s with the $(HTL)^1$ of the HTL curve for the matching NINEP at the same age. If the HCP is preventing occupational hearing loss the two (HTL)'s will be approximately equivalent.

One summary statistic useful to industrial management is the dollar value of potential savings in compensation costs for an on-the-job noise induced hearing loss as a result of an effective HCP. Due to the "learning effect", elimination of TTS contamination in audiometric data, more employees using HPDs, etc., the improvement in measured HTLs after acceptable HCP implementation will significantly reduce the company's potential compensation costs for occupational hearing loss.

The evaluation procedures recommended above have demonstrated consistency in assessing the effectiveness of the HCPs studied to date. Although these indicators appear to be reliable for the data available, the evaluator should exercise caution in applying them. For example, consider an INEP whose $\overline{HTL}$s at 4 kHz have approached a maximum hearing loss as a result of exposure to high noise levels over several years. The $(HTL)^1$ for such an INEP would be smaller than the value for a matching NINEP of the same age regardless of HCP effectiveness; therefore, the comparison of the (HTL)'s at 4 kHz for the two populations would not be a valid indicator in this case. An alternative approach to evaluating such an INEP would be to consider $\overline{HTL}$ changes at 2, 3 and 6 kHz.

Any deviation of the INEP under study from norms should warn the evaluator to consider whether additional potentially significant factors may be influencing the population's $\overline{HTL}$s. Changes in the race and sex composition of an INEP necessitate subgroup separation before analysis to prevent the $\overline{HTL}$ differences among subgroups from obscuring HCP effects. It is possible that INEPs from other geographic areas might exhibit HTLs different from those found in the currently available, regional data base. Critical thought by the evaluator would aid his recognition of such potential factors.

As additional INEP data sets are added to the data base and evaluated using these indicators, refined evaluation procedures and/or new indicators of HCP effectiveness hopefully will be developed. As HCP data from additional years of audiometric testing become available, criteria for assessing the effectiveness of HCPs during later stages of implementation may be identified.

REFERENCES

1. Driscoll, D.P., Royster, L.H., Comparisons Between the Median Hearing Threshold Levels for an Unscreened Black Nonindustrial Noise Exposed Population (NINEP) and Four Presbycusis Data Bases, J. Acoust. Soc. Amer., 66, Supp. No. I, S62.

2. Berger, E.H., Royster, L.H., Thomas, W.G., Hearing Levels of Nonindustrial Noise Exposed Subjects, J. Occup. Med., 19, 664-670.

3. Royster, L.H., Thomas, W.G., Age Effect Hearing Levels for a White Nonindustrial Noise Exposed Population (NINEP) and Their Use in Evaluating Industrial Hearing Conservation Programs, Amer., Ind. Hyg. Assoc. J., 40, 504-511, 1979.

4. Royster, L.H., Lilley, D.T., Thomas, W.G., Recommended Criteria for Evaluating the Effectiveness of Hearing Conservation Programs, Amer., Ind. Hyg. Assoc. J., 41, 40-48, 1980.

5. Royster, L.H., Driscoll, D.P., Thomas, W.G., Royster, J.D., Age Effect Hearing Levels for a Black Nonindustrial Noise Exposed Population (NINEP), Amer. Ind. Hyg. Assoc. J., 41, 113-119, 1980.

6. Robinson, D.W., Sutton, G.J., A Comparative Analysis of Data on the Relation of Pure Tone Threshold to Age, NPL Acoustics Report AC 84, 1978.

7. Royster, L.H., Royster, J.D., Thomas, W.G., Representative Hearing Levels by Race and Sex in North Carolina Industry, J. Acoust. Soc. Amer., 68, 551-566, 1980.

8. Royster, L.H., Royster, J.D., Industrial Hearing Conservation-- New Considerations, Hearing Instruments, 31, 4-5, 1980.

9. American Academy of Otolaryngology, Guide for the Evaluation of Hearing Handicap, J. Amer. Med. Assoc., 241, 2055-2059, 1979.

10. Royster, L.H., Thomas, W.G., Royster, J.D., Lilley, D.T., Potential Hearing Compensation Cost by Race and Sex, J. Occup. Med., 20, 801-806, 1978.

32 THE LONG-TERM EFFECTIVENESS OF A HEARING CONSERVATION PROGRAMME BASED UPON PERSONAL HEARING PROTECTION

S. Pell, T. A. Dear, and B. W. Karrh

INTRODUCTION

It is well documented that occupational noise exposure varies widely from industry to industry, within an industry, from worker to worker, and, for a given worker, throughout the working day. Measured exposure data varies exponentially in relation to the actual sound level due to differences in the capabilities of the instruments and methods used to record and analyze the data. Also, correlation of such data to worker hearing loss potential is highly variable. Yet, a key factor in the present and proposed workplace noise regulations is the "number" ... the stated sound level criterion. The occupational physician is much concerned about these criteria numbers because they permit that, once the specified level is reached, no further effort is required by regulation to protect unidentified employees whose hearing may still be at risk at or below the regulated level.

The present OSHA compliance hierarchy requires engineering controls first, both built-in and retrofit; secondly, administrative controls; and lastly, personal hearing protection.

Because of the Damage Risk Criteria upon which the criteria numbers are based and the limited availability and feasibility of engineering controls, the regulation is not designed to protect all workers.

The comprehensive hearing conservation program practiced at du Pont for more than 24 years has proven at least adequately effective in preventing noise-induced hearing impairment for all types of workers. The program calls for initial and follow-up audiometric testing; provision and fitting of personal protective devices (ear plugs or muffs); education, training, monitoring and supervision of personnel wearing the devices; and medical surveillance. Protection for all workers can be achieved by reliance on such a program and by restructuring government regulations to give first priority to engineering controls at the source (the point of original equipment manufacture and installation other than enclosures); second priority to hearing protection, followed by retrofit engineering controls and administrative-dose controls.

Some highlights and supporting details of this program and the claims for its success in terms of worker protection are presented here.

EVALUATION OF CURRENT DU PONT PROGRAMME

Pell, in a previous paper[1] evaluated and summarized the protocol, general results and conclusions of the du Pont programme as follows:

> "The effectiveness of a hearing conservation program was investigated by analyses of changes in hearing threshold levels over a 5-year period among 2,770 male employees of the du Pont Company. The study focused on 1,966 men in this group whose level of noise exposure did not change during the study period. Three categories of noise levels were established. One consisted of areas in which the level was below the hearing conservation criterion, approximately 90 dBA; the other two were above that level. The mean differences in hearing levels were essentially the same in the three noise level categories, at each test frequency, and regardless of the hearing level at the beginning of the study period. We therefore concluded that a hearing conservation program whose components include periodic audiometric testing and ear protection, and which utilizes a hearing conservation criterion of approximately 90 dBA, is capable of protecting the hearing of noise-exposed workers."

Efforts to protect the hearing of noise-exposed workers in the du Pont Company date back to the 1940's, when pure-tone audiometric testing was added to the routine periodic health examination in plants where noise levels were thought to be hazardous.

From the formal inception of du Pont's Hearing Conservation Program in

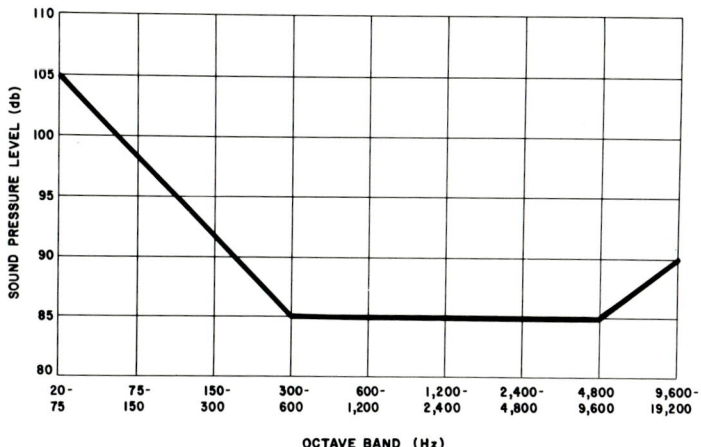

Figure 1.   Hearing conservation criteria.

1954 to the publication of the noise regulation amendment to the Walsh Healey Public Contracts Act in 1969, the hearing conservation criteria for this program was as shown in Figure 1. This criterion translates to approximately 92 dBA in terms of current noise regulation criteria. In accordance with the hearing conservation program, workplace noise level surveys are done routinely.

To analyze the data, we established three categories of noise levels, designated I, II, and III, shown in Table I. More specifically, Category I has an upper limit that translates to more than 91 dBA and in actual fact most of the employees in this group are office workers whose job exposures are usually less than 60 dBA. Category II limits translate to an exposure range of approximately 87 dBA to 97 dBA or more and Category III limits correspond to an exposure range of 97 dBA and up. In the pre-regulatory era, ear protection was required for all workers in Category III and most workers in Category II.

This emphasizes the fact that the study was not intended to assess effects of these noise exposure levels upon hearing acuity but represents an evaluation of the effectiveness of the current hearing conservation program involving the efficacy of personal hearing protection.

Table 1:   Sound pressure levels in each catetory.

Noise Level Category	Octave Bands (H_2)	
	20-75 to 150-300	300-600 to 4,800-10,000
I	All octave bands under 100 db	All octave bands under 85 db
II	All octave bands under 100 db	85-94 db in one or more octave bands
III	All levels	95+ db in one or more octave bands

Selection of the Study Population

The data in this were analyzed to determine whether changes in hearing threshold levels over a 5-year period, from 1966 through 1971, were related to the noise levels in the work areas. To accomplish this objective, it was necessary to limit the study to those subjects whose audiometric tests covered at least a 4½ year span.

Subjects were eliminated whose noise exposures varied throughout the day and from one day to the next; for example, maintenance and supervisory personnel who were not confined to a single work area.

When the project was started in 1966, the total male population at the seven participating plants were 18,758. After the primary eliminations, the number of subjects remaining in the study was reduced to 2,770 and subsequently to 1,966 as described later. This sample size was considered sufficiently large to accomplish the objectives of the study.

Table 2 shows the age distribution of the subject population according to the three exposure categories.

A trend toward lower exposure level category with increasing age is generally noted in these results. This aspect of worker mobility required that final analysis of the data be devoted to those whose noise exposure did not change during the study period - that is 1,173 in Category I, 394 in

Table 2: Age Distribution by Noise Level Category at the Beginning of the Study Period

Age (years)	Total	Noise Level Category I	Noise Level Category II	Noise Level Category III
Under 25	418	167	132	119
25-34	607	223	185	199
35-44	832	414	226	192
45-54	753	528	126	99
55-64	160	109	34	17
Total	2770	1441	703	626
Median Age	39.3	43.0	36.6	34.9

Category II and 399 in Category III, for a total of 1,966 subjects.

Statistical Analysis

For each subject, the hearing threshold levels obtained on the first audiogram taken during the study period were subtracted from the hearing levels obtained on the last audiogram. These differences were computed for each test frequency, and for the right ear only. For each of various subgroups categorized according to noise exposure, frequency polygons were constructed showing the distribution of these differences, and the mean difference and the standard deviation were calculated. Differences among the means were tested by analysis of variance.

RESULTS OF THE STUDY

The procedure involved comparison of mean differences by noise level category for each center frequency of noise as shown in Table 3. As expected, there was a positive mean increase in hearing threshold level over the 5-year period in each category and at all frequencies. In the lower frequencies (500 to 2000 Hz), the mean increases ranged from 0.6 to 2.7 dB, and in the higher frequencies, from 1.8 to 3.8 dB. There did not appear, however, to be any discernible positive association between the general increase in hearing loss and the categorized levels of noise in the

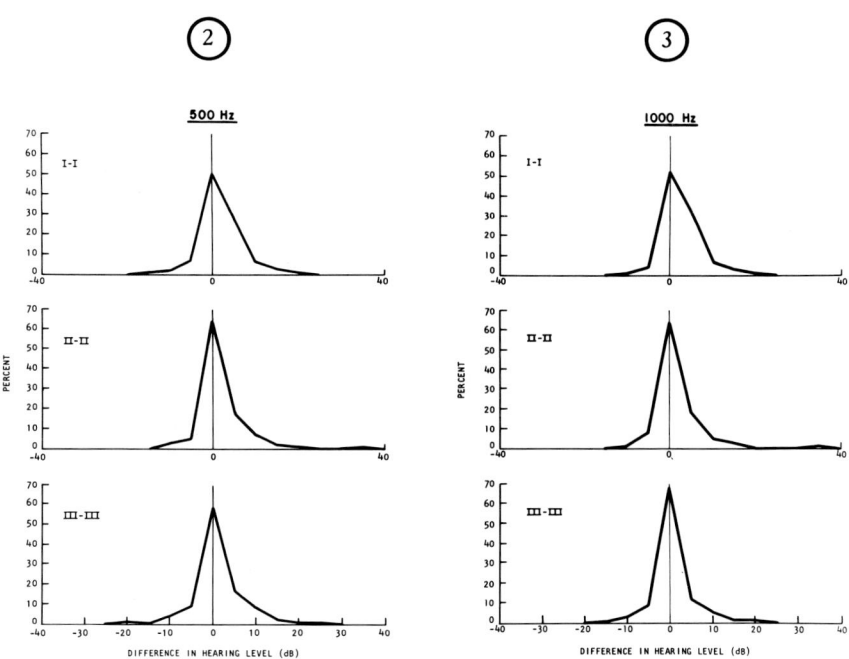

Figures 2-7. Compare statistical frequency polygons of the distributions of changes in hearing levels in three noise level categories at the noise center frequencies 500 through 6000 KZ. These polygons show that, for each test frequency, the size and shape of the distributions were about the same, and that the distributions tended to cluster about the same mean. If the noise was affecting the hearing of the workers, the polygons for categories II and III would have shown a noticeable, progressive shift to the right of the polygon for category I in each case.

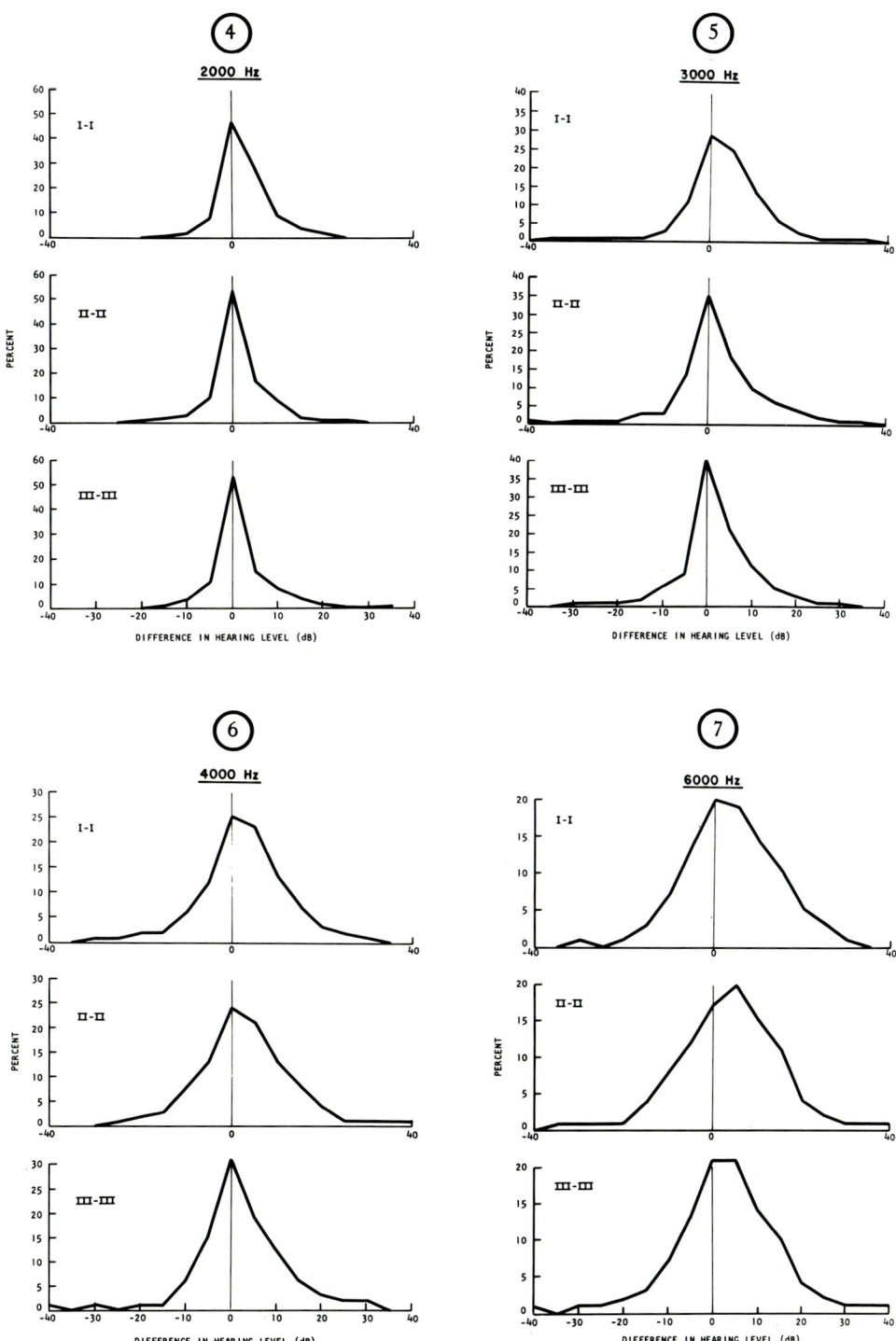

Table 3: Mean Differences in Hearing Threshold Levels over a Five-Year Period by Noise Level Category at the Beginning and End of the Period: Each Test Frequency - Males - Right Ear

Frequency (Hz)	Noise Level Category[a]	Mean Difference D	Standard Deviation s
500[b]	I	2.1	6.0
	II	1.6	5.8
	III	0.9	6.1
1000[b]	I	2.7	5.8
	II	1.8	5.6
	III	0.6	5.0
2000	I	2.4	6.7
	II	1.4	7.2
	III	1.5	7.0
3000	I	3.0	10.3
	II	2.4	10.2
	III	2.3	8.9
4000	I	1.8	11.7
	II	2.7	10.9
	III	2.9	10.1
6000	I	3.6	11.0
	II	3.8	11.4
	III	2.9	11.4

a   Noise level categories the same at beginning and end of the period.
b   Differences among means significant at 0.05 level (F test).

respective work areas. They are shown in greater detail in Figures 2-7.

Differences among means were statistically significant in the lower frequencies, but this could be expected with such a large sample size and the small variability of repeated threshold determinations in the low frequencies. The differences among the means were small, however, and the mean changes in the hearing threshold level tended to increase in the direction of the low rather than the high noise levels.

Table 4 shows mean differences in hearing levels of persons whose noise level category changed during the study period. These hearing changes were generally in the range found for those who remained in the same noise level category, and present no particular pattern that would indicate any adverse effects of noise exposure in the workplace.

Table 4: Mean Differences in Hearing Threshold Levels Over a Five-Year Period by Noise Level Category at the Beginning and End of the Period among Persons Whose Noise Level Category Changed during the Period: Each Test Frequency - Males

Noise-Level Category[a]		Frequency (Hz)					
First	Last	500	1000	2000	3000	4000	6000
I	II	1.8	2.7	3.1	2.8	2.9	5.1
I	III	2.3	2.7	3.2	3.9	4.0	3.3
II	I	1.8	1.6	1.1	1.2	-1.5	0.8
II	III	1.7	0.9	0.7	0.2	1.7	0.7
III	I	1.7	2.6	1.6	4.6	4.2	6.2
III	II	1.2	0.8	1.3	1.6	0.5	3.7

a The number of persons in each group is shown in Table II

Effect of Initial Hearing Threshold Level

The amount of sensorineural hearing loss that develops over a given period of time, as a result of either noise exposure or presbycusis, could depend, in part, on the hearing threshold level of the person at the beginning of the period. In fact, the data show that, as the amount of hearing loss increases, the rate at which additional hearing loss occurs, with respect to time, tends to decrease. Therefore, it was thought advisable to analyze the data according to the level of hearing loss at the beginning of the study period. In this way, changes that occurred among persons with the least amount of hearing loss and, therefore, probably most susceptible to the effects of noise could be seen. Since noise-induced hearing loss first becomes evident at the higher frequencies, this analysis was undertaken only for 3000, 4000, and 6000 Hz.

Mean differences in hearing threshold levels were computed for each of three classifications of hearing levels at the beginning of the period: 10 dB or less, 15 to 35 dB, and 40 dB or more. The results are shown in the frequency polygons for 4000 Hz, etc., in Figures 8, 9 and 10.

Additional comparisons among the three noise level categories show no indication of increased hearing loss among persons who work in defined noise areas, regardless of the initial hearing loss. Differences among the three noise level categories were generally small.

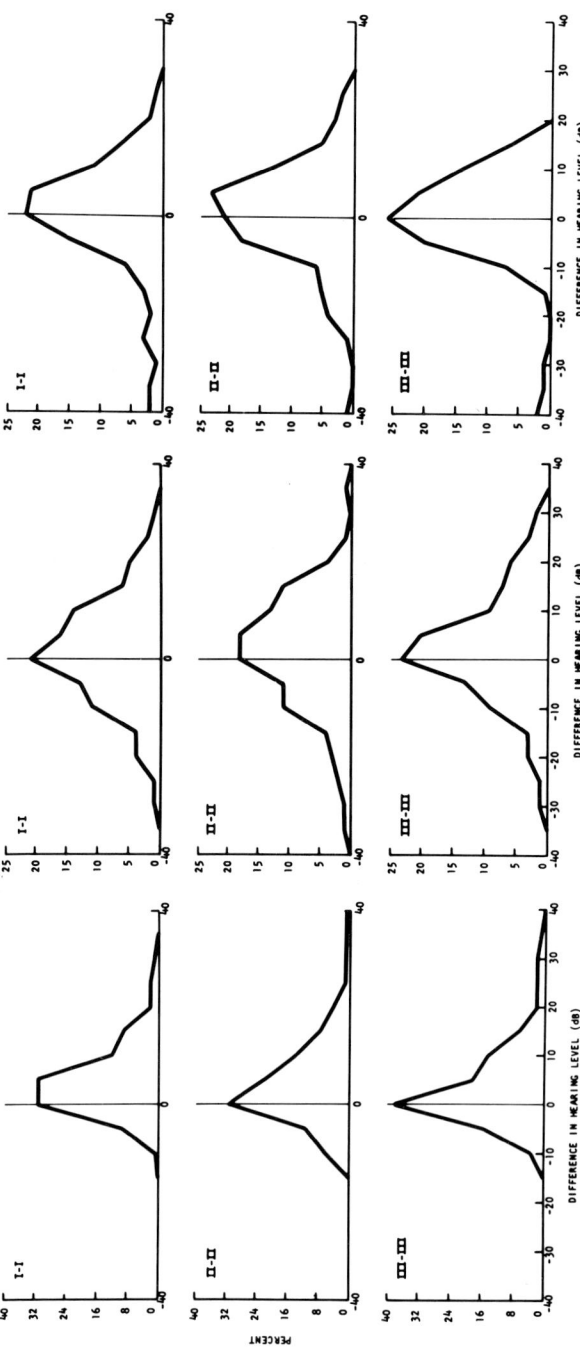

Figures 8,9,10. Hearing loss change according to initial hearing thresholds, at 3 kHz (Fig. 8), 4 kHz (Fig. 9) and 6 kHz (Fig. 10).

DISCUSSION

The analysis of changes in hearing threshold levels over a 5-year period has clearly indicated that persons who work in areas where noise levels exceeded 90 dBA showed hearing losses that were no greater than those experienced by persons who worked in areas where the noise levels were much less than 90 dBA. It is evident, therefore, that a hearing conservation program in which the hearing conservation criterion is approximately 90 dBA can successfully protect the hearing of noise-exposed workers. Since the men who work in areas that were above the criterion underwent close audiometric surveillance and were required to wear ear protection, there is no way of determining from this set of data the lowest noise level that would produce hearing loss, or what percentage of an exposed population would be affected by various levels of noise over various short and long term periods of direct exposure.

It is also important to bear in mind that category I, the control group, consisted mainly of persons with minimal workplace noise exposure. The comparisons of Categories II and III with Category I were comparisons between persons who worked in noise levels above 90 dBA with persons who worked in areas where the noise levels in most instances were between 50 and 70 dBA.

Significance of Changes Based on Test Variability

The data generated by the study provided an opportunity to assess the significance of changes in hearing threshold levels that occur as a result of test error. If the upper limit of normal is set at the mean plus two standard deviations, one can estimate the amount of hearing loss that should be considered significant over a 5-year period by referring to the data in Table 3, which shows the mean standard deviations of changes in hearing levels in each test frequency for persons working in relatively quiet areas (Category I). At 4000 Hz, for example, the upper limit would be 1.8 + 2 (11.7), or 25 dB. Thus, an increase in hearing loss over a 5-year period that is less than 25 dB need not be considered significant; that is, the loss was probably due to presbycusis and/or test error, and, therefore, not likely to be the result of occupational noise exposure.

About ten years have passed since the completion of the study discussed here. There has been a continued acquisition of data on a consistent basis. Incomplete analytical results of the additional data strongly support the findings of the original longitudinal study.

SOME DETAILS REGARDING THE DU PONT HEARING CONSERVATION PROGRAM

To avoid any misinterpretation of the program and the concerns upon which it is based, one must realize that, by definition, present regulations directed to noise in the workplace do not intend to protect all workers. The du Pont Company finds that insufficient approach and estimated degree of success unacceptable in the context of its long-standing successful safety programs, particularly since practical alternatives that drastically reduce reliance on damage risk based criteria are readily available.

The use of hearing protectors as a means of compliance where reasonable and appropriate is often equal to or superior to engineering and administrative controls in protecting the hearing of noise-exposed workers by providing noise attenuation well below 90 dBA. Personal protection also has demonstrated maximum benefit-to-cost ratios for any compliance methods presently available.

Extensive programs, initiated in the 1950's, in engineering controls directed to the source of noise continue.

A comprehensive hearing conservation program calls for 1) initial and follow-up audiometric testing; 2) supplying and fitting, personal protective devices, such as earplugs or muffs; 3) training and monitoring of personnel wearing the devices; and 4) medical surveillance. Cooperation of the worker and supervision is essential to an effective hearing conservation program, as is the case in any worker safety program. This cooperation can only be achieved by insuring that each participant understands the importance of the program and his or her duties, responsibilities and benefits. This is best accomplished through on-going education and training programs through line organization.

Our experience has shown that maximum effectiveness of hearing conservation results when employees understand the reasons for the program and cooperate and take initiative in its implementation and conduct on a daily basis. This cooperation is accomplished by educating them regarding the potential effects of exposure to high-noise levels, whether encountered at work or during leisure hours. A short movie or appropriate presentation by the local plant doctor and safety specialists which explains how excessive noise can impair hearing and how hearing protective devices work and should be worn, contributes markedly to the cooperation received. This training is also presented to new employees reporting to work, and at any other time that is considered appropriate.

Supervisors are responsible for monitoring worker compliance with all safety rules and personal protective equipment requirements. This includes such items as safety glasses, hard hats, hearing protective devices, etc. If an employee is not using any designated protective equipment or not using it properly, the supervisor discusses this with the employee and re-explains the reasons for the equipment and how it should be used. Plant medical personnel will assist the supervisor if requested. If necessary to gain compliance with the requirements for personal protective equipment, regardless of the type, appropriate disciplinary action will be taken.

Audiometric Testing
An essential part of the hearing conservation program is audiometric testing and this starts prior to placement. All applicants are given pre-placement physical examinations which include an audiometric test, usually using a self-recording audiometer calibrated to the proper standard. All employees receive periodic examinations which include an audiogram. After being hired, if their assignment is to a designated noise area, they are then included in the hearing conservation program. This means that they are given an audiometric test immediately prior to being assigned to a noise area, three to six months after the onset of exposure,

one year after the onset, and annually thereafter. This helps to assess individual susceptibility at an early stage.

Hearing Protection
Employees are fitted with hearing protective devices at the time of the preplacement audiometric test. These devices are fitted by registered nurses who have been adequately trained in this procedure and are under the supervision of a physician. Training in their use and care is emphasized.

USE OF HEARING CONSERVATION BY SMALL COMPANIES
Questions have been raised concerning the ability of smaller manufacturers and businesses to conduct successful hearing conservation programs and supervise effective use of hearing protectors. We believe that faced with the choice between the uncertainties and expense of an engineering control program and hearing conservation, the smaller employer can and will establish a program of hearing protection and audiometric testing. To learn more about the specific problem, du Pont engaged Hearing Conservation and Noise Control Inc. (HCNC) to survey small business from this standpoint. HCNC concluded that the industries sampled did not make significant use of engineering controls because of a lack of expertise and the high cost of such solutions. HCNC found that hearing protection and audiometry are the most useful and effective methods for the small employer.

COST EFFECTIVENESS OF HEARING PROTECTION
VS. ENGINEERING CONTROLS
The cost of our hearing conservation program, involving use of hearing protective devices, is less than $20 per worker per year. This is far more cost effective than BBN's estimated $267,000/man as a cost of achieving protection for the additional 30,000 workers estimated to be at risk of material impairment due to industrial noise exposure between 90 and 85 dBA. It is also more cost effective than BBN's extremely low estimate of $10.5 billion for a program to reduce workplace noise levels to 90 dBA.

Table 5: COMPLIANCE MONITORING COMPARISON

		Engineering Controls	Hearing Protection	Administrative/Dose Controls
1.	Visual Evidence	Hardware	Devices in place	None
2.	Measured Evidence	Area levels and audiometric testing	Audiometric testing (with margin of safety)	Exposure estimates and statistical analysis audiometric testing (with risk)
3.	Documented Evidence	Straight forward compliance plan (survey)	Straight forward compliance plan and medical records	Complex statistical complications and medical records
4.	Supervision	Annual check (survey)	Spot checking	Employee surveillance (location - task) timing
5.	Medical	Audiometric testing	Training, fitting, audiometric testing action (as required)	Audiometric testing (with risk based on dose estimate)
6.	Communication	Some benefit	Some benefit	No benefit
7.	Enforcement	Straight forward	Straight forward with margin of safety	Complex methodology
8.	Reduce noise level at the ear	Yes	Yes	No
9.	Protection inside enclosures	No	Yes	Not unless included in dose
10.	Protection from hearing	Adequate	Adequate with margin of safety	Inadequate due to potential risk
11.	Time for implementation	Long-term	Immediate	Short-term, if not dependent on engineering controls to some lower level
12.	Cost	Very high, unproductive	Low approximately $20 per year, low risk	High cost, high risk

The relevance of this dramatic cost differential is supported by our experience that the use of hearing protectors as a means of compliance, where reasonable and appropriate, is equal to or often superior to engineering and administrative controls in protecting the hearing of noise-exposed workers by providing attenuation on the order of 25 dBA. Where equivalent protection of employee health is available by various methods, the question of relative costs and benefits of these methods is extremely relevant. The diversion of resources to meet unnecessary compliance requirements by infeasible engineering controls utilizes scarce capital and expertise for unjustifiable, nonproductive costs.

Thus the hearing of employees can be preserved while the debate over other less relevant issues continues and while noise control technology evolves to reduce potentially-damaging levels of noise at the source, where this is possible. In light of this proven effectiveness and economy, we urge that hearing protectors, used in the context of a hearing conservation program, be recognized as the present cost-effective means of compliance, at least equal to engineering and administrative controls in protecting the hearing of noise-exposed workers and preventing potential impairment.

Additional perspectives regarding the alternative means and their potential for worker protection can be evaluated by the comparison of Table IV.

CONCLUSION

In summary, du Pont's confidence in the 90 dBA (or higher)/8 hour criteria and audiometric testing at 85 dBA is based on more than 20 years of experience in administration of a hearing conservation program which includes the use of personal protection devices as described earlier. These findings are corroborated in a similar study from the Ingersoll-Rand Company[2].

The authors suggest (see Table 5) that a detailed hearing protection program is more effective than dose-administrative controls. Where equal protection of health is available by various methods, relative cost effectiveness should be heavily weighed in selection of the best alternative. The cost of our hearing conservation program, on a unit worker basis is 1/400 of the cost estimated by BBN for industry to meet a 90 dBA standard. It is therefore urged that hearing protectors, as used in a hearing conservation program of the type described in the preceding discussion, be recognized as a means of compliance at least equal to engineering and administrative-dose controls in protecting the hearing of noise-exposed workers in industry.

Safety procedures and environmental controls for the safety and health of employees, customers and the public have long been a well defined part of du Pont operations and are a company tradition. Because the control of employee exposure to the potential hazard of industrial noise through prevention is and has been an integral part of the du Pont employee safety program, this study offers useful perspective and common sense recommendations on the issues of industrial noise control and protecting the health of individual workers.

REFERENCES
1. Pell, S., An Evaluation of a Hearing Conservation Program -a Five-Year Longitudinal Study. Amer. Indust. Hyg. Assoc. J., 34, 82-91, 1973.

2. Gosztonyi, R.E., The Effectiveness of Hearing Protective Devices. J. Occup. Med., 17, 569-580, 1975.

33 HEARING CONSERVATION BASED ON HEARING PROTECTORS: A PROVINCIAL PROJECT

David Y. Chung, R. Patrick Gannon, Margaret E. Roberts, and Keith Mason

INTRODUCTION

In a hearing conservation program the method of choice in noise control is engineering controls at source. In such a type of control the hazard is eliminated altogether. Other methods such as hearing protection, administrative dose control, and retrofit engineering control are secondary in priority. However, engineering control at source is often technically infeasible and economically impractical. Any regulatory agency which attempts to make engineering control at source the only allowable method would likely end up unsuccessful in providing hearing protection to workers. The most acceptable and probably the most effective way to control noise at present is, we believe, the use of hearing protectors. It is likely to stay so for many years to come. There are various reasons for this:

(1) Efficient hearing protectors can provide workers with more than 20 dB of attenuation when they are fitted properly.

(2) Often engineering noise control procedures cannot reduce noise to a non-hazardous level. In such cases a program of personal hearing protection still has to be implemented.

(3) The cost of a hearing conservation program that involves the use of hearing protectors is usually far less than one that employs engineering control.

Results from several studies have indicated that hearing protectors are effective in hearing conservation programs [1,2,3,4]. Like most remedies, personal hearing protection is not perfect. There are problems such as the reluctance of some workers to use hearing protectors and the improper use of hearing protectors by some others. Most of the criticism made of noise control programs with hearing protectors can be overcome by proper education and supervision.

In British Columbia hearing conservation is under the jurisdiction of the Worker's Compensation Board. There are basically two divisions which deal with hearing conservation programs: (1) the Prevention Services and (2) the Medical Services. The former is involved in the enforcement of regulations related to noise and the latter the monitoring of the programs with audiometry and medical surveillance and the rehabilitation of the hearing-impaired workers.

Industrial Health and Safety Regulations of the Workers' Compensation Board of British Columbia state that companies where workers are exposed to a steady-state noise of Leq 90 dBA for eight hours (Appendix I) or impact noise that exceeds the values shown in Appendix II are required to have a hearing conservation program which includes engineering controls, personal hearing protection and audiometric testing. When there is a hearing conservation program then all workers routinely exposed to a Leq of 85 dBA or more for 8 hours have to have a pure-tone audiogram done annually.

Hearing protectors are classified according to CSA standard Z94.2 -1974 into A, B, and C (Appendix III). The minimum CSA class of hearing protector to be worn at a particular noise level is shown in Appendix IV. Exemptions to the wearing of hearing protectors by the individual may be granted by the WCB for medical reasons. It is incumbent upon the workers to fit their hearing protectors effectively.

Industrial audiometric technicians employed by industries are trained by the WCB in a 3-day training program, during which they are instructed in basic anatomy and physiology of the auditory system, the techniques of pure-tone audiometry, the proper use of hearing protectors and the counselling of the hearing-impaired. Refresher courses are also offered and periodic attendance is required of the technicians. If companies prefer to use mobile audiometric contractors they may do so as long as technicians are certified by the WCB. An audiometric inspection officer goes out to each company annually to ensure that the audiometric equipment and testing booth meet the standard required by the WCB (ANSI S3.6-1969 and ANSI S3.1-1977).

With the industrial audiometric program the WCB requires a copy of all audiograms from the industries. It is expected the number of workers to be tested under this program will reach 250,000 when all industries comply with the regulations. All workers under this program will be tested annually. Depending on the situation, workers with abnormal changes in hearing level will be either counselled or referred to their attending physicians. To accomodate and utilize the information, optical scan forms, to be completed by technicians, have been designed so that information can be stored in the computer directly. Along with the audiometric data the optical scan forms also contain information on medical, shooting, noise and smoking history, noise control, etc. Questions on the noise control section are shown in Appendix V. It consists mainly of questions related to hearing protectors.

RESULTS

Data obtained to date from these industrial audiometric optical scan forms were analysed. At the time of analysis there were 61,074 entries. Unfortunately, not all questions on the forms were completed. Thus the N in each category analysed is less than the total N.

Figure I depicts the percentage of entries wearing each class of hearing protection. The N analysed here was 31,243. These include only those who answered the question "noise level of job". This is one of the questions that the workers were advised specifically not to answer when they were not sure of their job noise level. Approximately half of the entries did not answer this question. Since presently no ear-plug is given an A-Class according to CSA standard Z94.2 - 1974, and very few workers use a C-Class hearing protector, only B-Class hearing protectors are subdivided into B-Class muffs and B-Class plugs in the analysis. One third of the entries stated that they did not wear hearing protectors regularly.

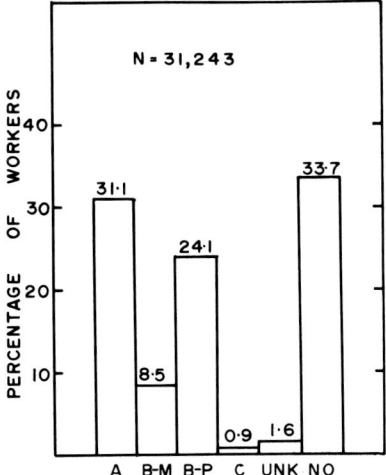

Figure 1.   Percentage of workers wearing different class of hearing protector. N includes some workers working at noise level less than 90 dBA. A: A-Class, B-M: B-Class muffs, B-P: B-Class plugs, C: C-Class, UNK: unknown, and NO: nonwearers.

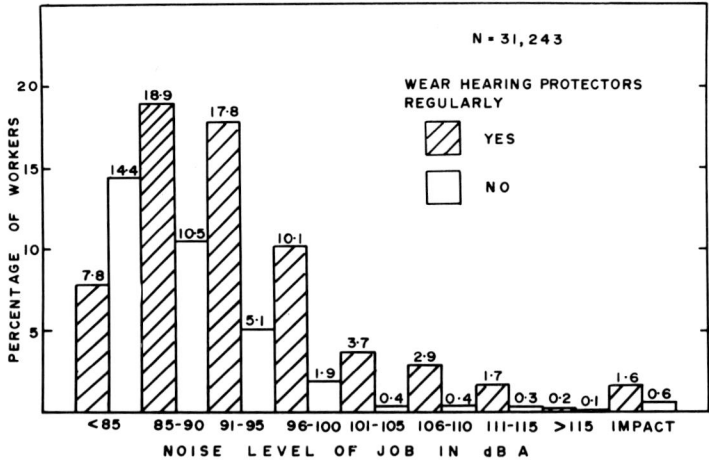

Figure 2.   Percentage distribution of hearing protector wearers versus nonwearers as function of job noise level.

Of course, some of these workers actually worked in noise levels of less than 90 dBA. Figure 2 shows the percentage distribution of hearing protector wearers versus non-wearers as a function of job noise level. If only workers working in noise levels exceeding 90 dBA were considered,

19% claimed that they did not wear hearing protectors regularly. A further breakdown of the analysis can be seen in Figure 3 which shows the percentage of workers wearing different classes of hearing protectors as a function of job noise level.

There are a few points which deserve to be mentioned here:

(1)   The percentage of workers wearing C-Class protectors is practically negligible at all noise levels.
(2)   At noise levels above 105 dBA most workers wear A-Class earmuffs as required by the regulations of the WCB, and
(3)   The percentage of workers who do not wear hearing protectors decreases with increase in noise level.

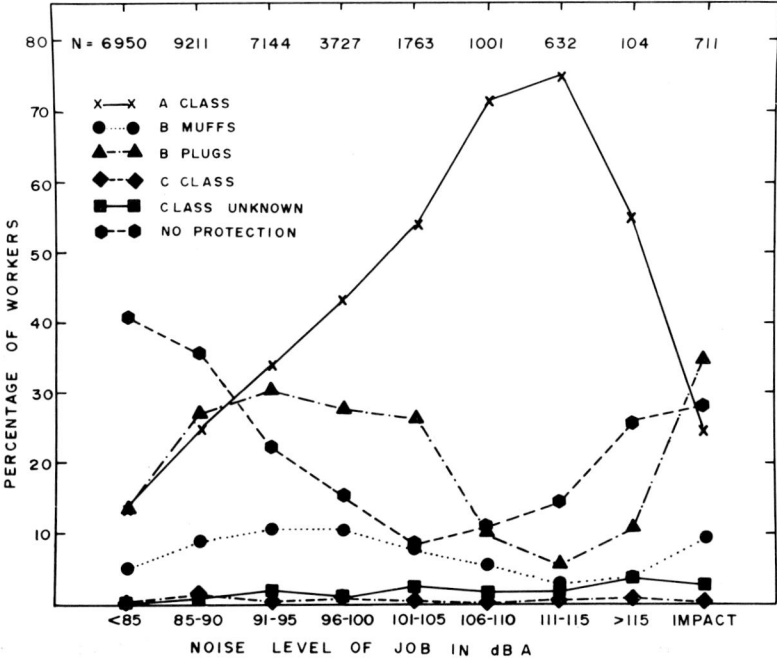

Figure 3.   Percentage of each hearing protector wearer classification as a function of job noise level.

The explanations for the deviations from these observations for levels above 115 dBA and impact noise are probably due to the small sample size

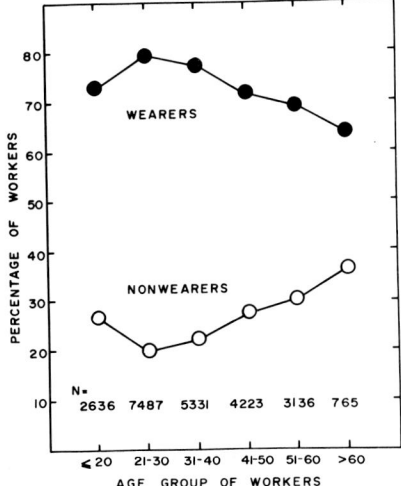

Figure 4. Percentage of hearing protector wearer versus nonwearer as a function of age.

in the former category, the lack of understanding of impulse/impact noise by workers and audiometric technicians in the latter category. In addition, at 115 dBA and above some workers use both plugs and muffs.

One comment we often hear from safety supervisors is that older workers are more reluctant to wear hearing protectors. Figure 4 shows that there is certain validity in such a statement. The same trend persists even when the workers were divided into groups with similar amount of noise exposure. The trend that appears in Figure 4, however, does not seem to be as positive as the impression that one gets from industry.

Conclusions

One of the many goals of this computerized audiometric program is to find out whether hearing protectors are effective in preventing noise-induced hearing loss. The answer to this question is not as simple as it appears. There are many factors which also affect the amount of hearing loss. Attempts were made to assess the protective function of hearing protectors with the industrial audiometric data. Since the program has been in operation for only one and a half years, the number of repeat audiograms obtained was less than 3,000. It was not possible to demonstrate the effectiveness of personal hearing protectors by correlating the change of hearing in one year and the regular use of hearing protectors. The results should not be construed as evidence against the effectiveness of hearing protectors in hearing conservation. More likely, it shows that the proper assessment of the effectiveness of personal protection requires a period of more than one year. Hopefully, in five years a proper assessment of the effectiveness of personal hearing protection can be made with the province-wide computerized audiometric program.

An effective province-wide hearing conservation program requires a regulatory role played by a central agency. The task is a formidable one since (1) it needs the co-operation of both labour and management and (2) it involves industries of various sizes and types, and which are located in different areas. This takes time, patience and expertise. In British Columbia a firm foundation has been laid for the conservation of hearing with the hope of the eventual elimination of occupational noise-induced hearing loss.

REFERENCES
1. Summar, T.M., Industrial Hearing Conservation (a report on a longitudinal survey), Nat. Safety News 100, 52-54, 1969.

2. Gosztonyi, Jr., R.E., The Effectiveness of Hearing Protective Devices. J. Occ. Med. 17, 569-580, 1975.

3. Axelsson, K., Axelsson, A., Jonsson A., Aspects on Personal Noise Protection. Scand. Audiol. 7, 247-253, 1978.

4. Dear, T.A., Karrh, B.W., An Effective Hearing Conservation Program - Federal Regulation or Practical Achievement? Sound and Vibration, Vol. 13, No. 9:12-19, 1979.

Appendix I. Criteria for the requirement of a hearing conservation program for steady state noise.

Noise Level (dBA)	Maximum Daily Exposure Time Without Hearing Protection (hours)
87	16
90	8
93	4
96	2
99	1
102	½
105	¼
over 105	0

Appendix II. Criteria for the requirement of a hearing conservation program for impact noise.

Peak Sound Pressure Level (dB)	Maximum Number of Impacts per 24 Hour Period
118	14,400
121	7,200
124	3,600
127	1,800
130	900
133	450
136	225
139	112
140	90
over 140	0

Appendix IV. Minimum CSA class of hearing protector which has to be worn.

Steady State Noise for 8 Hrs. (dBA)	*Minimum CSA Class of Hearing Protector
85 - 95	C
96 - 105	B
106 - 115	A
over - 115	A muff and B plug
Impact Noise	A

* CSA Standard Z94.2-1974

Appendix III. CSA standard Z94.2 - 1974. Classification criteria for hearing protectors.

Frequency (Hertz)	CLASS A		CLASS B		CLASS C	
	Minimum Single Frequency Attenuation (dB)	Minimum Sum of Frequency Group Attenuations (dB)	Minimum Single Frequency Attenuation (dB)	Minimum Sum of Frequency Group Attenuations (dB)	Minimum Single Frequency Attenuation (dB)	Minimum Sum of Frequency Group Attenuations (dB)
125	None	25	None	18	None	6
250	None		None		None	
500	29		None		None	
1000	35	185	25	135	15	85
2000	35		25		15	
3000	35		25		15	
4000	35		25		15	
6000	None	60	None	50	None	40
8000	None		None		None	

Note: Attenuation measurements made according to ANSI Z24.22 (1957).

Appendix V. Questions on Noise Control section in optical scan form.

NOISE CONTROL			NOISE LEVEL OF JOB d BA	
DO YOU WEAR EAR PROTECTORS	YES ----	NO ----	< 85	----
CLASS	WORN REGULARLY	BEFORE TEST	85-90	----
			91-95	----
A	----	----		
			95-100	----
B-MUFF	----	----		
			101-105	----
B-PLUG	----	----		
			106-110	----
C	----	----		
			111-115	----
CLASS UNKOWN	----	----	116-120+	----
ENCLOSURE	YES ----	NO ----	IMPACT	----
MEDICAL EXEMPTION	----	----		

34 PLANNING A PROVINCIAL HEARING CONSERVATION PROGRAM

P. L. Pelmear and M. J. Pike

The Advisory Council on Occupational Health & Occupational Safety (Ontario) in a recent report[1] concluded that the overall percentage of employees at risk to some noise above 85 dBA was between 7-10 per cent of the workforce, and that twice as many employees are exposed to 85 dBA as are exposed to 90 dBA. Assuming the workforce in Ontario to be 4.3 million it is estimated that at 90 dBA 215,000 workers and at 85 dBA 430,000 workers are at risk. Thus, the number of workers exposed to noise is larger than the total number exposed to any other hazardous physical agent or toxic substance.

Table I Claims Set up by Five Year Periods

	Industry Schedule I			Schedule II	Totals I & II
	A Mining	B Non-Mining	Total	C	A & B & C
1949-1953	2	2	4	1	5
1954-1958	10	18	28	3	31
1959-1963	31	151	182	3	185
1964-1968	224	387	611	17	628
1969-1973	794	901	1,695	49	1,744
1974-1978	4,174	3,731	7,905	182	8,087
TOTAL	5,235	5,190	10,425	255	10,680

Source: Workmen's Compensation Board Industrial Noise Deafness Report, Claims Reported by Year Claim Set Up and Rate Number, January 1980, Table 2.

This is a matter for concern as are The Workmen's Compensation Board's statistics for Ontario on compensation claims. By the end of 1979, The Workmen's Compensation Board (W.C.B.) had received 14,094 claims for noise induced hearing loss with mining and non-mining industries contributing almost equally to the total (Table I). The high risk industries accounting for the non-mining claims filed include steel making, metal manufacturing and forestry. These industries are much the same as those identified as high risk by American sources, which include amongst others, steel making, metal product manufacturing, forestry and logging, car manufacture and construction.

Another concern is the increasing cost to industry resulting from industrial hearing claims. The average total value medical aid for permanent disability settlements rose to $6,448.20 in 1978, with an average lifetime payout per award of approximately $16,000. It is by no means certain that the backlog of claims has been cleared and a large reservoir of cases is likely to be uncovered by many companies, both large and small, when hearing conservation programs are fully instituted. This likely conse quence is often a powerful deterrent to management and is one which requires considerable education to overcome.

For these several reasons provincial governments through regulations in the past, have specified requirements to attenuate noise and prevent hearing loss. Unfortunately the record shows that they have not been entirely successful. There is clearly a need for more positive legislation, health education and medical surveillance.

HEARING CONSERVATION
Many companies have designed and implemented effective hearing conservation programs[2,3] and the essential features include:
- (a) Noise measurement to identify sources and evaluate the hazard
- (b) Noise reduction
- (c) Provision of appropriate hearing protection
- (d) Health education
- (e) Periodic monitoring   - environment
                            - personnel by audiometry

The key issue has been and continues to be the sound level at which hearing conservation programs should be introduced: 85 or 90 dBA? The powerful industrial lobby has always argued very strongly that 90 dBA should be accepted because of the economic implications - the cost of noise reduction primarily and, to a lesser extent, the cost of hearing protection and monitoring audiometry.

The philosophy in Ontario for health protection at work as indicated in the gazetted occupational health hazard regulations August 1978 requires the adoption, application, installation and institution in progressive stages of engineering controls, work practices, and administrative controls to eliminate, control, limit or reduce a hazard to below the threshold limit value (TLV). This requires action if it is feasible and economically practical, to a degree which is effective. Surely a very reasonable requirement. It is therefore difficult to understand why there should be such resistance to adopting a TLV of 85 dBA for noise, since this is the safe level for the majority. Furthermore if the 90 dBA TLV should be retained those industries operating below 90 dBA but above 85 dBA will have no incentive to eliminate the hazard which as mentioned earlier, puts over 200,000 workers at risk in Ontario. Monitoring audiometry should be instituted at 85 dBA and preferably at 80 dBA, if the hyper-susceptible are to be identified and counselled.

The International Standard ISO 1999[4] reports that 8 per cent of workers exposed to 85 dBA for 30 years could experience a 25 dB hearing loss in the speech frequencies (0.5, 1 and 2 kHz) compared with 18 per cent of workers exposed to 90 dBA for thirty years. Thus an 85 dBA exposure level protects about 92 per cent of those at risk, while a 90 dBA exposure level protects only 82-85 per cent. Even allowing for data errors in selection and calculation[5] this must be a compelling reason for action to protect workers at the lower level. Enlightened employers will surely realize the folly of ignoring practicable safe work practices, and legislators should stand firm so that the requirement for safe practices will prevail.

ONTARIO LEGISLATION
Under regulations made under the Construction Safety Act 1973, Industrial Safety Act 1971, and the Mines Act 1970, where workers were

exposed to a sound level of 90 dB or greater, measures had to be taken to reduce the sound level to below 90 dB. Where such measures were not practicable workers had to wear 'hearing protection'. These requirement still apply under the industrial establishments regulations of our new Occupational Health and Safety Act 1978. However the incidence of hearing loss and subsequent compensation indicates that our legislation has not been entirely successful and that something more is necessary.

Our new Occupational Health and Safety Act requires that management and unions should jointly adopt a policy of internal responsibility through consultation and safety committees, to identify and resolve health and safety problems. Good practices should follow. Basic requirements stipulated in regulations and guidelines are required to guide them. However, only the safety regulations that apply to industrial establishments, construction projects, mines and mining plants have to date been issued. Occupational health service and specific toxic substance regulations are pending, but it would be unwise to anticipate the date.

Meanwhile, when biological, chemical or physical agents are used and are likely to endanger the health of workers, the Occupational Health and Safety Act, Section 20 (part 4 on toxic substances - see appendix) permits an inspector to order conditions for administrative control, work practices and engineering control, and to set time limits for compliance.

Part 3 of the act also specifies the duties of a constructor, employer, supervisor, worker, owner and supplier. If so prescribed the employer shall establish an occupational health service, accurately keep and maintain records, monitor, and comply with threshold limit values (section 15, see appendix). Such prescription must await the implementation of the proposed occupational health service and specific toxic substance regulations (including noise), which were initially gazetted in July/August 1978. The nature of their contents, revised in the light of comments received, will be of vital importance.

A NOISE REGULATION

Most regulations require a definition of the hazard. With respect to noise, 'unwanted sound' is quite inadequate. It is much more satisfactory in a regulation to choose a level, for example 80 dBA, and to require initial noise surveys when this level is likely to be exceeded so that the hazard, if it exists, may be identified. Thereafter a monitoring program should be established and maintained to monitor noise levels at intervals of not greater than 3 years where they exceed 85 dBA, and within 60 days of any change to or modification of existing equipment, machinery, processes or methods which might affect the noise levels.

Where a worker is exposed to a noise level of 85 dBA or greater, measures should be taken to reduce it to below 85 dBA. Where the measures prescribed cannot be promptly and effectively adopted, applied, and installed, personal hearing protection sufficient to attenuate the sound level to below 85 dBA should be provided and used. Some people would have regulations define the grade of ear protectors for specific noise levels. Although obviously intended to be helpful, this recommendation is not practical. Graded ear protectors would give workers a false sense of security since on occasions the grading may be inappropriate, or may be inadequate for the hyper-susceptible individual. The onus should be on the employer to provide the most appropriate and acceptable ear protectors that workers can wear to protect their hearing.

Clearly visible warning notices should be posted at entrances to hazardous work places. There has been much academic debate about maximum allowable durations of exposure to sound levels without hearing protection. Proponents of the equal energy principle, demand the use of the 3 dB halving-doubling rule, while others feel that the equal energy rule is too conservative and prefer a 5 dB trading relationship. It is important to realize that few workers in industry are going to be permitted restricted exposure without wearing ear protectors unless they are working in isolation because their presence among workers required to wear ear protectors would demand too much explanation. If workers see others not wearing safety equipment they will tend to do likewise. In practice, hazard areas have to be defined, and all who enter regardless of time exposure, need to use ear protectors to conform to regulations. In view of this there would appear to be little justification for including exposure tables in regulations because their application and use would be rare. Their publication should be restricted to data sheets and text books.

Personal exposure records should be maintained for workers, and an audiometric screening program should be established and maintained for workers in areas where noise levels exceed 85 dBA. This should include audiometric tests on employment, either annually or at such times as an inspector may order.

The tests should be undertaken by a qualified industrial audiometric technician. This means a person qualified by training or experience in audiometry. In Ontario short courses of instruction have been available in several centres, and large numbers of personnel have already been trained.

The audiometric tests should consist of threshold measurements at least at .5,1,2,3,4 and 6 kHz. The audiometer should be calibrated annually to Canadian Standards Association standard, Z 107.4-1975, and the maximum background noise levels for audiometry rooms should not exceed the American National Standards Institute Standard S3.1-1977. These requirements are obvious since to perform audiometric examinations otherwise is to waste time and money for both employer and employee.

Workers should be required to submit to such tests if at risk to noise, and they should be advised of the results. Furthermore a worker should be advised to consult a physician if the threshold measurement in either ear averages 25 dB or more at .5,1,2 and 3 kHz; or there has been a confirmed shift from the previous audiogram of 15 dB or more at any frequency; or has sustained an average loss of 5 dB or more over any 3 adjacent frequencies. This is to ensure accurate diagnosis by a physician, and to provide more effective health education to prevent further loss and subsequent workmen's compensation.

The occupational health medical service of the ministry of labour in Ontario has always had the responsibility of auditing medical surveillance programs, and such a regulation if adopted here, would require the results of all audiometric tests showing impairment to be submitted to the chief, occupational health medical service, to a physician designated by the worker, and to a physician designated by the employer. for the ministry to deal effectively with the data and to audit and evaluate the information the medical service of the ministry will require the data to be submitted in a format suitable for easy handling and computer analysis. The work load, both in the occupational health medical services of industry and the ministry could be considerable.

CONCLUSION

The introduction of legislative requirements on such an elaborate scale can be justified without doubt because of the extent of the hazard in industry, the social consequences of hearing loss to workers, the magnitude of Workmen's Compensation Board liability and the need for positive action to conserve workers' health. Without legislation only enlightened industry seeks to resolve its health and safety problems. With legislation all will do so if the ministry of labour directs effectively and is vigilant in its auditing. The preparation and implementation of feasible regulations is a legislative exercise, essential for the common good, and one to which all parties can contribute.

REFERENCES

1. Report of the Advisory Council on Occupational Health and Occupational Safety. Advisory Memorandum 79-111. Occupational Hearing Loss: Prevention, Compensation and Rehabilitation, Ontario Ministry of Labour, Toronto, 1980.

2. Pelmear P.L., Hearing Conservation. J. Soc. Occup. Med. 23, 22-26, 1973.

3. Pelmear, P.L., Industrial Noise. The Practitioner 221, 668, 1978.

4. International Organization for Standardization. Recommendation R 1999: Assessment of Occupational Noise Exposure for Hearing Conservation Purposes, 1975.

5. Ward, W.D., Gloring, A., Exhibit I: A critique of Research Data

Relating Hearing Level to Exposure to Noise below 90 dBA. J. Occup. Med. 17, 21, 776, 1975.

APPENDIX

OCCUPATIONAL HEALTH AND SAFETY ACT, 1978

Section
15. (1) In addition to the duties imposed by section 14, an employer shall,
- (a) establish an occupational health service for workers as prescribed;
- (b) where an occupational health service is established as prescribed, maintain the same according to the standards prescribed;
- (c) keep and maintain accurate records of the handling, storage, use and disposal of biological, chemical or physical agents as prescribed;
- (d) accurately keep and maintain and make available to the worker affected such records of the exposure of a worker.

20. (1) Where a biological, chemical or physical agent or combination of such agents is used or intended to be used in the work place and its presence in the work place or the manner of its use is in the opinion of a Director likely to endanger the health of a worker, the Director shall by notice in writing to the employer order that the use, intended use, presence or manner of use be,
- (a) prohibited;
- (b) limited or restricted in such manner as the Director specifies; or
- (c) subject to such conditions regarding administrative control, work practices, engineering control and time limits for compliance as the Director specifies.

35 SUMMATION OF INTERNATIONAL SYMPOSIUM ON HEARING PROTECTION IN INDUSTRY

W. Dixon Ward

This conference provides an illustration of how a previously simple situation has become considerably more complex. When I first got into the area of ear protection about 26 years ago, we had only two objectives: to make employees aware of a hazard to hearing, and to get employers to furnish ear protectors. Their effective use was up to the employee. Now, however, with 1984 just around the corner, Big Brother insists that we be protected from all harm whether we like it or not, so we have discussions of extra-scientific problems such as: how to persuade workers to use protectors (by force if necessary); whether or not ear protection is even permissible (at best a last resort if noise cannot be reduced at the source); how great a margin of safety one should have on attenuation figures; and the like. On the other hand, since bureaucrats demand simplicity in assessment of hazard, despite a patent complexity of subject matter, we find ourselves involved with the question of rating hearing protectors by a single number, a rating that has been achieved in the United States only by postulating that A-weighting of all sounds is an adequate measure of hazard, that everyone works in pink noise, and that "everyone" constitutes 97.5% of the exposed workers.

Beyond this extension of problems farther into the political realm, however, we find ourselves addressing the same questions now as earlier. I shall try to review the specific questions and the evidence presented here to answer them, in approximately the same order as the order of presentation as organized by our astute Chairman, Dr. Alberti, and our super systematizer, Dr. Shaw.

WHAT IS THE GOAL OF HEARING PROTECTION?

The quick answer to this question is always "prevention of damage to hearing." The traditional measure of damage, and the easiest the measure, is a loss of auditory sensitivity, i.e., an increase in Hearing Threshold Level (HTL), and this was taken for granted in most of the presentations. However, Dr. Henderson reminded us that tinnitus is a separate distressing symptom of noise damage, and that auditory acuity may also be affected by noise exposure to a degree not completely predictable from threshold measurements, so that frequency and intensity difference limens, processes responsible for temporal integration, and even speech discrimination ability, may be abnormal in the presence of apparently normal thresholds. Possible physiological correlates of stages of this "subliminal damage" were discussed by Dr. Hunter-Duvar and illustrated with his incomparably beautiful slides; it is apparent that in the future many investigators will be studying the cilia of the hair cells closely. At the moment, however, we still have no method of proven validity for inferring damage in an ear with normal thresholds, so HTLs will probably continue to be the indicator of choice for some time.

We must seek, therefore, the threshold of damage -- that exposure that just produces, in some specified fraction of those exposed, a measurable hearing loss. Although the relation between exposure to steady noise and resultant loss is becoming fairly well established, the importance of intermittence and high crest factor is still being scrutinized. Both the paper of Dr. Voigt* and my own imply that crest factor may be even more important than previously believed. It is interesting that Voigt et al. found an increase in handicap over control values not in those exposed to even 86-100 dB of continuous noise, but only in 100-dB-equivalent but "strongly fluctuating" noise, which meant that the peaks were well over 100. Everyone certainly agrees that plenty of problems still face us in adequately measuring impulse noise; Mr. Rasmussen summarized this situation*, reiterating the problem of the size of the microphone and its orientation, especially when dealing with such short-duration transient events. I was brought back to the old days by his demonstration of the use of the toy cricket as an impulse source, the noise source we used to study temporary threshold shift 20 years ago[1].

Dr. Atherley* told us that the 3-dB versus 5-dB controversy would be solved if we could find out what would be the result if 200 people were given daily exposures of 15 minutes at 115 dBA for 10 years. The newspaper account of our meeting says there are about 200 people at this conference; I wonder how many of the people here would volunteer for this experiment? Now, the whole question of tolerable acoustic dose becomes irrelevant if we go to protection of areas rather than of people, as is apparently happening nowadays. The evidence is almost overwhelming that not only here but in the United States, rulemakers are going to do what our Congress mandated: determine those <u>levels</u> the attainment and maintenance of which are necessary to protect the public health and welfare. Thus, the <u>duration</u> of exposure is going to become an academic issue, as Dr. Pelmear correctly indicated. As soon as this occurs, the trading relationship does not matter: when the level gets above a certain point, it is judged to be potentially hazardous if continued long enough, and thus noise control measures must be instituted.

Should exposures be limited through noise reduction or by use of protection? This is a topic that I thought was going to be soft-pedalled, although it does have to be discussed sooner or later. Mr. Menzies pointed out that we should be measuring exposures rather than place levels if we want to obtain an adequate representation of the noise exposure that people are getting; I suspect that most of us still think this is well worth doing even if it does become an academic issue. Mr. Tengling reminded us how fast L_{eq} increased with just a short period of non-use of hearing protectors. That of course is the nature of decibels; it is just bound to go that way. If you don't use your ear protectors even for very short periods, the L_{eq} goes up. This perhaps highlights one of the chief shortcomings of L_{eq}: the effect of temporal pattern is completely ignored.

HOW DO HEARING PROTECTORS WORK AND HOW IS PROTECTION MEASURED?

This received a lot of attention, as it should. Dr. Shaw's "old ideas" were

---

* Manuscripts not published.

shown to be not so old after all: we still have the in-the-ear versus over-the-ear, passive versus active, and linear versus nonlinear classifications. The bulk of the evidence is that ordinary ear plugs are linear. Although we have had a little bit of argument to the contrary, I believe that, by and large, the evidence, especially from Dr. Martin's cadavers, is overwhelming, and one should look very closely for artifacts in experiments that claim nonlinearity for protection, especially in levels over 90 and 100 dB. It does not appear that it is necessary to use "realistic" levels to establish the degree of protection afforded by all but deliberatly nonlinear protectors, although one can use procedures such as those described by Dr. Damongeot and Dr. Humes: any characteristic that is unique to a given effective level will serve --reflex threshold, MCL, aural overload threshold, etc. At the moment, however, there appears to be no real need for such somewhat indirect tests.

In the analysis of performance, the types of tests can be classified as real-ear, semi-objective or objective; all of the methods should ultimately agree. The big problem is making the objective devices closely resemble the response of the real ear and head in order to achieve comparability of results of different techniques. Dr. Chillery emphasized the importance of all the characteristics of the head and ear: resonances, reflections, bone conduction, and the effect of real skin and hair.

This leads us to the single-number-rating controversy, whose proponents seem to be winning despite some solid evidence that Dr. Chung presented showing that you get quite different results in different noises. I had the uneasy feeling that Dr. Tobias and Dr. Michael feel that a single-number rating must be possible because it is necessary; I have never understood that logic, though it is becoming familiar enough. If different protectors, in different noises, lead to different numbers, then you are doing an injustice to one protector or another by using the single-number scheme that assumes a pink-noise environment. However, it appears that OSHA inspectors need a single predetermined number, and so it has come to pass.

The problem of testing nonlinear devices has not really been solved by the use of artificial or cadaver ears or by the temporary threshold shift reduction (TTSR) procedure that we employed^2 although they do provide means of evaluating hearing protectors such as the Gunfender at high noise levels. The problem is how to standardize such procedures; I do not expect ANSI to go along with writing specifications for TTSR or cadaver studies. But at least the procedures do exist and do indicate whether nonlinear devices accomplish anything at all. At any rate, we should insist that nonlinear devices be judged by some procedure other than the real-ear threshold shift procedures that have been standardized.

The use of miniature microphones to evaluate ear protectors actually in situ is a new development described by Dr. Rood. It might even be useful to get three microphones in order to measure the successive effect of the protectors in a double-protection scheme. I think this is one of the ways that we may be able to find out why we don't get closer to the bone-conduction limit by adding over-the-ear and in-the-ear protectors; the results might give us a clue as to how this might be improved.

The desirability of having standard procedures, as Dr. Nixon presented it, is unquestioned. His list of "standards needed", however, sounds to me more like a list of "research that needs to be done" in at least half of his specific examples. Apparently he is much surer of the state of the facts in these areas than I am.

In regard to the correction of attenuation by substracting N standard deviations, I am surprised that Dr. Shaw was all that incensed over it, although I am a little worried myself about arbitrarily modifying a perfectly legitimate test result. However, in a sense of allowing "corrections" for careless workers in the field, I fear that, pragmatically, this is something we can't fight successfully and so laboratories that select their test subjects carefully in order to get small SDs will continue to do a land office business.

Dr. Brinkmann provided us with a fascinating account of the thoroughness with which protectors can -- and should -- be investigated, including effects of temperature, humidity, headband tension, and especially aging processes. Someone asked if the distance they had to survive a drop was dependent upon the height of his outstretched arm, but I did not hear the answer to that.

Double protection came up again and again. We were informed by Ms. Cruchley that it is required under certain conditions in the Armed Forces not only in the United States but also in Canada. In view of the fact that as one eyeballs the curves of single vs. double protection one wonders whether it is really worth the effort, it may be worth emphasizing that if you have two protectors, either of which has a probability of being misfit or misworn of say 0.3, then the probability of <u>both</u> being ineffective is only 0.09. That is, the chief value of double protectors is as a safety factor.

One type of ear protection not discussed is that provided by turbans. Because of the type of material that is used, you don't have to have a Gunfender or another ear plug with a hole in it to get as much as a 20-dB limiting of impulse noise[3]. In view of the propensity for the people in the northwest part of India and in Pakistan to shoot a lot, it is probably good that they wear such protectors.

WHAT ARE THE UNWANTED SIDE EFFECTS OF EAR PROTECTION?

Comfort was discussed at length by Dr. Damongeot, who showed us some examples of how one should go about assessing the comfort and acceptability of hearing protectors. He emphasized, as did Mr. Berger, that we have to study comfort over a long period of time, although there is evidence that subjective judgments are relatively constant over a period of half an hour or so. The relation between protectors and ear disease was brought up but no one could point to any statistics, so I guess that it is a dormant issue at the moment.

The ability to hear and to respond to a warning siren was discussed by Dr.

Wilkins. His research showed a slight decrement in the actual percentage of response, although not in detectability, apparently because there is a slight effect here that comes because the <u>absolute</u> level of sound has been reduced. How you compensate for that is not clear. As long as there is only a 6% reduction in frequency of response, it is perhaps a hazard that we can live with, but if we can figure out a way of negating it, so much the better. I think we were all glad to hear from Dr. Michael that perception of the ubiquitous "roof talk" in mines has finally been attacked experimentally. It is gratifying to learn that it is nothing mysterious --its snap, crackle and "speed" can be recognized in the absence of drilling noise but not in its presence. The advantage of an active defender in such a situation becomes even more obvious.

As a corollary to the ability to hear warning signals, the ability to hear speech in levels that are at all hazardous has no relation to the problem of trying to carry out casual conversations; under those conditions what is involved is just instructions or warnings that are shouted. So, as Dr. Tobias points out, we should really be studying shouts in such a situation and not PB's spoken in a normal conversational voice. The results that Dr. Abel got seem to reflect this pretty accurately, showing that under certain conditions, where marginal comprehension already exists, then a further disruption of the information transmission in the form of wearing hearing protectors, thereby reducing everything, is enough to provide a clear decrement in intelligibility scores from people with a sensorineural hearing loss, although not from people with normal hearing. I am sure that you can create conditions, if you want to, in which everyone would show a drop in speech perception, but on the other hand there are several articles in the literature, one quite recent[4], that find no changes even for people with sensorineural hearing loss: it depends upon the conditions. So that when Dr. Abel says there is a 15% reduction due to wearing protection, this is a useless statistic because it only applies to the individual situation she studied and would be different in other conditions.

All in all, the discussion of unwanted side effects was quite restrained. At least nobody exposed us to an account of all the psychological hazards we heard about at the OSHA hearing in Washington four or five years ago, where workers were getting up and telling us all about the nausea, dizziness, headaches and insomia "caused" by ear plugs and muffs. One psychologist even inveighed against the "feeling of psychological isolation" that allegedly accompanied the wearing of a hearing protector. I thank you all for your silence on such will-o-the-wisps.

WHAT ARE THE PROBLEMS OF USAGE?
Leakage, due to an imperfect seal, seems to be the number one problem, although deterioration of materials was running a close second, especially when Dr. Royster told us that V51R's would degenerate in just a few days under some conditions. Leakage is a problem with all protectors except apparently the E.A.R. It is apparently of little help to buy custom molded ones, because their material is not as flexible as the skin. This is Dr. Tobias' explanation for why molded plugs, which at first glance sound so great because of the individual fitting, turn out to be not as good or at any rate not better than the regular issue. Everyone emphasized that the right and left ears may be of different sizes, necessitating a careful fit for each.

The problem of the attachment of muffs to a helmet was raised when Dr. Acton mentioned the requirement that the helmet must be able to move an inch up and down. What does that do to the hearing protector? We were assured that nobody's ear had yet been cut off. The question of multiple protection devices seems to be confused but is at least being handled.

The spectre of carcinogenic materials and the restriction of their use was mentioned. There is a general belief in our society today that if an injection of a substance in massive doses will cause cancer in mice, then you don't want it rubbing against the skin, even in low concentrations. Where one can find a ready substitute, there is nothing wrong with this timidity, but if it means a big sacrifice in the effectiveness of a protective device, then it seems a pity; but probably nothing can be done about it. The effect of ozone and other substances, particularly skin acid in some individuals, in inducing rapid deterioration, has been well promulgated at this meeting.

Finally, we come to the problem of deliberate misuse, which was described in detail by Miss Riko. She regaled us with many of the things that can be done to hearing protectors to make them ineffective. One wonders how much this sort of thing may louse up longitudinal studies, especially when the use of protectors is mandatory; apparently some people will go to any lengths to sabatoge doing anything they have been told that they must do. I believe, though, that this is the sort of reaction that disappears with time. When the worker is first ordered to do it he figures out ways to circumvent the protection, but then as time goes on he decides it is not worth the effort -- everyone else seems to be accepting it, so he decides to accept it himself. Do you suppose that this might account for some of the "learning effect" that is found in serial audiograms? I think we ought to think of alternative explanations for this phenomenon. I really can't believe that any learning effect takes place over a period of a year, so I keep looking for other explanations for Dr. Royster's "learning effect" such as acceptance of hearing protection. Of course this theory would not apply to the learning effect in non-exposed people, but in that case the fact that they are in an audiometric program may make them more aware of their sociacusic exposures. However, there is no way that I can think of to establish this either.

WHEN IS THE PROGRAM WORKING?
Dr. Else gave us an excellent set of questions that, in essence, delineates the specific steps in determining why there may be a problem, why ear protection is the best solution, and how effectiveness of the program can be monitored. The complex interaction between the mere existence of the program itself and the use of protectors that Dr. Karmy described is fascinating; it makes one wonder to what extent these instructions, the propaganda, are having effects somewhat indirectly, in unexpected ways, as I just mentioned in regard to "learning effect." I suppose that Dr. Royster would argue that DuPont's program, as described by Mr. Dear, is not working because it did not demonstrate any improvement and indeed,

showed additional loss over five years. I would still contend that if the additional loss is no greater than in the general population (i.e., due to presbyacusis, nosoacusis and sociacusis) then the program is indeed working.

I was pleasantly surprised to hear Dr. Martin emphasize that effects of noise are caused by doses and not by levels -- I thought I was the only one who believed that[5]. The study of mining noises is particularly difficult, and the contribution to this topic by Mr. Savich should have a great influence in helping the professionals in this field, who have always had a great deal of difficulty because of the reluctance of miners to wear protectors. I was glad to hear that they had somehow been persuaded in Sweden, which brings us to the next question.

HOW DO YOU GET WORKERS TO WEAR EAR PROTECTORS?

The excellent evaluation of psychological factors by Bilsom reported by Mr. Lofgreen of course makes sense: some sort of reward (positive reinforcement) is more likely to produce results than the negative effect of losing hearing in 40 years. Their general approach apparently works; at least it has been successful in several places. Group dynamics -- peer pressure -- also has something to do with successful use, as was reflected in the study by Zohar et al.[6] that Dr. Nixon told us about. One thing that he did not mention about this study (the one where they gave the workers feedback about their TTS at the end of the day) was that they tried, with a control group, to use the threat of withholding wages to increase the use of hearing protectors; this was completely ineffective.

Is 60% use some sort of limiting value? This figure appeared a couple of times, not only in the Bilsom experience, but also in Dr. Karmy's studies. Would 60% of the population, when pressured a little bit, protect their hearing, 40% not? I tend to think that this is just a coincidence, not any magic number, because in the highest intensities, such as around jet aircraft, compliance is better because the noise is just so unpleasant. So then, how do you get 100%? The use of force can work; if everyone in a given work area is forced to wear protection, then at least it is a nondiscriminatory situation. However, as a Libertarian I dislike that course of action. Besides, it is in the mandatory-use places that workers sabotage their protectors.

WHAT IS THE BEST PROTECTOR?
The apparent winner at this Symposium is the E.A.R., although I regret seeing it come out this way. I would much prefer a dead heat between Bilsom and E.A.R., because both are such good contributors to our societies and in particular to our meeting here. Indeed, I am not as sure as Dr. Royster is that his 3-dB difference in temporary threshold shift is meaningful. The debate over the effectiveness of plugs vs. muffs will continue, I am sure, for years to come, as inconclusively as it has been here. As Dr. Aram Glorig always says, "The best protector is the one that is worn."

HOW CAN PROTECTORS BE IMPROVED?
Bone conduction remains the limit, everyone agrees; no one has modified Zwislocki's classic analysis to show that anything better is possible. The question is, how can one get closer to it? Mr. Gorman showed us two muffs, designed by mathematical analysis, then constructed according to the analysis, that were able to provide a better low frequency attenuation. This is the approach that should be exploited in depth. It was interesting when the question of tuned protectors arose; although Dr. Shaw neatly side-stepped the issue by saying they were misused anyhow, the question remains how effective they could become.

Then there is the question I raised during one of the discussions.

SHOULD EVERYONE USE HEARING PROTECTORS?
Schori and McGatha[7] showed that the typical noise exposure for people who do <u>not</u> work in noise is an $L_{eq(8h)}$ of 80 dBA with a standard deviation of 5 dB. If this is indeed the highest innocuous exposure then we should probably all be walking around with protectors. But then what do we do when we talk? Even when our ears are covered, our voice gets to our ears by bone conduction at a level that requires 110 dB of noise to mask and

therefore must have a very high effective intensity.

I would like to continue with a few topics that were not mentioned in this symposium. For example, consider differences in age and protection requirements. Do older people need more protection, or perhaps less? This probably wasn't brought up because there really is no good evidence one way or another. In analyses that have been made recently, the progression of hearing loss in a given noise seems to be the same irrespective of age, so that age per se doesn't seem to make you more susceptible[9,10]. A related question is whether the damaged ear requires more protection than the undamaged. The answer is that we are not sure; but how could we verify a posture answer anyway? The insuperable obstacle is getting agreement on what consitutes "equal further damage" in a normal and damaged ear. Is going from 40 to 50 dB HL, in an already-damaged ear, equivalent to a change of from 0 to 10 dB, or perhaps instead from 0 to 30, in a normal ear? People with slight pre-existing high-frequency losses do not seem to be any more susceptible to TTS in the high frequencies, relatively speaking, than they are at the low frequencies where their thresholds are normal. However, Burns and Robinson[11] did show a small but significant correlation, in industrial workers, between temporary threshold shifts in the 1-and 2-kHz region and Hearing Threshold Levels at 3 and 4 kHz. It is likely, therefore, that to some extent the existence of a loss indicates that the ear is usually susceptible to damage, in which case greater protection would be required, rather than that the ear concerned had merely been subjected to an unusually severe exposure that would have caused the observed amount of damage in any ear.

I was surprised that no one brought up the question of something other than hearing protectors that we might use to reduce noise-induced hearing loss. I was prepared to say something about all the cocktails of vitamins A and E, nicotinic acid, nylidrin, gingko-biloba extract, Hydergine, dextran, etc., that are given to people to reduce hearing loss from acoustic trauma. So I shall say it anyway: there is no convincing evidence that they do any more good than a placebo, although it gives the patient the impression that the doctor is doing <u>something</u>.

Having briefly reviewed the presentations, I shall now try to point out where it seemed we had agreement on where research was most urgently needed, where we should encourage people to work. We should continue studying the concept of the "safe noise dose" for both steady and impulse noise, with emphasis on the importance of peak factor. The possibility of the existence of a "critical" intensity or dose should be kept in mind in such studies. The problem of the effectiveness of ear plugs after several hours of wearing needs further work (with more than an N of 2, which is the number of people that were involved in a recent published study). The use, in dosimeters, of miniature microphones small enough to be placed at the eardrum can be developed for analysis of the effectiveness of various protectors in the same way as they are being used to study how well hearing aids are performing. This technique would appear to be particularly well suited to an attack on the double-protector question. In some work areas, especially in the mines, this miniaturization can at last indicate how well people are wearing their protectors and we will also have a better idea of what mining exposures actually are.

An interest in building better dummy heads continues to exist, and the question of what constitutes good artificial skin will still occupy us for quite a while.

Do we need new designs? Yes, there is a need for greater attenuation for protectors against the impulse noise of high intensity weapons, a major military problem. When repeated impulses of around 185 dB are involved, even double protection may not protect the most susceptible ears from developing TTSs that last more than a few hours, and so may be hazardous. It is therefore good to continue to look for attenuators with greater effectiveness, either because they are intrinsically better or because they are more easily and reliably used. The development of active attenuators is sure to increase in pace; as all the controls and circuits become smaller, it should become possible to produce an active device that will weigh no more than the present passive ones.

We should also, it appears, develop new laws of physics so that the single-number rating scheme will apply to all protectors irrespective of the noise spectrum in which they will be used.

We may as well continue to gather longitudinal exposure data, for only in this way will we be able to relate hearing loss to <u>actual</u> noise exposure; by "actual" I imply that we indeed measure the noise that is getting through the protector and thus know the true exposure. I can see no other way of studying the effect of noise on hearing in humans, now that protection is used, unless we study in undeveloped countries where they don't yet have hearing conservation programs.

Finally, we must continue to develop better means of persuasion. I don't like the thought that if I want to walk through Times Square I must put ear plugs in because the level is over 90 dBA. That is where we are headed if we accept the concept of mandatory use in industry. Mandatory wearing can be successful, as Dr. Royster points out; I just don't like it. This point has, I guess, taken us from the scientific arena to the political, so let me just restate some of the political problems that will probably continue to be bandied about. Under what conditions is noise reduction to be preferred over ear protection, and vice versa? How much over protection ("margin of safety") should we have? What are the cost considerations? (Although this appears to be a quantitative question, it ultimately becomes a value judgement.) Whose responsibility is hearing protection? Is it any part of the worker's responsibility or not?

I can't help closing with a political comment on the situation outlined by Dr. Pelmear here in Ontario - a comment I make not as a scientist but merely as a normal taxpayer and consumer. Where it is "feasible," noise levels must be reduced not to 90 dBA but to 85; Oh happy noise control engineers! There is going to be a requirement of another audiometric examination in case of a 15 dB change at any frequency or a sum of 15 dB at any 3 adjacent frequencies; Oh happy audiologists! All this repeat audiometry is of course to be under medical supervision; so, Oh happy doctors! But alas, poor employers, alas poor taxpayers, alas poor consumers, especially in view of the fact that all these costs could be eliminated, together with industrial hearing loss, by the proper use of hearing protectors.

REFERENCES

1. Ward, W.D., Selters, W., Glorig, A., Exploratory studies on temporary threshold shift from impulses. J. Acoust. Soc. Amer. 33, 781-793, 1961.

2. Ward, W.D., Lupberger, A., Evaluation of two nonlinear ear protectors using a constant temporary threshold shift technique shift technique. J. Acoust. Soc. Amer. 53, 315(a), 1973.

3. Singh, D., Marhija, I.J., Protection against blast injuries of the ear. J. Laryngol. Otol. 86, 949-953, 1972.

4. Rink, T.L., Hearing protection and speech discrimination in hearing-impaired persons. Sound and Vibration 13(1), 22-25, 1979.

5. Ward, W.D., Noise levels are not noise exposures! Proc. NOISEXPO Conf. 170-175, 1974.

6. Zohar, D., Cohen, A., Azar, N., Promoting increased use of ear protectors in noise through information feedback. Human Fact. 22, 69-79, 1980.

7. Schori, T.R., McGatha, E.A., A real-world assessment of noise exposure. Sound and Vibration 12(9), 24-30, 1978.

8. Howell, R.W., A seven-year review of measured hearing levels in make manual steelworkers with high initial thresholds. Brit. J. Indust. Med. 35, 27-31, 1978.

9. Welleschik, B. and Raber, A. Einfluss von Expositionszeit und Alter auf den lärmbedingten Hörverlust. Laryng. Rhinol. 57, 1037-1048, 1978.

10. Burns, W. and Robinson, D.W. Hearing and Noise in Industry. London, Her Majesty's Stationery Office, 1970.

Subject Index

Subject Index

A-weighted sound levels
  C-weighted vs, 267–268
  computation of, 223, 229
  in hearing protection, 83–84
  and Short Method, 226
  in single-number factors, 232
Acoustic trauma
  in auditory temporal summation, 24–25
  clean up process after, 12
  in inner ear damage, 1–13; *see also* Inner ear damage from acoustic trauma
Acoustical degradation, 95–96
Acoustical performance, as standard attribute, 95
Acoustical Society of America, 91
Acoustical Standards Board, 72
Advisory Council on Occupational Health & Occupational Safety (Ontario), 569
Age and hearing protection requirements, 588
Air leakage, 59–61, 584
  in circumaural hearing protector, 104
  in earcushion, 433
  in earmuffs, 472
  in earplugs, 59–61
  obstacles as cause of, 61
  slot for, 61
American National Standards Institute (ANSI) 92, 222, 237, 574
American Optical Eargage, 301
American Standards Association, 91, 411
Anechoic chamber in testing, 165
ANSI, *see* American National Standards Institute
Artificial heads
  attenuation and, 117–119, 138
  circumaural hearing protectors and, 108, 109
  design of, 120–124
  earmuffs in, 119, 138
  endplates in, 124
  pinna in, 119
Attenuation
  artificial heads and, 117–119, 138
  bond conduction in, 211–219, 294, 428–429, 432–440
  circumaural contour in, 105–117
  in circumaural hearing protector, 101–128, 429–432
  clarity in, 443
  cross-modality matching in, 200–205
  cup mass in, 107
  decrease in, 202–203
  earcushion in, 428
  earmuffs and, 117, 134–140, 306–308, 342, 374–376, 412–414
  in mines, 417–420
  objective procedure in, 136–140
  physical method of testing, 415–417
  subjective procedure in, 134–140
  earplugs and, 342, 374–376
  flat response in, 443
  formula in low frequency, 430
  free-field hearing thresholds in, 316, 318
  as function of wearing time, 263–271
  glasses in, 328, 412–414
  hair in, 104, 182, 328
  in high noise levels, 199–209
  in HPD, 304–306
  ideal, 323–324
  impulse-noise measurement in, 287–291
  impulse-noise stimuli in, 285
  insertion loss in, 283
  ISVR objective test facility in, 124–128

Attenuation (contd.)
  of left and right earshells, 194
  linearity in, 278-291
  manikin in estimating, 200-201
  masked bone-conduction threshold in, 205-206
  measurement methods in, 440
  miniature microphones in measurement of, 175-196; see also Miniature microphones in attenuation measurement
  noise spectrum in, 169
  objective measurement of, 441
  open-ear measurements in, 284-285
  physiological noise in, 278-291, 294, 296-297
  real-ear probe-microphone measurements in, 207-208
  replications in, 194-196
  semi-objective measurement of, 441-442
  skin/flesh stimulation in, 115-117
  in speech intelligibility, 374-375, 379-385
  standard deviations in, 170, 245, 310, 318
  standard subjective test methods in evaluating, 273-297
  standard test data in, 291
  steady-state noise measurement in, 286-287
  steady-state stimuli in, 291, 295
  subjective free-field threshold measurement in, 294
  subjective threshold shift in, 440-441
  superliminal methods of measuring, 211
  as term, 284
  transmission loss in, 283
  uncorrelated data in, 237
  of unoccluded ear, 284
  user fitting of HPD in, 315-322
  volume in, 107
  in work place, 321
Audiometer-headset test, 167-168
Audiometry
  in du Pont's HCP, 553-554
  and education in hearing protector usage, 501-503, 505-506
  and employee attitudes toward hearing protection, 491-508
  in HCP, 574
Auditory nerve, after noise exposure, 20-21
Auditory system, as phonon collector, 35
Average Speech Frequency (ASF), 250

Bone conduction, 51, 434, 435
  in attenuation, 211-219, 294, 428-429, 432-440
  in circumaural hearing protector, 106
  ear prominences in, 436-437
  earcushion in, 435-436
  earmuffs in, 438-439
  earplugs in, 438-439
  in improvement of HPD, 587
  mastoid processes in, 436-437
  miniature microphones in, 439
  and pathway to cochlea, 294-295
  pinna in, 435
Bone conduction testing
  airborne sounds in, 213
  in attenuation measurment, 211-219
  background noise in, 212
  bone sound in, 213-214
  measurement chain in, 214
  measurement file in, 217
  principles of, 211
  procedure in, 214
  sound level in, 218
  testing site in, 211-212

C-weighted sound levels, A-weighted sound levels vs, 267-268
C-weighted unprotected level, in single-number factors, 232
C-weighted values in hearing protection, 84
Cadaver ears in testing, 279-280
  equipment used in, 281
  methods in, 280-283
  sound levels in, 281
  standard subjective procedures vs, 293
Canadian Forces (CF), 387-400
  flight personnel in, 390-391
  hearing categories in careers in, 389-390
  otitis externa in, 394-395

Canadian Forces Hearing Conservation Program, objectives of, 388–391
Canadian Hearing Standards, 389
Canadian mines, 403–423
   earmuff attenuation in, 420–422
      clamping force in, 419–420
      comfort in, 419–420
      hydrofore drill operator and, 419
      jaw crusher operator and, 419
      jumbo (three drills) operator and, 418
      laboratory tests of, 410–417
      participants in tests of, 418
      percentage of usage of, 403
      practical recommendations on, 423
      technical and attenuation data on, 404–410
   earplugs in, percentage of usage of, 403
   major benefit of noise control in, 403
Canadian Standards Association, 574
   classification of hearing protectors in, 91–96
   earmuffs and, 92
   historical review of, 91–94
   laboratory measurements and field performance in, 94–95
   sound attenuation requirements for, 99
Carcinogenic materials in hearing protection devices, 584–585
Circumaural hearing protectors, 428, 429, 430–436, 438
   artificial heads and, 108, 109
   in attenuation, 101–128, 429–432
   in bone conduction, 106
   characteristics of, 106–108
   concha in, 105
   ear canal in, 105–106, 109–115
   experimental work in, 109–119
   head geometry in, 104
   head surface covering in, 104–106
   headband force in, 107
   leakage in, 104
   parameters of, 102
   pinna in, 105
   protector cushions in, 107
Climatic tests, in earmuffs, 146
Combat Arms School at CF Base Gagetown, 399–400

Comfort in hearing protectors, 151–161, 457
   adaptation pressure in, 157
   application force of cups on head and, 155
   in earmuffs, 151, 404–409
   in earplugs, 151
   evaluation of physical characteristics of, 154–157
   global, *see* Global comfort
   heat and, 154–155
   questionnaires on, 154
   subjective evaluation of, 151–154
   tightness of spring in, 155
Concha, in circumaural hearing protector, 105
Construction Safety Act 1973, 571
Construction test, of earmuffs, 140
Consumer Reports on hearing protection devices, 165–166
"Critical" level, 42, 48
Cross-modality matching, 200–205
   in attenuation, 200–205
   convergence in, 201–202
   unprotected and protected, 201–202
Cup mass, in attenuation, 107
Custom-molded plugs
   deliberate abuse to, 333
   failure of, 328
   maintenance of, 331
   placement of, 325
   sizing in, 328

Deiter cells in inner ear damage, 6
"Delayed recovery," as term, 48
Detection response condition (DR), 348
Detection response difference, 350–351
Disposable earplugs, fitting, 473
Disposable mineral fiber inserts, 332
Dosimeters
   accuracy of, 258
   ear-borne sound level, 245–246
   introduction of personal, 251
   miniature microphones in, 589
   static measurements compared with, 252–255
   at Stelco plants, 251–252
Dosimetry
   "noise dosimeter vest" in, 417–420
   in noise measurement, 255–258

Dosimetry (*contd.*)
  single-number noise-reduction
    factor in, 239–246
  static measurements vs, 256
du Pont's Hearing Conservation
    Program
  audiometric testing in, 553–554
  evaluation of, 542–545
  HTLs in, 545–549, 551
  present regulations and, 552
  selection of study population in,
    544–545
  statistical analysis in, 545

Ear canal, in circumaural hearing
    protector, 105–106, 109–115
Ear canal resonances, earmuff in,
    113–115
Ear canal size, 329
  race and, 457–459
  sex and, 392, 457–459
Ear cushion
  in attenuation, 428
  in bone conduction, 435–436
  glasses in, 433
  hair in, 433
  leakage in, 433
Earmuffs
  adjustment in, 406
  application force in, 140–142, 146
  in artificial heads, 119, 138
  attenuation and, 117, 134–140,
    306–308, 342, 374–376,
    412–414
    characteristics of, 166
    in mines, 417–420
    objective procedure in, 136–140
    physical method of testing,
      415–417
  bizygomatic diameter data in,
    409–410
  in bone conduction, 438–439
  in Canadian mines, *see* Canadian
    mines, earmuff attenuation in
  Canadian standards and, 92
  characteristics of, 54–56
  clamping force in, 406, 414–415
  climatic tests in, 146
  and combat helmets, 391–392
  comfort in, 151, 404–408
    tests of, 408–409
  construction tests of, 140

cup motion in, 59
cushion seals in, 414–415
deliberate abuse to, 333
dropping, 145
in ear canal resonances, 113–115
ear cushion seals in, 422
earplugs vs, 161, 266, 271,
  318–319, 334–335, 382, 396
evaluating, 239–246
failure of, 325–328
fitting, 245, 473
glasses in, 472
global comfort in, 152–154
guidelines for, 388–389
hair in, 414–415
hats and, 420
head size in, 409–410
headband in, 142–146, 331
heat and, 467
humidity effects in, 146
inattention in, 354
leakage in, 472
maintenance of, 331
mass of, 155
mechanical tests in, 140–146
in military, 391–392, 584
pinna in, 473
placement of, 325–327
replacement of, 477
in ships' engine and boiler rooms,
  396–397
sizing of, 327–328
softness in, 406
in speech intelligibility, 395–396
"super," 266
temperature in, 146
transmission loss in, 54, 58–59
type approval tests in, 147
"ventilation aperture" in, 60
in warning sounds, 357
weight in, 408
white noise and, 372
Earplugs, *see also* Custom-molded
  plugs, Foam-type plugs, Pre-
  molded plugs
air leakage in, 59–61
attenuation in, 342, 374–376
in bone conduction, 438–439
in Canadian mines, percentage of
  usage of, 403
characteristics of, 56–58
in circumaural protector, 438–439
comfort in, 151

earmuffs vs, 161, 266, 271, 318–319, 334–335, 382, 396
failure of, 324–325
fitting, 473
free-field hearing threshold in, 380
guidelines for, 388–389
Gunfender (Gundefender) amplitude sensitive, 397
inserting, 392–393
insertion loss in, 289–291
maintenance of, 477–478
in military, 392–395
non-linear, 62–65, 163–165, 287–291
polymer foam cylinder, 392–395
rapid removal of, 467
re-usable, 473
in ships' engine and boiler rooms, 396–397
signal-to-noise ratio in, 371
in speech intelligibility, 395–396
transmission loss in, 54, 289–291
Education
   in hearing protector usage, 366, 462, 478–479, 501–503, 505–506, 553
   initial training in, 479
   for maintenance and cleaning staff, 479
   for new employees, 479–480
   refresher training in, 479
   for selector of hearing protectors, 478
   in serial audiometry, 494–495
   for storeman, 479
   for supervision and management, 479
"Effective level," definition of, 36
Effective quiet, definition of, 36
Effective response condition (ER), 348
Effective response difference, 350–351
Electronic sound absorption, 65–67
Engineering controls vs hearing protection, 554–556, 559
EPA, see United States Environmental Protection Agency
"Equivalent level," 36
Evaluation methods for hearing protection devices, 76–83
   air-to-air loudness balance in, 78

aural reflex method in, 80
bone-to-air comparison in, 78
insert receiver to air comparisons in, 78–79
laboratory vs field performance in, 89
loudness balance methods in, 77–78
masked-threshold method of, 81–82
miniature microphones in, 81
octave band method in, 83
subjective comparison methods in, 81
subjective-objective methods in, 81
temporary threshold shift methods in, 79–80
total protector evaluation in, 90
warning and communication signals in, 88–89
Executive Standards Board, 72
Exposure duration, and hearing protection, 475, 578, 579
"Eyeglass leakage," 61; see also Glasses

Flat loss, in speech intelligibility, 378
Flat response, in attenuation, 443
Foam-type earplugs
   cleaning, 394–395
   placement of, 325
   in speech intelligibility, 396
Free-field air-conduction to body-conduction ratio, 51
Free-field hearing threshold
   in attenuation, 316–318
   in earplugs, 380
   in speech intelligibility, 373, 384

Germany, standards in, 133–148
Glasses
   in attenuation, 328, 412–414
   in earcushions, 433
   in earmuffs, 472
   and HPD, 244
Global comfort
   adaptation pressure to local contour in, 160
   application force of cups and, 158

Global comfort (contd.)
    application pressure of flap in, 160
    in earmuffs, 152–154
    mass in, 157–158
    and physical characteristics of HPD, 157–160
    tightness of spring and, 158–160
Gunfender (Gundefender) amplitude sensitive earplug, 397

Hair
    in attenuation, 104, 182, 328
    in earcushions, 433
    in earmuffs, 414–415, 420
HCP, see Hearing conservation program
Hearing Conservation and Noise Control Inc. (HCNC), 554
Hearing conservation program, 447–469, 559–568
    audiometric data bases in, 511–539
    audiometric tests in, 453, 574
    characteristics of effective, 448–450
    cost effectiveness of, 554–556
    damage risk criteria in, 541
    du Pont's, see du Pont's Hearing Conservation Program, 542–543
    education in, 553; see also Education
    effectiveness of, 553, 585–586
        evaluating, 448, 521–531
        survey of, 450–455
    employees in
        and attitudes toward hearing protection, 258–260, 339, 465, 491–508
        hearing loss in, 466
        and misuse of HPD, 323–324
        physician conflict with, 466–467
    essential features in, 570–571
    factors in comprehensive, 552
    graded ear protectors in, 573
    hazard areas in, 573–574
    hearing protection phase of, 447–469
    hearing protector effectiveness in, 565
    HTLs in evaluating, 522

    impact noise in, 566
    long-term effectiveness of, 541–557
    management in
        commitment of, 481–482
        and fitting procedures, 468
        legal aspects of, 466
        problems of, 452–453, 464–468
        replacement policy of, 467–468
        selection of HPDs by, 465–466, 472
    monitoring, 480–481
    noise regulations in, 573–575
    personal exposure records in, 574
    planning provincial, 569–575
    potential compensation cost in, 534–536
        calculating, 535
    race and, 536–537
    at Selco plants, 250–261
    sex and, 536–537
    in small companies, 554
    steady state noise in, 566
    test-retest comparisons in, 522–531
    threshold limit value (TLV) in, 571
    unionization due to, 465
Hearing loss
    and actual noise exposure, 590
    and cochlear tuning, 21–24
    in mining and non-mining industries, 567–570
    occurrence time of, 422
Hearing protection
    classification criteria for, 567
    crest factor in, 578
    in damaged vs undamaged ears, 588
    engineering controls vs, 554–556, 559
    goal of, 577–579
    single vs double, 582
    "strongly fluctuating" noise in, 578
Hearing protection devices (HPDs), see also Earmuffs, Earplugs, Foam-type earplugs
    acoustical model of, 52–54
    carcinogenic materials in, 584–585
    characteristics of, 54–59
    classification of, 64
    cleaning, 332–333, 476–478

SUBJECT INDEX

cosmetic effects of, 462
dangers associated with use of, 482–483
difficulties in achieving usage of, 471
evaluation of, see Evaluation of hearing protection devices
"experimenter best fit" in, 274–276
failure of, 323–337
   custom-molded plugs, 325, 328
   earmuffs, 325–328
   foam-type plugs, 325
   placement technique, 324–327
   pre-molded plugs, 324–325, 327–328
   proper fit, 327
   sizing, 327–328
fitting, 274–276, 457–459, 472–473
health and safety problems in wearing, 453
in-the-field evaluations of, 463–464
inserting user-moldable, 460–461
irritation of ear canal lining in wearing, 459–460
maintenance of, 330–331, 476–478
mandatory use of, in industry, 590
measuring, 579–582
medical problems created by, 455
misuse of, 333, 585
multiple safety gear, 333–335
new designs for, 427–444, 589
nonlinearity in, 62–65, 580
performance descriptor of, 83–85
physician education on use of, 467
practical effectiveness of, 266–268, 323–324, 474–476
problems associated with, 453–457, 584–585
   sources of information on, 447
psychoacoustical basis of effects of, 361
removal of, 265–266, 474–475
selecting, individual problems in, 335–336
side effects of, 582–584
"subject fit" in, 274–275
testing insert, 167
worn by talker in noise, 396
Hearing protection standards, see Standards for hearing protectors

Hearing threshold levels (HTLs)
   in du Pont's HCP, 545–549, 551
   in INEP, 514–519, 520–521
   "learning effect" of, 514, 515, 519–520, 531, 535, 537
   as measure of hearing damage, 578
   in NINEP, 514–519, 520–521, 531–534
   in noise exposed employees vs reference population, 513
   in presbycusis, 513, 516, 517, 549
   race and, 514–519, 520–521, 535, 536
   sex and, 514–519, 520–521, 535, 536
   test variability in, 557–558
HPD, see Hearing protection devices
HTLs, see Hearing threshold levels

Impulse noise
   in attenuation, 285, 287–291
   hearing protectors in, 86–87
Industrial hearing claims, 570
Industrial noise exposed population (INEP)
   HTLs in, 514–519, 520–521, 531–534
   prior audiometric testing in, 518
   race in, 535
   sex in, 535
Industrial Safety Act 1971, 571
Industry
   accidents and incidents in, relative occurrence of, 364
   government legal confrontations vs, 465
INEP, see Industrial noise exposed population
Inner ear damage from acoustic trauma, 1–13
   cilia in, 4–6
   Deiter cells in, 6
   organ of Corti in, 2, 6, 12
Insert protectors, physical measurement method for, 86
Insertion loss
   in attenuation, 283
   definition of, 102
   in earplugs, 289–291
   REAT method in, 182

Insertion loss (*contd.*)
 transmission loss vs, 184–187
Intermittent exposure, 45
 problems in studying, 42
Intermittent sound, 42–43
International Standard ISO 1999, 571
International symposium on personal hearing protection in industry, summation of, 577–591
ISO 4869, status of, 74–75
ISO test fixture, 138–140

Leakage, *see* Air leakage
"Learning effect"
 of HTLs, 514, 515, 519–520, 531, 535, 537
 in serial audiometry, 585
Liquid filled cushion, 427
Long Method
 Short Method vs, 225
 in single-number performance factors, 221

"Magenta" noise, definition of, 38
Masked bond-conduction threshold, in attenuation, 205–206
Military, 387–400
 earmuffs in, 391–392, 584
 earplugs in, 392–395
 hearing conservation program in, purpose of, 387
 hearing protection requirements in, 391–395
 noise attenuating helmets in, 398
 presbycusis in, 390
 special hearing protection devices for, 397–400
Mines Act 1970, 571
Miniature microphones
 in attenuation measurement, 175–196
  broad band and sequential band in, 191–193
  broad band noise vs one-third octave data in, 195
  difference between left and right ears in, 188–190
  equipment in, 177–180
  in evaluating HPDs, 81
  method of, 176
 noise field in, 184
 noise-generating in, 180
 one-third octave data vs broad band noise in, 195
 sequential band and broad band in, 191–193
 subjects in tests of, 180–182
 testing of, 182–184
 in bone conduction, 439
 in dosimeters, 589
 in evaluating ear protectors, 581
Mining, "roof talk" in, 339, 583
Mining Congress Meeting in Cleveland in 1972, 222
Mining Enforcement and Safety Administration (MESA), 226
Molded plugs, deliberate abuse to, 333
Motivating people to use hearing protectors, 485–490, 586–587
 campaign in, 488–490
 case example of, 486–488
 force in, 586–587
 group dynamics in, 586
 reward in, 485, 586
 withholding wages in, 586

N.C. Department of Labor, 511
N.C. State University, 512
National Academy of Science-National Research Council Committee on Hearing, Bioacoustics, and Biomechanics (CHABA), 387
National Acoustic Laboratories (NAL) in Australia, 304
National Institute for Occupational Safety and Health (NIOSH), 200, 226, 268, 270, 323
National Research Council, Ottawa, 404
National Safety Council, 92
Neural adaptation, psychological temporal integration and, 24–25
Neural behavior, from noise-treated units, 24–25
Neural input-output functions, recruitment and, 26–28
Neurons
 characteristic frequency of, 16
 spontaneous activity (S.A.) in, 16–17, 20

SUBJECT INDEX

threshold shift of, 20-21
tuning curve in, 17-18
NINEP, see Nonindustrial noise exposed population
NIOSH, see National Institute for Occupational Safety and Health
NIPTS, see Noise-induced hearing loss
Noise, defining, 573
Noise damage, noise exposure vs noise level in, 238
"Noise dosimeter vest," 417-420
Noise exposure, dosimeter in measurement of, 238-239
Noise-induced hearing loss (NIPTS)
   VIII nerve in, 16-20
   neurological symptoms in, 15-31
   problems in studying human, 15
   subjective tinnitus in, 28-31
   susceptibility to, 389
Noise level, noise exposure vs, 238
Noise measurement
   dosimeter measurements in, 255-258
   steady noise, 253
   of varying noise, 253-254
   varying product mix, 255
Noise Reduction Rating (NRR), 226-228
   computation of, 227, 233
   determining, 232
   standard deviation in, 310
Nonindustrial noise-exposed population (NINEP)
   HTLs in, 514-519, 520-521, 531-534
   prior automatic testing in, 518
   as reference population, 513
Non-linear (amplitude-dependent) hearing protectors, 62-65
Non-linear ear protector evaluation, 87

Objective testing, 177
"Occlusion" effect, in body-conducted sound, 51
Occupational deafness risk, 263-265
Occupational Health and Safety Act 1978, 572, 576
Occupational Safety & Health Administration, 511
Octave band measurements, difficulties of, 221

One-third octave bands
   in standard subjective tests, 277
   in warning sounds, 342, 344
Ontario Regulations for protection against excessive noise, 250
Open-ear measurements in attenuation, 284-285
Organ of Corti, 2, 6, 12
Otitis externa, 394-395
Overprotection, potential dangers of, 269-271

Permanent threshold shift (PTS), 35-36
Personalized sound, history of, 249-252
Personalized sound exposure analysis, 249-261
Physikalisch-Technische Bundesanstalt (PTB), 134
"Pink" noise, 93
   definition of, 225
Pinna
   in artificial heads, 119
   in bone conduction, 435
   in circumaural hearing protector, 105
   in earmuffs, 473
Plane-wave radiation, 277
Polymer foam cylinder earplugs, 392-395
Pre-molded plugs
   on band placement, 325
   failure of, 327-328
   maintenance of, 330-331
   placement of, 324-325
   sizing of, 328-329
Presbycusis
   HTLs in, 513, 516, 517, 549
   in military, 390
Protection, definition of, 474
Pure-tone stimuli, 276-277
   in testing, 175
   in warning sounds, 357

Race
   and ear canal size, 329
   in HCP, 536-537
   and HTLs, 514-519, 520-521, 535, 536
   in INEP, 535

Rating factor K, definition of, 93
Real ear attenuation at threshold
    (REAT), 70-71, 76, 77
  current standard and, 296
  disadvantages of, 175-176
  in insertion loss, 182
  physiological noise in, 296-297
  as realistic assessment of attenuation, 297
  replications in, 187-188
  semi-objective method vs, 193-195
  as term, 274
Real-ear probe-microphone measurements, 207-208
Real world performance of hearing protectors, 299-311
  data comparisons in, 305-310
  in laboratory setting
    experimental procedure in, 300-302
    results in, 302-303
    standard deviation in, 302
    test sequence and description in, 301
    validity of, 299
REAT, see Real ear attenuation at threshold
Recruitment, 15
  and neural input-output functions, 26-28
Reissner's membrane, 2
Re-usable earplugs, fitting, 473
"Ringing of the keys," 339
Rockefeller Foundation, 512
"Roof talk" in mines, 339, 583

"Safe noise dose," 589
Semi-objective testing, 177
Serial audiometry, see also Audiometry
  attitude questionnaires in, 497
  audiometric tests in, 495-497
  in control plants, 501
  education in, 494-495
  and employee attitudes toward hearing protection, 491-508
  experimental design in, 492-494
  in hearing protection usage, 497-500, 503-506
  "learning effect" in, 585
  measuring success of, 497-500

Sex
  and ear canal size, 392, 457-459
  in HCP, 536-537
  and HTLs, 514-519, 520-521, 535, 536
  in INEP, 535
Short Method, see also Single-number performance factors
  A-frequency weighting in, 226
  calculations from, purpose of, 225
  first proposal of, 224-225
  O.B. level in, 226
Single-number noise-reduction factor (SNNRF)
  in dosimetry, 237-246
  methodology in, 239-243
  noise spectra in, 238, 244
  obtaining, 238
  octave band analysis in, 238
  results in, 244-246
Single-number performance factors, 221-234, 580
  A-different procedures in development of, 226
  development of, 225-228
  EPA method and, 232-234
  importance of, 329
  Long Method in, 221
  MESA/MSHA Method in, 230-232
    computation of, 231
  NIOSH method in, 228-230
    calculation of, 229
  noise exposure spectrum in, 225
  Noise Reduction Rating (NRR) in, 226-228
  in real world data, 310-311
  simple calculation of, 227
  Short Method in, 221
Speech intelligibility, 371-385, 583
  age in, 378, 383-384
  attenuation in, 374-375, 379-385
  bilateral flat loss in, 372
  bilateral noise-induced high frequency loss in, 372
  bilateral sensori-neural hearing loss in, 383
  earmuffs in, 395-396
  earplugs in, 395-396
  flat loss in, 378
  fluency vs non-fluency with language spoken and, 372, 384
  foam-type ear plugs in, 396
  free-field hearing threshold in, 373, 384

SUBJECT INDEX

hearing impairment and, 371
hearing level and, 384
helmets in, 400
HPD in, 347, 460
masked threshold in, 383
methodology in, 373-374
noise background in, 383
normal subjects vs subjects with hearing loss in, 380
protected vs unprotected listening in, 383-384
signal-to-noise ratio in, 383
speech-to-noise ratio in, 383
Spontaneous activity (S.A.), tinnitus and, 28-31
Standard deviations, 170
  American National Standards Institute and, 222
  in attenuation, 170, 245, 310, 318
  in NRR, 310
  in real world performance of HPD in laboratory setting, 302
  size of, 85
  subtracting N, 581
Standard subjective tests
  in attenuation, 273-297
  cadaver ear tests vs, 293
  one-third octave bands in, 277
  plane-wave radiation in, 277
  procedures in, 274
  protector fitting in, 274-276
  pure-tone stimuli in, 276-277
  sound field in, 276-277
  stimuli in, 276-277
Standards for hearing protectors
  concept of, 69-71
  development of, 71-73
  evolution of, in United States, 70-71
  intended purpose of, 73
  international, 73-76
  measurement methods for, criteria in, 82-83
  need for, 85-90
  updating of, 75-76
Standards Committee for Hearing Protection, 92
Standards Review Board, 72-73
Static measurements, dosimetry compared with, 252-258
Static noise analysis measurements, 249-261
Steady-state noise measurement, in attenuation, 286-287, 291, 295

Stelco plants
  dosimeter system at, 251-252
  employee co-operation at, 258-260
  furnace operation at, 256
  HPC at, 250-261
  mobile equipment at, 257-258
  operator's station at, 253, 255
  primary rolling mill at, 253-254
Stereocilia in acoustic trauma, 12, 13
"Strongly fluctuating" noise, 578
Subjective free-field threshold measurement in attenuation, 294
Subjective testing, 177, see also Standard subjective tests
Subjective threshold shift
  in attenuation, 440-441
  predicting average, 442

Temporary threshold shift (TTS), 36, 38, 40-41, 46-47
  burst duration in, 40
  hearing damage reversibility of, 35
  steady noise vs industrial noise in, 39
Temporary threshold shift reduction (TTSR), 581
Testing hearing protectors, see also Cadaver ears in testing, Standard subjective tests
  selecting hearing protectors for, 171-172
  selecting subjects for, 171-172
  standard vs nonstandard methods of, 163-173
"Threshold" dose, 43
Tinnitus, 578
  spontaneous activity and, 28-31
  tonotopic boundary in, 30
Tone burst, pattern of response to, 24
Tonotopic boundary, in tinnitus, 30
Total-energy theory of auditory system, 35
  and cumulative effect of exposure, 45-46
  definition of, 45
  and single continuous exposure, 45
Transmission loss
  in attenuation, 283

Transmission loss (*contd.*)
  in earmuffs, 54, 58–59
  in earplugs, 54, 289–291
  insertion loss vs, 184–187
Tuning curve in neurons, 17–18
  bandwidth of auditory nerve fiber, 24
  tips and tails of, 27–28
  "U" shaped, 23
  "V" shaped, 21–22
  "W" shaped, 23
Turbans, as hearing protectors, 582
Tympanic membrane, average behavioral threshold at, 18–19
Tympanomanometry, 80

U.S. Bureau of Mines, 222
U.S. Construction Safety Act of 1969, 92
U.S. Department of Labor (OSHA), 222, 511
U.S. National Institute for Occupational Safety and Health (NIOSH), 222
United States Environmental Protection Agency's hearing-protector labelling procedure, 170–171, 226–228, 310
University of Lund, 271
User fitting of hearing protectors, 315–322
  methodology in, 315–316
  subjects in, 315

"**V**entilation aperture" in earmuffs, 60

Walsh Healey Public Contracts Act in 1969, 543
Warning sounds
  acoustical characteristics of, 357
  acoustical effectiveness of HPD in, 341
  ambient noise in, 359
  attention demand of, 340, 341, 347–352
  audibility of, 340–345, 347
  auditory filter in, 347
  in broad-band noise, 347
  combined recognition and attention demand of, 352–361
  detection of, 341–347
    methodology in, 341–345
  detection response condition in, 348
  detection response difference in, 350–351
  earmuffs in, 357
  effective response condition in, 348, 365–366
  effective response difference in, 350–351, 358–360
  failure of perception of, 362–363
  hearing protection in, 339–367
  inattention and, 354, 359
  intensity of, 365
  irrelevant sounds and, 359
  masked thresholds of, 341, 345–347
  mean occluded and unoccluded ear conditions in, 345–346
  methodology in studies on, 354–358
  in noise, audibility of, 347
  non-linear growth in masking and, 347
  one-third octave band in, 344, 357
  over-protection and, 364
  perception of important, 347–348
  pure tones in, 357
  recognition of, 340, 341, 359, 365–366
  recognition response (RR) in, 352
  recognition response difference (RRD) in, 358–359
  reduced loudness of, due to acoustic attenuation of HPD, 360
  risks associated with, 363
  "risk pyramid" in, 366
  selection of intentional, 365
  sensory process in perception of, 339–340
  sigmoid shape of psychometric functions in, 349–350
  signal level above masked threshold in perception of, 362
  signal-to-noise ratio in, 341, 347, 362

SUBJECT INDEX

single metric "evaluation of threshold" vs, 348
simple sounds vs complex sounds as, 359
split-plot factorial design in, 349, 353–354
visual or vibro tactile signals in, 365–366

Wearing time, occupational deafness risk and, 263–265
White noise, earmuffs and, 372
Workers' Compensation Board of British Columbia state, 560–564
Workman's Compensation Board of Ontario, 306, 315